FUNDAMENTALS OF
OBSTETRIC & GYNECOLOGIC ULTRASOUND

FUNDAMENTALS OF OBSTETRIC & GYNECOLOGIC ULTRASOUND

E. Albert Reece, MD
The Abraham Roth Professor and Chairman of
Obstetrics, Gynecology and Reproductive Sciences
Professor of Internal Medicine
Director, The Division of Maternal-Fetal Medicine
Temple University School of Medicine
Philadelphia, Pennsylvania

Israel Goldstein, MD
Director of Ultrasonography
Department of Obstetrics and Gynecology
Rambam Hospital
B. Rapport Medical School
Technion High Institute of Technology
Haifa, Israel

John C. Hobbins, MD
Professor and Chief of Obstetrics
Director, Prenatal Diagnosis & Genetics
Department of Obstetrics and Gynecology
University of Colorado Health Sciences Center
Denver, Colorado

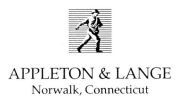

APPLETON & LANGE
Norwalk, Connecticut

Notice: The author(s) and the publisher of this volume have taken care that the information and recommendations contained herein are accurate and compatible with the standards generally accepted at the time of publication. Nevertheless, it is difficult to ensure that all the information given is entirely accurate for all circumstances. The publisher disclaims any liability, loss, or damage incurred as a consequence, directly or indirectly, of the use and application of any of the contents of this volume.

Copyright © 1994 by Appleton & Lange
Simon & Schuster Business and Professional Group

94 95 96 97 98 / 10 9 8 7 6 5 4 3 2 1

Prentice Hall International (UK) Limited, *London*
Prentice Hall of Australia Pty. Limited, *Sydney*
Prentice Hall Canada, Inc., *Toronto*
Prentice Hall Hispanoamericana, S.A., *Mexico*
Prentice Hall of India Private Limited, *New Delhi*
Prentice Hall of Japan, Inc., *Tokyo*
Simon & Schuster Asia Pte. Ltd., *Singapore*
Editora Prentice Hall do Brasil Ltda., *Rio de Janeiro*
Prentice Hall, *Englewood Cliffs, New Jersey*

Library of Congress Cataloging-in-Publication Data
Reece, E. Albert.
    Fundamentals of obstetric and gynecologic ultrasound / E. Albert
Reece, Israel Goldstein, John C. Hobbins.
        p.   cm.
    Includes index.
    ISBN 0-8385-9247-3
    1. Ultrasonics in obstetrics.   2. Fetus—Ultrasonic imaging.
3. Generative organs, Female—Ultrasonic imaging.   I. Goldstein,
Israel, M.D.   II. Hobbins, John C., 1936–   .   III. Title.
    [DNLM: 1. Ultrasonography, Prenatal. 2. Fetal Diseases—
ultrasonography. 3. Obstetrics—methods. 4. Gynecology—methods.
WQ 209 R322f 1993]
RG527.5.U48R435   1993
618'.047'543—dc20
DNLM/DLC
for Library of Congress   93-19569
                                                            CIP

Production Editor: Sondra Greenfield
Designer: Michael J. Kelly

ISBN 0-8385-9247-3

90000

9 780838 592472

To my wife Sharon and our children Kelie, Brynne and Sharon-Andrea with love and gratitude for being supportive, patient and long-suffering.

E. Albert Reece

With boundless love and deep respect, for my dear wife, Vered. She has given me encouragement, support and confidence to pursue my dreams and meet my goals. Without her, this work could never have been completed.

With pride, for my four sons and daughter.

With gratitude, for my late cherished father and my late adored mother.

With great affection and admiration, for my brother and his family.

With deep appreciation and esteem for my beloved parents-in-law, who believe in me and in my dreams, and have given me opportunity and determination to succeed.

But always and forever—for Vered.

Israel Goldstein

Contents

Preface

Ultrasound technology has revolutionized modern gynecologic and obstetric care. It now plays a major role in the treatment of normal and complicated pregnancies, not only in estimating the age and size of the fetus, but also in assessing fetal well-being, in detecting congenital anomalies, in identifying deviant fetal growth, and in guiding the performance of a number of prenatal diagnostic procedures. The introduction of transvaginal ultrasound has especially enhanced our ability to diagnose a variety of gynecologic problems.

With this text we hope to provide the inexperienced user of ultrasound with the essentials of this technology for obstetric and gynecologic practice. Previous texts have targeted the more advanced audience, consequently the needs of the less experienced or beginning practitioner of ultrasound have not been met.

This book was designed to provide a comprehensive view of ultrasound from the very basic techniques to sophisticated applications. We begin with a simple description of the setup of an ultrasound room along with image reading and interpretation, and eventually provide a detailed discussion on the detection and management of congenital anomalies. Based on current trends, the majority of gynecologists and obstetricians will, to some degree, perform ultrasound examinations in clinical practice. Therefore, the ultimate goal of this book is to supply the clinician with sufficient knowledge so he or she may provide excellent care.

Although this textbook is designed to contain the essentials in obstetric and gynecologic ultrasound, the overall balance in scope, content, and design should serve the needs of clinicians in practice, house staff physicians, sonographers, and junior subspecialists.

E. Albert Reece
Israel Goldstein
John C. Hobbins

Acknowledgments

The authors wish to thank Arnon Wiznitzer, MD, Carol Homko, RN, MS and Susan Koch, MS for the tremendous amount of time and effort they invested in assisting us in the preparation of this book. We also want gratefully to acknowledge Gianluigi Pilu's conceptual and substantive contributions, especially in the chapters on fetal dysmorphology syndromes, skeletal deformities, fetal echocardiography, and the central nervous system. Our sincere appreciation goes to our secretaries, especially Roz Robinson, for their many hours of typing, retyping, and correcting the several versions of this book. We are grateful also to Virginia Simon, Director of the Yale BioMedical Communication Library, for her beautiful illustrations and annotations.

We are particularly grateful to Craig Percy, former medical editor of Appleton & Lange, who nurtured this project from an idea to an approved book proposal. We remain grateful to others at Appleton & Lange who took this project over and carried it to fruition, namely Edward Wickland, publisher and Sondra Greenfield, managing editor. Their patience and forbearance allowed us to complete this book in good spirits. Once again, a very big thank you to all who have collectively participated in this project.

Fundamentals of
Obstetric &
Gynecologic
Ultrasound

Basic Principles of Ultrasound

INTRODUCTION

The use of ultrasound during pregnancy has become an important obstetric tool for assessing a variety of factors. There are two types of obstetric examinations: the common or basic examination and the targeted examination of a fetus suspected of anatomic or functional defects. Other applications of ultrasound include the assessment of fetal well-being or the adjunctive use of ultrasonography when performing invasive procedures. This chapter reviews the basic principles of ultrasound.

BASIC PHYSICS

Sound is a wave characterized by frequency, wavelength, amplitude, intensity, and propagation speed. Frequency, amplitude, and intensity are determined by the source of the sound. For ultrasound, the frequency is above that audible to the human ear and is described in units called hertz (Hz), defined as 1 cycle per second. Audible sounds may be between 20 and 20,000 Hz, while diagnostic ultrasound for fetal imaging is usually 3 to 7.5 million cycles per second (megahertz, or MHz). Because frequency is defined as the number of waves per second and is determined by the length of each wave, the wavelength and frequency are inversely related.

The generation of the ultrasound signals used for fetal imaging depends on the piezoelectric phenomenon of certain materials, such as resins, crystals, or ceramics. Electrical stimulation induces mechanical deformation, which stimulates the generation of waves at ultrasonic frequencies. The phenomenon also operates in reverse: the echoed mechanical waves generate electrical signals. Thus we can stimulate the ultrasound carrier frequency electrically and then generate an electrical signal from the returning echoes.

All ultrasound transducers rely on similar princi-

ples. Sound is generated as a pulse; then the same crystal that transmitted the sound listens for the returning echoes. Although the speed of sound varies as it passes through soft tissue, bone, and the like, the average speed of sound as it passes through the body is uniformly calculated at 1,540 meters per occ. This allows the distance to the source of the returning echoes to be calculated. The intensity of the echo determines the brightness of the dot at that point on the screen.

Accumulation of the returning information allows the signal processor to paint an image and update it at very brief intervals. To create the illusion of a moving image, the frame rate, that is, the rate at which the image is updated, must be greater than the flicker–fusion rate of the eye, which is about 15 cycles per second—the speed at which rapidly updated pictures appear to be moving rather than flickering.[1]

Ultrasound Transducers

While the operating principles or the physics of ultrasound transducers may be similar, the mechanical designs may vary. The type most often used for obstetric sonography is the *linear-array transducer*, so-called because its numerous crystals are arranged along a straight, flat surface and are fired electronically in a predetermined order. The image thereby generated is rectangular. Currently available linear-array transducers typically have 64 or 128 elements (Fig. 1–1).

Mechanical-sector transducers use either moving crystals or rocking mirrors to create the image. In the former design, the crystal(s) rotate on a wheel or rock back and forth. In the latter design—less frequently used at present—the crystal remains stationary, while a mirror rocks and reflects the sound. Both types create a sector image, which looks like a wedge whose apex is at the tip of the transducer (Fig. 1–2).

A third type of transducer is the *phased-array sector.* This type of transducer has no moving parts. In-

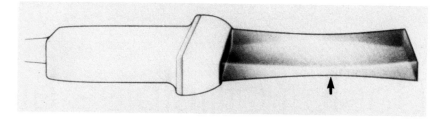

Figure 1–1. Schematic diagram of a linear-array transducer demonstrating the parallel (arrow) emission of sound waves from the transducer. (*Reprinted with permission from Reece EA, Copel J. Basic principles of ultrasonography. In: Reece EA, Hobbins JC, Mahoney MJ, et al, eds. Medicine of the Fetus and Mother. Philadelphia: JB Lippincott Co, 1992: 490*).

stead, it has many elements that are fired in very precise ways to "steer" the beams. A wedge-shaped image is produced, which also features a small "footprint" (Fig. 1–2). The most recent variation in transducer technology has been the introduction of curvilinear transducers, which combine the advantages of both linear and sector designs (Fig. 1–3).

The advantage of the linear-array transducer is that it is easier to learn, since whatever is being imaged is directly under the portion of the transducer that is imaging it. The obvious disadvantage is that it is more cumbersome than the other transducers, which, because of their smaller footprints, allow more angle flexibility in approaching the object of interest. For example, the use of linear array is limited in early pregnancy or gynecologic examinations because much of the pelvis is shadowed by the symphysis pubis, while with sector-type transducers, the symphysis pubis can be completely circumvented by an angled view.

On the other hand, the distinct disadvantage of a sector scanner is that its strength (the small footprint) becomes its weakness if one is interested in information from the near field, since its near field is so narrow. For example, not all of a third-trimester fetal head can be imaged with a sector scanner so, although a biparietal diameter (BPD) measurement can be obtained, an occipital frontal diameter may not be measured.

The curvilinear transducer incorporates the best features of both transducers, allowing the operator the ability to angle, while producing an image that actually is wider at the best focal distance than a standard linear array.

In the first trimester, patients having vaginal sonography need not have full bladders—a definite advantage from their point of view. In fact, a full bladder may unacceptably displace the uterus out of the focal plane of the transducer. Vaginal probes can also be useful for examination in late pregnancies of the fetal head in the vertex presentation or the spine of fetuses in the breech position with suspected anomalies.

Resolution

All transducers produce an ultrasound beam focused through some type of lens. As the beam leaves the transducer, the signal is not infinitely thin, but rather has a thickness known as its *azimuthal resolution*. Any echo sources within the beam reflect back to the transducer, becoming superimposed on the screen image; thus, two adjacent objects within this plane may appear superimposed. The lens portion of the transducer serves to focus the beam at a depth that may be controlled by the operator, providing optimal resolution (ie, the thinnest slice) at a desired portion of the image. The further the beam travels, however, the more it diverges, causing deterioration in the image quality. In mechanical-sector transducers, the thickness of the ultrasound beam is the same as the lateral resolution and generally has a fixed optimal depth. In linear, curved, and annular-array transducers, this thickness is determined by a lens and can be manipulated by the operator.

The ultrasound image is characterized by two other types of resolution, known as *axial* and *lateral*. These can be thought of as the ability of the scan to distinguish between two separate objects; the closest juxtaposition at which they can be differentiated defines the resolution. Axial resolution (parallel to the direction of the sound waves leaving the transducer)

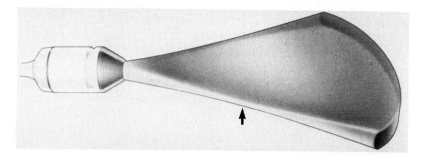

Figure 1–2. A schematic diagram of a mechanical-sector ultrasound transducer demonstrating the pie-shaped emission of sound waves from the transducer (arrow). (*Reprinted with permission from Reece EA, Copel J. Basic principles of ultrasonography. In: Reece EA, Hobbins JC, Mahoney MJ, et al, eds. Medicine of the Fetus and Mother. Philadelphia: JB Lippincott Co, 1992: 490*).

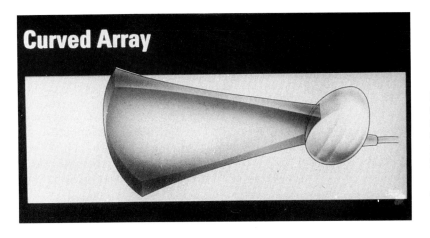

Figure 1–3. Schematic representation of a phased-array, or curvilinear, ultrasound transducer. Note the emission of sound waves from the transducer is somewhat similar to both the linear and the sector, giving a pie-shaped, yet, at the same time, greater thickness to the ultrasound beam. (*Reprinted with permission from Reece EA, Copel J. Basic principles of ultrasonography. In: Reece EA, Hobbins JC, Mahoney MJ, et al, eds.* Medicine of the Fetus and Mother. *Philadelphia: JB Lippincott Co, 1992: 491*).

is related to the length of the ultrasound pulse, which, in turn, is related to the distance of the fetus from the transducer.

Lateral resolution (perpendicular to the axial) is inevitably poorer than axial and is related in part to how highly focused the beam is. For mechanical-sector transducers, this resolution is equal to the beam diameter in millimeters, increasing with depth, and equivalent in millimeters to the azimuthal resolution.

The optimal lateral resolution in linear, annular, phased, and convex-array transducers is determined by the operator, based on the focal requirements of the scan. The optimal depth of focus can be found, and several depths may be obtained with electronically steered transducers. Although selecting multiple depths will provide better resolution at those levels in the scan and can be useful for obtaining selected still images, it also slows the frame rate significantly, resulting in a very discontinuous image—similar to

watching movement under a strobe light. This can detract from the quality of the fetal image and outweigh the advantages of multiple focal depths.

Optimal resolution is generally obtained by using the highest possible transducer frequency. For prenatal diagnosis by abdominal sonography, this is best accomplished with 5 MHz crystals. The improved resolution of higher-frequency transducers comes at the cost of decreased tissue penetration, and they have generally proved inadequate for abdominal sonography. With term pregnancies or obese patients in the second trimester it may be necessary to use even lower-frequency (3 or 3.5 MHz) transducers, which enhance tissue penetration but decrease resolution.

The depth of minimal beam diameter will be the area of optimal resolution. On many systems, the operator can select this by setting the focal depth. When desired, several bands of depth can be selected, but at

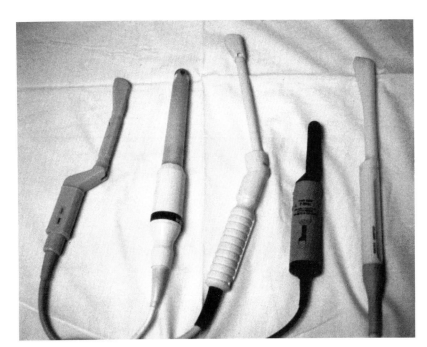

Figure 1–4. This picture demonstrates the variety of transvaginal ultrasound transducers. As you will note in some cases the transducers are straight, while others have either a bent shaft or bent tips. (*Reprinted with permission from Reece EA, Copel J. Basic principles of ultrasonography. In: Reece EA, Hobbins JC, Mahoney MJ, et al, eds.* Medicine of the Fetus and Mother. *Philadelphia: JB Lippincott Co, 1992: 491*).

the expense of a significant slowing of the frame rate. In obstetric sonography, one or at most two focal points are usually sufficient.

Since there is substantial dissipation of ultrasound as it traverses through tissue, there are basically two ways to counter this phenomenon. Returning echoes can be artificially amplified through adjustment of the gain. Since those echoes returning from the far field need more help, ultrasound machines have a built-in mechanism to amplify echoes according to how long it takes them to return. Echoes from the far field are automatically amplified more than those from the near field. This feature of virtually every machine is called time-gain compensation (TGC). Most machines allow the user to adjust gain across the entire field to selectively amplify near- or far-field echoes.

The only other way to counteract tissue attenuation is to "muscle" ultrasound through the body by increasing the intensity (or ultrasound energy). This can be done by increasing the output. Although this method can enhance images, especially in obese patients who transmit sound poorly, it does subject the fetus to higher intensity levels. Despite the fact that no independently confirmed evidence of bioeffect in tissue has been demonstrated at the time of this writing in any experimental setting, or at intensities delivered by today's equipment (this does not include some Doppler machines), it is still prudent to use an output setting that is as low as possible to obtain the best image. The ALARA principle (as low as reasonably achievable) is one that every practitioner should keep in mind when approaching a pregnant patient.

A final control common to most obstetric ultrasound systems is *dynamic range*. This control defines the way the returning echoes are assigned shades of gray on the screen. A wide dynamic range produces a gray image; a narrow range results in a high contrast image. Operator preference is important in setting this control.

REFERENCES

1. Kremkau FW. *Diagnostic Ultrasound: Principles, Instruments, and Exercises*. 3rd ed. Philadelphia, Pa: WB Saunders Co.; 1989.

The Safety of Diagnostic Ultrasound

INTRODUCTION

It has been estimated that more than one half of all pregnant women in the United States are examined with ultrasound.[1,2] This widespread acceptance, due in part to its clinical utility, convenience, and noninvasiveness, has led investigators to question whether potential health risks may be associated with its use. Initial concerns regarding ultrasound safety were raised by MacIntosh and Davey,[3] who suggested that chromosomal aberrations could be induced by an ultrasonic fetal-pulse detector. Subsequently, Liebeskind et al[4] reported sister chromatid exchanges (SCE) in human lymphocytes after exposure to diagnostic ultrasound. Neither of these findings, however, has been replicated by other investigators.[5,6]

A number of experiments has been conducted to study the safety of ultrasound. The results, however, have led to confusion, because not only were small mammals used, but also insects, plants, and cell suspensions. It is almost impossible to extrapolate from the inconsistent positive findings of such experiments to humans.[2]

In both animal experiments and therapeutic applications that use very-high-intensity levels of ultrasound, modification of biologic structures and functions does occur.[1] However, no confirmed ultrasonically induced adverse effects in humans have yet been reported when diagnostic levels of ultrasound are used.[2,7] Furthermore, the acoustic outputs, carrier frequencies, and pulse lengths of diagnostic ultrasound are all significantly less than those used for the reviewed experiments.

ULTRASONICALLY INDUCED BIOLOGIC EFFECTS

Ultrasound in higher intensities than those used for diagnostic purposes can produce biologic effects, mainly via thermal changes and the induction of microcavitation.[8]

Thermal Changes

As ultrasound propagates through tissues, its energy is absorbed and converted into heat. This heat is dissipated by adjacent tissues and by blood flowing through the insonated area. During a normal diagnostic scan, tissue temperature will rise less than $1°C$[1]; such aberrations occur normally during the human diurnal cycle, while $3°$ to $4°C$ increases can occur in febrile states. It is therefore unlikely that tissue damage would be caused by such minor increases in temperature.[1,2] There is no significant tissue heating during diagnostic ultrasound, because of the very low average intensity to which the tissue is exposed—less than 20 milliwatts per square centimeter.[2] Computer modeling suggests that such exposures do not cause temperature rises above $1°C$. In the same way, the continuous-wave Doppler devices used externally to monitor fetal heart rate operate at these same intensities and would therefore seem equally unlikely to produce hazardous increases in temperature.

Presently, there are no studies of adverse effects to living mammals from increases in body temperature of $1°C$ or less.[1,2] A recent report by Miller and Ziskin uncovered no effects to animals at temperatures below $39°C$. These authors also showed that the generation of heat-shock protein may be protective against tissue injury at certain elevated temperatures.[9] A recent study by Soothill and colleagues, using a thermocouple probe during ultrasound exams in humans, revealed that the mean fetal muscle temperature was $36.9°C$ and the mean amniotic fluid temperature was $36.6°C$.[10]

From the information available thus far, a few conclusions can be drawn regarding fetal temperature elevation in utero and its relationship to fetal anomalies: 1) there seems to be an association between elevated temperatures and fetal anomalies; 2) this elevated temperature must be several degrees above normal and depends on the duration of exposure; the higher the temperature, the shorter the exposure time required to induce adverse effects; 3) this relationship (elevated temperature and adverse effects) is stronger and reproducible in animal models; 4) a similar relationship has not been clearly demonstrated in humans, as evidenced by the lack of adverse effects during febrile states; and 5) current ultrasound equipment is almost incapable of inducing significant thermal effects in the human fetus.

Microcavitational Changes

Cavitational mechanism refers to the interaction of sound with the microscopic gas bubbles that preexist in tissues, causing the bubbles to increase and decrease rapidly in size. Plant and insect tissues contain these gas bubbles, and there is evidence that diagnostic ultrasound can produce adverse effects in these lower organisms. Mammalian tissues also contain such gaseous nuclei, but little is known about conditions under which they occur or produce biologic effects.[11] In humans, there is no direct evidence to suggest that, under clinical conditions, ultrasound-induced microcavitation produces biologic effects.[11] Diagnostic ultrasound involves short pulses with long intervals between adjacent pulses.[12] Andrews et al[13] found that the median exposure time was 105 microseconds. They also found that the median maternal exposure time was 131 microseconds and the exposure to the fetus was even less. The combination of low intensity and minimum exposure time suggests that adverse effects on the human fetus would be unlikely.

The potential deleterious effects of ultrasound on sensitive cell functions have been tested by many investigators. Particular attention has been given to experiments relating to SCE.[4,14–17] This phenomenon involves the exchange of portions of two chromatids in the same chromosome, which may be enhanced by ionized radiation, chemicals, alcohol, and carcinogens. SCE can occur spontaneously; however, an increase in SCE frequency may indicate a risk of other types of chromosomal crossover, as well as abnormal exchanges.[14,15]

Liebeskind et al[4] described a small but statistically significant increase in the SCE rate in human lymphocytes after exposure to diagnostic levels of ultrasound, but these results have not been subsequently corroborated. In a recent review,[16] Gross examined 14 papers dealing with ultrasound and SCE; 11 of these papers concluded that diagnostic ultrasound did not cause an increase in SCE rates.

Additionally, the results of MacIntosh and Davey[3] indicating an increase in chromosomal aberrations in human lymphocytes exposed to ultrasound were later retracted.[18] Although an initial report by Sanada et al[19] did observe pseudopod formation in platelets (an early sign of activation) after in vivo exposure to pulsed Doppler, their finding has not been corroborated by a number of investigators after exposure of platelets to therapeutic intensities of continuous-wave ultrasound.[18–21]

ULTRASOUND RISK AND HUMAN EPIDEMIOLOGY

Human epidemiologic data have been used to evaluate potential adverse effects of ultrasound. Table 2–1 summarizes a number of studies examining possible effects of ultrasound exposure in utero. The majority of the reports fail to identify specific adverse outcomes related to ultrasound exposure.

Scheidt et al[21] did, however, find neurologic abnormalities in neonates exposed to diagnostic ultrasound in utero. In this study, data from the Amniocentesis Registry of the National Institute of Child Health and Human Development were analyzed for possible effects of diagnostic ultrasound exposure in the second trimester of pregnancy. The first group, 297 newborns of mothers who had undergone both amniocentesis and diagnostic ultrasound, was compared with 661 newborns of mothers who had amniocentesis only, and with 949 newborns whose mothers had undergone neither ultrasound nor amniocentesis. The investigators initially studied the neonatal outcome for weight, length, head circumference, and detailed neurologic examination. They found a significantly higher rate of abnormal grasp and tonic neck reflexes among neonates exposed to ultrasound; however, a year later they reevaluated the data for infections, abnormal hearing, convulsions, and neurologic development and found no difference among the three groups. The authors therefore suggested that the initial findings in the ultrasound group could have been coincidental.

The potential relationship of ultrasound exposure to childhood malignancies has been investigated by Kinnier-Wilson and Waterhouse.[22] The mothers of 1,731 children who died of cancer in the United Kingdom between 1972 and 1981 and the mothers of 1,731 matched control children were asked about exposure to diagnostic ultrasound during pregnancy. There was no difference in ultrasound exposure between the sick and control children. Although a difference between cases and controls exposed during the earlier years of ultrasound use was found, it was felt to be the result of the selective application of ultrasound to abnormal pregnancies.

In another study, Cartwright et al[23] analyzed information obtained by interviewing the parents of 555 children with malignancies diagnosed between 1980 and 1983. The parents of 1,110 healthy children were used as a control group. They found no significant

TABLE 2–1. STUDIES OF ULTRASOUND EXPOSURE IN UTERO

Author	Type of Study	No. of Subjects	Findings
Bernstine (1969)[26]	Retrospective	720 Newborns exposed to Doppler in utero	No significant abnormality rate
Hellman et al (1970)[27]	Retrospective	1,114 fetuses exposed to ultrasound	2.7% Incidence fetal anomalies
Serr et al (1971)[28]	Retrospective	150 newborns	No difference in abnormality rates
Falus et al (1972)[29]	Retrospective	171 Newborns exposed to ultrasound in utero	No significant developmental disorders at ages 6 months to 3 years
Scheidt et al (1978)[21]	Retrospective and follow-up	297 Ultrasound and amniocentesis; 661 amniocentesis; 949 neither	Abnormal grasp and tonic neck reflexes; no difference for 122 other outcomes
Kinnier-Wilson and Waterhouse (1984)[22]	Retrospective	1,731 Mothers whose children died of cancer; 1,731 matched controls	No difference in ultrasound exposure duration between sick and control subjects
Cartwright et al (1984)[23]	Retrospective	555 Children with malignancy; 1,110 control children	No significant association between exposure to ultrasound in utero and cancer risk
Bakketeig et al (1984)[30]	Retrospective	510 Ultrasound; 499 controls	No adverse short-term biologic effects
Stark et al (1984)[24]	Retrospective and follow-up	425 Ultrasound exposed; 381 not exposed	Increased risk of dyslexia; no difference for any other neurologic outcomes
Lyons et al (1988)[25]	Retrospective and follow-up	149 Sibling pairs of the same sex; 1 exposed and 1 not	No growth difference between siblings at birth and at 6 years of age

From Reece EA, Assimakopoulos E, Zheng X, et al. The safety of obstetric ultrasonography: concern for the fetus. Obstet Gynecol. 1990;76:139–146, with permission.

association between exposure to ultrasound in utero and risk for childhood cancer.

A long-term epidemiologic study by Stark and associates[24] examined outcomes such as growth, immunologic and neurologic maturation, and childhood behavior after exposure in utero to diagnostic ultrasound. Gestational age, Apgar scores, birth weight, length, head circumference, congenital anomalies, and congenital and neonatal infections were also scrutinized. The children were later examined between 7 and 12 years of age, when they were tested for hearing performance, visual acuity and color vision, cognitive function, behavior, and neurologic status. No significant biologic differences between the two groups were found, although there was a higher incidence of dyslexia in the exposed group. Many children in the exposed group had low birth weights. In many cases, the low birth weights were probably the reason for the ultrasound examination itself, making it difficult to interpret the results.[1]

A more recent epidemiologic study[25] analyzed 149 sibling pairs of the same sex with one child exposed to diagnostic ultrasound in utero and one not exposed. It found no statistically significant difference in head circumference, height, weight at birth, or weight at 6 years of age. Furthermore, there was no difference in the pattern of growth between the two groups over the 6-year postnatal evaluation period.

Conclusion

The available information reveals that although ultrasound at high intensities is associated with biologic effects, similar biologic effects are not reproducible at diagnostic levels. Therefore, although the possibility exists that such biologic effects may be identified in the future, current data indicate that the benefits to patients exposed to prudent levels of diagnostic ultrasound outweigh the risks, if any, that might be present.

REFERENCES

1. American Institute of Ultrasound in Medicine. Bioeffects consideration for the safety of diagnostic ultrasound. J Ultrasound Med. 1988;7(suppl):53–56.
2. Reece EA, Assimakopoulos E, Zheng X, et al. The safety of obstetric ultrasonography concern for the fetus. Obstet Gynecol. 1990;76:139–146.
3. MacIntosh IJC, Davey DA. Chromosome aberrations induced by ultrasonic fetal pulse detector. Br Med J. 1970;4:92–93.
4. Liebeskind D, Bases R, Mendez F, et al. Sister chromatid exchanges in human lymphocytes after exposure to diagnostic ultrasound. Science. 1979;205:1273–1275.
5. Meire HB. The safety of diagnostic ultrasound. Br J Obstet Gynaecol. 1987;94:1121–1122.
6. Wells PNT. The safety of diagnostic ultrasound: report

of a British Institute of Radiology Working Group. *Br J Radiol.* 1987;20S:1–43.

7. Thompson HE. Introduction: First Symposium on Safety and Standardization of Ultrasound in Obstetrics. *Ultrasound Med Biol.* 1986;12:679–684.

8. Williams AR. *Ultrasound: Biological Effects and Potential Hazards.* London: Academic Press Inc; 1983.

9. Miller MW, Ziskin MC. Biological consequences of hypothermia. *Ultrasound Med Biol.* 1989;15:707–722.

10. Soothill PW, Nicolaides KH, Rodeck CH, et al. Amniotic fluid and fetal tissues are not heated by obstetric ultrasound scanning. *Br J Obstet Gynaecol.* 1987;94:675–677.

11. Carstensen EL. Acoustic cavitation and the safety of diagnostic ultrasound. *Ultrasound Med Biol.* 1987;13:597–606.

12. Taylor JWK, Dyson M. Experimental insonation of animal tissues and fetuses. In: Sanders CR, James AE, eds. *The Principles and Practice of Ultrasonography in Obstetrics and Gynecology.* New York: Appleton-Century-Crofts; 1980;15–24.

13. Andrews M, Webster M, Fleming JEE, et al. Ultrasound exposure time in routine obstetric scanning. *Br J Obstet Gynaecol.* 1987;94:843–846.

14. Gebhart E. Sister chromatid exchange (SCE) and structural chromosome aberration in mutagenicity testing (review article). *Hum Genet.* 1981;58:235–254.

15. Wolff S. Sister chromatid exchange. *Annu Rev Genet.* 1977;11:183–185.

16. Gross AS. Sister chromatid exchange and ultrasound. *J Ultrasound Med.* 1984;3:463–470.

17. Barnett SB, Barnstable SM, Kossoff G. Sister chromatid exchange, frequency in human lymphocytes after long duration exposure to pulsed ultrasound. *J Ultrasound Med.* 1987;6:637–642.

18. MacIntosh IJC, Brown RC, Brown RC Jr, et al. Ultrasound and in vitro chromosome aberrations. *Br J Radiol.* 1975;48:230–232.

19. Sanada M, Hattori A, Watanabe T, et al. The in vivo effect of ultrasound upon human blood platelets. *Nippon Choompa Igakukai. Koen-Rombunshu.* 1977;37:149–150.

20. Hawkins SD, Weinstock A. The effect of focused ultrasound on human blood. *Ultrasonics.* 1970;8:174–176.

21. Scheidt PD, Stanley F, Bryla DA. One year follow-up of infants exposed to ultrasound in utero. *Am J Obstet Gynecol.* 1978;121:742–748.

22. Kinnier-Wilson LM, Waterhouse JAH. Obstetric ultrasound and childhood malignancies. *Lancet.* 1984;2:997–998.

23. Cartwright RA, McKinney PA, Hopton PA, et al. Ultrasound examinations in pregnancy and childhood. *Lancet.* 1984;2:999–1000.

24. Stark CR, Orleans M, Haverkamp AD, et al. Short and long-term risks after exposure to diagnostic ultrasound in utero. *Obstet Gynecol.* 1984;63:194–200.

25. Lyons EA, Dyke C, Toms M, et al. *In utero* exposure to diagnostic ultrasound: a 6-year follow up. *Radiology.* 1988;166:687–690.

26. Bernstine RL. Safety studies with ultrasonic Doppler technic: a clinical follow-up of patients and tissue culture-study. *Obstet Gynecol.* 1969;34:707–709.

27. Hellman LM, Duffus GM, Donald I, et al. Safety of diagnostic ultrasound in obstetrics. *Lancet* 1970;1:1133–1135.

28. Serr DM, Padeh B, Zakut H, et al. Studies on the effects of ultrasonic waves on the fetus. In: Huntingford PJ, ed. *Proceedings 2nd European Congress on Perinatal Medicine.* Basel: Skarger AG. 1971;302–307.

29. Falus M, Koranyi G, Sobel M, et al. Follow-up studies on infants examined by ultrasound during fetal age. *Orv Hetil.* 1972;113:2119–2121.

30. Bakketeig L, Eik-Nes SH, Jacobsen G, et al. Randomized controlled trial of ultrasonographic screening in pregnancy. *Lancet.* 1984;2:207–211.

3

Physical Examination of the Fetus

INTRODUCTION

Ultrasound examination of the gravid uterus has evolved over the last two decades from an attempt to observe only the fetal heart rate and detect large fetal abnormalities to detailed evaluation of fetal structure and functions. The ultrasound study in many cases has become an essential part of obstetric management. The majority of pregnant women throughout the world today have the opportunity to have ultrasonic visualization of their developing fetuses performed in outpatient clinics.

Equipment differs in image quality, transducer frequency, transducer size and shape, and the ability to focus to a desired depth. Examiners vary in their degree of experience and formal training. The ability to detect malformations of the fetus, placenta, umbilical cord, and uterine body and cervix depends on the level of skill, knowledge, and experience of the operator. For each routine ultrasound examination, however, there are guidelines the examiner should follow, including the site of the exam, patient preparation, and specifics on the exam itself.

THE "MECHANICS" OF THE ULTRASOUND EXAMINATION

The Ultrasound Room

Only the essential equipment necessary to perform the examination should be included in the ultrasound room. The size of the room should be in relative proportion to the size of the ultrasound machine, with a patient bed, computer setup, and a desk for the examiner. The ultrasound room should also contain all the incidentals needed to perform invasive procedures, such as amniocentesis, chorionic villous sampling, or percutaneous umbilical cord sampling.

The ultrasound examination is often performed in semidarkness. However, since the examiner becomes fatigued after only a few hours in that setting, ultrasound examinations should be done in semidaylight, with blinds that allow the operator to adjust the amount of light entering through the window.

The examiner should be seated on the right side of the patient during the examination, if he or she is right-handed, and should hold the transducer in his or her right hand while using the left hand to operate the ultrasound machine dials, computer, camera, and video camera. The examining table must be positioned so that the end containing stirrups (for transvaginal scanning) is not facing the door. The examiner should also warm the ultrasound gel prior to use, as the warmth may add to the patient's comfort.[1]

Patient Preparation

The first and perhaps the most important step in patient preparation is to explain to the patient the aim of the ultrasound examination. Sometimes patients are referred for an examination to check the location of the placenta, while others may be referred for fetal biometry. The reason should be explained to the patient. The limitations of ultrasonography should also be explained, in some circumstances, so that the patient develops a realistic impression of the technology and understands what can be accomplished and what cannot. The information that is given must be tailored to the circumstance and to the individual patient.

Many pregnant women with full bladders waiting to be examined complain about their discomfort from bladder distention and feelings of urgency. Now, most if not all ultrasound examinations can be done without full bladders. This is especially true with transvaginal examinations, as a full bladder distorts the pelvic anatomy by compressing pelvic organs and may occupy most of the screen, displacing important target organs.[2]

Prior to the examination the pregnant woman should be interviewed for essential demographic information, obstetric history, information about any structural or genetic abnormalities in the family, and the present pregnancy. This information should be recorded.

Conducting the Examination

The various types of transducers have been described in detail in Chapter 1, "Basic Principles of Ultrasonography." In brief, there are three main types of transducers: The linear, sector, and curvilinear (Fig. 1–1, Fig. 1–2, Fig. 1–3, and Fig. 1–4). The linear and curvilinear transducers are usually used in the second or third trimesters for measuring long bones, fetal head, and abdominal circumferences. The sector transducers are used for transvaginal examinations, for gynecologic and infertility studies, and in first-trimester examinations.

When the technician is approaching the patient with a transducer, orientation of the image produced is important. In sagittal scans of the patient's lower abdomen the left side of the image should represent its most cephalad portion. That is, the left side points toward the patient's umbilicus and the right side toward the symphysis pubis.

Transducers come in all sizes and shapes. The connecting cable may insert on one side or in the middle in linear or curvilinear arrays. The "end-cabled" transducer should be applied to the abdomen so that the end of the cable is facing cephalad. Most machines will "fire up" when they are turned on, so the first image produced automatically is oriented in the standard way if the cabled end is pointing cephalad. When the cable is in the middle, try to find a distinguishing mark on one end of the transducer to aid in the initial orientation. It is easy for the operator to get back on track, if temporarily lost, by inserting a finger under one end of the transducer to see where the acoustic shadow appears on the screen. If the operator wants to change the orientation of the image by 180 degrees without changing the position of the transducer, almost every machine has a readily available switch labeled "image reverse" that will accomplish this. Mechanical, phased array, and annular arrays will have a groove or ridge on the portion of the transducer that is meant to face cephalad. The operator can instantly visualize the orientation of the wedge-shaped image by rocking the transducer from side to side.

It is important that the beginner not press too hard on the patient's abdomen. There is a natural tendency to attempt to use strength to get more information from the transducer by pushing it toward the object(s) of interest. Patients with full bladders are particularly appreciative of a gentle transducer application.

The transducer tip is covered with transducer gel and placed into a protective rubber sheath (condom) or glove in transvaginal ultrasound. After the transducer is covered, trapping air beneath the rubber sheath should be avoided, as it may create unwanted artifacts on the screen. An ample amount of gel needs to be placed on the transducer and some on the outside of the glove or sheath to facilitate vaginal penetration and to enhance contact between the transducer and the surface tissue inside the vagina.[3] Some operators gently spread the labia apart with a gloved hand, to aid in the gentle introduction of the transducer.

ESSENTIAL COMPONENTS

Sonographic Examination of the Fetus

Technical Bulletin No. 116 from the American College of Obstetricians and Gynecologists[4] states that a basic ultrasound examination should include evaluation and documentation of the following:

1. Fetal number
2. Fetal presentation (in second and third trimesters)
3. Fetal position
4. Placental location
5. Amniotic fluid volume
6. Gestational dating (preferably by multiple parameters)
7. Detection and evaluation of maternal pelvic masses (best done in the first trimester)
8. Survey of fetal anatomy for gross examinations (in second and third trimesters)

The optimal time for an ultrasound exam is determined by its purpose; further, the timing affects its accuracy in achieving different goals. An ultrasound exam for gestational dating is best done as early as possible in the pregnancy because that is when fetal biometry is most accurate. A targeted ultrasound to exclude congenital anomalies would have its best yield in midgestation, when organogenesis is complete and the structures of interest are large enough to permit accurate evaluation. Assessment of fetal well-being should be done in the third trimester, after extrauterine fetal viability is reached.

First-Trimester Physical Examination of the Fetus
In normal pregnancies the earliest sonographic evidence of pregnancy is the gestational sac, which is usually strategically placed in the middle of the uterus. The gestational sac can be measured by using the longitudinal diameter and then rotating the tranducer 90 degrees to obtain the anterior–posterior and transverse diameters (Fig. 4–2 and Fig. 4–5).

The embryo represents the second sign of a normally developing pregnancy with abdominal scanning. The heartbeat and fetal movements can be seen at 6 weeks and 4 days and at 8 weeks, respectively. The above milestones can be observed about 6 days earlier with transvaginal approach. The crown–rump length is a measurement used to compute fetal age. Attention should be given at this time to the shape of the gestational sac, the heartbeat frequency, the characteristic movements of the embryo, and the size of the yolk sac. The number of the fetuses, location of the placenta, and any retroplacental echo-free areas beneath the placenta should be noted.

It is easy to identify some fetal structures by the end of the first trimester of pregnancy. The fetal head with its typical ellipsoid shape in the axial plane, the abdomen with the intra-abdominal sonolucent structures of the stomach and the bladder, the external fetal morphology of the spine, the anterior abdominal wall, and the site of cord insertion are visible. The upper and lower limbs can also be identified.

Ultrasound is most commonly used in the estimation of gestational age, thus circumventing the use of indirect means such as fundal height measurement, fetal heart tone auscultation, or the recording of fetal movement. Ultrasound permits noninvasive measurement of embryonic and fetal structures.[5]

Crown–Rump Length. Fetal crown–rump length is the most accurate single measurement for estimating gestational age (Fig. 4–11). Chervenak and colleagues have suggested that ultrasound measurement of crown–rump length can be more accurate in estimating gestational age in the first trimester than measurement of human chorionic gonadotropin (HCG).[6] The strength of the crown–rump length as a useful biometric parameter is in its consistent reproducibility up to about 12 weeks' gestation, after which the measurement is no longer useful.

Other Parameters. It is now possible to measure biparietal diameter (BPD), head circumference, abdominal circumferences, and trunk circumference with transvaginal scanning. These correlate well with gestational age. One study, for example, found the circumference of the trunk, measured perpendicular to the long axis and at a point below the cardiac pulsation, to be highly accurate in estimating gestational age, with an error rate of ± 3 days.[7]

Second- and Third-trimester Physical Examination of the Fetus
The fetus is examined during the second and third trimesters for two main reasons: 1) to evaluate fetal growth, and 2) to assess the normal development of the fetal organs and structures. The amniotic fluid, placenta, and umbilical cord are also evaluated. The relationship of the long axis of the fetus to the maternal abdomen provides sonographic orientation.

The fetal position is determined in order to ascertain whether it is vertex, breech, oblique, or transverse. The fetal head, spine, anterior abdominal wall, and lower limbs should next be surveyed and biometric measurements of the fetal organs performed. It is preferable to begin with head measurements, BPD and occipitofrontal diameter (OFD), transverse cerebellar diameter, and lateral ventricular measurements. The cephalic index (BPD/OFD × 100) and head circumference $(D_1 + D_{2/2})$ (3.14) are calculated from the BPD and OFD.

Head. The oval outline of the fetal head should be sought in all examinations. A fetal head may present deep in the pelvis, and, on rare occasions, a cursory examination might suggest that the head measurement is unobtainable, when, in fact, the fetus is anencephalic. The intracranial anatomy should also be examined to ascertain that midline structures are present. The BPD can be obtained as early as the late first trimester. This versatile measurement is commonly used in both early and late pregnancy, though its accuracy decreases with advancing gestation. The accuracy of the BPD measurement is ± 6 days in early pregnancy. When the second-trimester BPD and first-trimester crown–rump length are combined, there is 20% less variability in predicting gestational age than when either parameter is used independently.[8] Other head measurements aside from BPD, include: orbital distances, OFD, and head circumference. The transducer is then moved in a cross-sectional plane toward the thorax and the abdomen. The circumferences of these structures are measured by calculation. The long bones (the femur, humerus, tibia, and ulna) are measured directly. It is important to visualize both upper and lower limbs; measurements of one upper and one lower limb, however, are acceptable for routine ultrasound examination. The estimated fetal weight can be calculated from these measurements.

The fetal organs must also be assessed, starting from the head and moving toward the lower limbs, with each of the areas evaluated separately. The shape of the fetal head, the relationship of the lateral ventricles to the hemispheric width, and the position of the choroid plexus within the ventricle are also assessed. The midline structures of the fetal head are evaluated: the third and fourth ventricles, the cisterna magna, and the septum cavum pellucidum.

Fetal Spine. The fetal spine ossifies as early as 10 weeks and is seen as parallel sets of echoes representing the articulation facets. These facets can be seen from the cervical region through the sacral spine, where the converging facets come to a point. The spine should be examined in both longitudinal (coronal) and transverse planes in targeted examinations for neural tube defects. (Fig. 3–1). The fetal spine is examined by passing the transducer from the upper spine toward the lower spine in both longitudinal and cross-sectional planes. The ossification of the vertebrae and the presence of skin covering are markers for normal and complete vertebral development. The spine is also scanned in sagittal and coronal planes. The spine should be scanned a few times from the cervical vertebrae toward the sacrum to be sure no subtle abnormalities are missed.

Heart. A four-chambered image of the fetal heart should be part of all ultrasonic examinations after 18 to 20 weeks of gestation. Major structural anomalies of the heart, which can distort the normal four-chamber view, may be excluded by demonstrating ventricles and atria of equal and appropriate sizes on either side of a normal-looking ventricular septum. Although some significant lesions that result in critical neonatal illness may not be detected with this approach (eg, transposition of the great vessels), it is a rapid and easy-to-perform screen for congenital heart disease. The fetal heart rate should also be evaluated. It is important to confirm that the apex of the heart is on the same side as the fetal stomach. Echocardiography is used for a more detailed sonographic evaluation of the fetal heart when necessary.

Abdomen. The fetal abdomen and stomach can be visualized as early as 12 weeks' gestation, and the kidneys can often be observed at that time as well. Ventral wall defects can be excluded by the demonstration of an intact abdomen in the area of the umbilical cord insertion (Fig. 3–2). Other normal structures that should be sought are the single cystic area representing the stomach, on the left side of the abdomen, and the umbilical vein, which hooks toward the right in the liver. The gallbladder may be occasionally seen, inferior to the liver on the right. The fetal bladder is usually visible as a fluid-filled structure in the midline, low in the pelvis, during a routine examination. The bladder may visibly fill and empty over the course of the examination. The normal size of the stomach, kidneys, and bladder should be observed in the abdomen. The hepatic portion of the umbilical vein is continued in the axial plane into the portal sinus. The portal sinus is deviated to the right side of the fetus, away from the fetal stomach, is located at the same level as the stomach, and is seen as a sonolucent structure on the left side. In the axial plane, the fetal kidneys are located on either side of the fetal spine. The differences in echogenicity between the lung and liver can be visualized in the upper part of the abdomen, and the diaphragm can be observed as an echogenic line between upper and lower trunk. The small intestine with the motion typical of peristalsis in the fetal colon can be visualized between the two main echo-free structures of the fetal abdomen. The normal insertion of the umbilical cord into the anterior abdominal wall should also be noted.

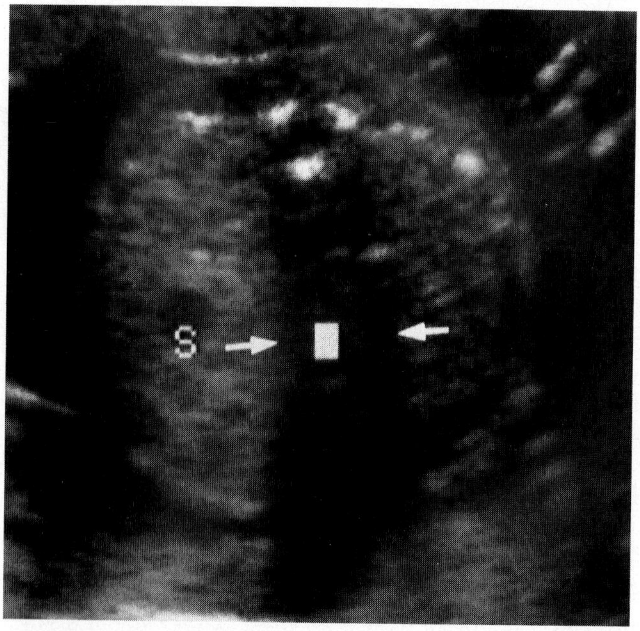

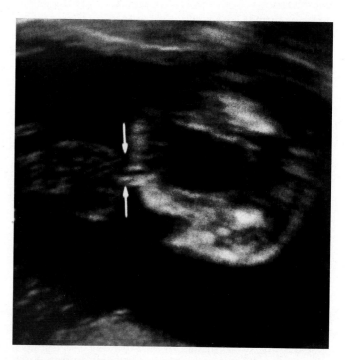

Figure 3–1. Transverse section of fetal spine (S) demonstrating a neural tube defect (arrows and box).

Figure 3–2. Transverse scan of fetal abdomen demonstrating an intact abdomen with normal cord insertion (arrows).

Extremities. The four fetal limbs should routinely be identified during any second- or third-trimester examination. Standard growth curves are available for the proximal and distal segments of the bones in the upper and lower extremities. While it is not necessary to measure all six tubular bones in every fetus, the sonologist should measure at least one or two segments. The relative size of the long bones bilaterally in comparison with each other should be assessed. The angle between the lower limbs and both feet should be seen, and an effort should be made to count the fingers on both hands. The amount of amniotic fluid should be noted; the presence of bands inside the amniotic fluid should be excluded.

The location, age of the placenta, and the three umbilical vessels in the umbilical cord should also be evaluated. A routine ultrasound examination is not complete without noting fetal behavior, body and breathing movements, and fetal tone.

The BPD remains the gold standard for gestational age determination in midtrimester, because it is easily identifiable and highly reproducible. The BPD cannot always be measured, unfortunately, even in early gestation, because of certain fetal positions, such as direct occiput anterior or posterior, fetal compression, fetal crowding, multiple gestation, or even fetuses that are deep in the pelvis. Bear in mind also that the BPD may be distorted as part of any fetal structural anomaly.

To circumvent these problems another intracranial landmark, the transcerebellar diameter (TCD), has been used.[9,10] The TCD can be obtained from the latter part of the first trimester onward (Fig. 5–46). The corresponding gestational age is easy to remember since the gestational age is the same as the TCD in millimeters up to 24 weeks. Later in pregnancy, however, this close relationship no longer holds. Measuring the TCD allows gestational dating independent of the shape of the fetal head, making it extremely useful when the fetal head is compressed. The TCD is also useful in the evaluation of intrauterine growth retardation because it remains relatively unaffected, even when growth as measured by other fetal parameters has been compromised.

Other parameters that may prove useful during this period are the clavicular length and the foot length.[11–13] Foot length measurement may be useful in select circumstances, such as in fetuses with hydrocephaly or limb dysplasia.[14,15]

Fetal gestational-age assignment from biometry becomes more difficult in the late third trimester, due to the normal biologic variation, which is most prominent in later gestation. The size of the fetus can be accurately evaluated, on the other hand, by estimates of fetal weight derived from various combinations of abdominal circumference and BPD, femur length, and head circumference (see Chapter 14, Estimated Fetal Weight). Gestational age in the third trimester may also be estimated by nonbiometric parameters, which can be tied to fetal maturation.

A high degree of correlation between gestational age and fetal intestinal appearance has been reported.[16,17] Goldstein and coworkers[17] demonstrated that colonic echogenicity and colonic diameter correlated with gestational age and, in some instances, may even be superior to BPD or femur-length measurement.

Correlations have also been observed between fetal lung maturation and the ultrasonic detection of epiphyseal ossification centers in the fetal long bones.[18,19] Goldstein and colleagues[19] reported that sonographic detection of lower limb epiphyseal ossification centers was an accurate indicator of gestational age during the third trimester. A significant correlation was observed between the distal femoral epiphyses, the proximal tibial epiphyses, and the lecithin-to-sphingomyelin (LS) ratio in nondiabetics. For example, a distal femoral epiphysis greater than 3 mm and the presence of a proximal tibial epiphysis of any size was seen with LS ratios indicative of fetal lung maturity in almost all cases. This combination of findings may acceptably substitute for amniocentesis in selected cases when pulmonic maturity should be assessed but amniocentesis is contraindicated.

Goldstein and associates[20] demonstrated in another study that a highly accurate estimation of term gestation could be obtained by combining the colonic grade with the detection of proximal humeral epiphyses. Proximal humeral epiphyses equal to or greater than 3 mm and a mature colonic pattern (grade 3), for example, indicated a 95% probability that the fetus was full term.

The Report

All the above-mentioned normal or abnormal findings should be documented, and recommendations made to the referring physician in a formal report. Any picture or videotape should be kept as a documentation of the fetal examination.

REFERENCES

1. Kurtz AB. The basic ultrasound examination of uncomplicated pregnancy. *Radio Clin North Am.* 1990; 28:1–17.
2. Timor-Tritsch IE, Rottem S. How transvaginal sonography is done. In: *Transvaginal Sonography.* New York, NY: Elsevier; 1988.
3. Kremkau FW. *Diagnostic Ultrasound: Principles, Instruments, and Exercises.* 3rd ed. Philadelphia: WB Saunders Co; 1989.
4. ACOG Technical Bulletin. American College of Obstet-

rics and Gynecology Technical Bulletin No. 116. May 1988: 1–3.

5. Reece EA, Gabrielli S, DeGennaro N, et al. Dating through pregnancy: a measure of growing up. *Obstet Gynecol Survey.* 1989;44:544–554.

6. Chervenak FL, Brightman RC, Thornton J, et al. An analysis of sonographically determined fetal crown–rump length and human chorionic gonadotropin as predictive of gestational age (abstract). Proceedings of the 33rd Annual Meeting of the Society of Gynecologic Investigation, Toronto, Ontario, Canada. March 26–29, 1986.

7. Reece EA, Scioscia AL, Green J, et al. Embryonic trunk circumference in the estimation of gestational age. *Am J Obstet Gynecol.* 1987;156:713–715.

8. Bovicilli L, Orsini LF, Rizzo ON, et al. Estimation of gestational age during the first trimester: real-time measurement of fetal crown–rump length and biparietal diameter. *J Clin Ultrasound.* 1981;9:71–75.

9. Goldstein I, Reece EA, Pilu G, et al. Cerebellum measurements with ultrasonography in the evaluation of fetal growth and development. *Am J Obstet Gynecol.* 1987;156:1065–1069.

10. Reece EA, Goldstein I, Pilu G, Hobbins JC. Fetal cerebellum growth unaffected by intrauterine growth retardation: a new parameter for prenatal diagnosis. *Am J Obstet Gynecol.* 1987;157:632–638.

11. Yarkoni S, Schmidt W, Jeanty P, et al. Clavicular measurements: a new biometric parameter for fetal evaluation. *J Ultrasound Med.* 1985;4:467–470.

12. Jeanty P, Dramaix-Willmet M, Van Kem J, et al. Ultrasonic evaluation of fetal limb growth: part II. *Radiology.* 1982;143:751–754.

13. Hadlock FP, Harrist RB, Dieter RL, et al. Fetal femur length as a predictor of menstrual age: sonographically measured. *Am J Obstet Gynecol.* 1982;138:875–878.

14. Mercer BM, Sklar S, Shariatmader A, et al. Fetal foot length as a predictor of gestational age. *Am J Obstet Gynecol.* 1987;156:350–355.

15. Goldstein I, Reece EA, Hobbins JC. The sonographic appearance of the fetal heel, ossification centers and foot length measurements provide independent marks for gestational age estimation. *Am J Obstet Gynecol.* 1988;159:923–926.

16. Zilianti M, Fernandez S. Correlation of ultrasonic images of fetal intestine and gestational age in fetal maturity. *Obstet Gynecol.* 1983;62:569–573.

17. Goldstein I, Lockwood CJ, Hobbins JC. Ultrasound assessment of fetal intestinal development in the evaluation of gestational age. *Obstet Gynecol.* 1987;70:682–686.

18. Tabsh KMA. Correlation of ultrasonic epiphyseal center and lecithin: sphingomyelin in ratio. *Obstet Gynecol.* 1984;64:92–96.

19. Goldstein I, Lockwood C, Belanger K, et al. Ultrasonic assessment of gestational age with the distal, femoral and proximal tibial ossification centers in the third trimester. *Am J Obstet Gynecol.* 1988:158;127–130.

20. Goldstein I, Reece EA, Hobbins JC. Estimating gestational age in the term pregnancy using a model based on multiple indices of fetal maturity. *Am J Obstet Gynecol.* 1989;161:1235–1238.

4

First-Trimester Ultrasound

INTRODUCTION

Ascertainment of fetal well-being in utero has interested an increasing number of clinicians during the last three decades. Efforts have also been made to make prenatal diagnoses earlier in gestation. Sonographic images have not only become an informative means of defining the state of fetal health, but they are also of prognostic value for future pregnancies. First-trimester evaluation is desirable, since it can provide information on embryonic/fetal development. Evidence of congenital malformation at this stage reduces the waiting period for information, and if parents choose termination of pregnancy, maternal morbidity is less if the procedure is done in the first trimester. When a viable fetus is documented by ultrasonography at 8 to 12 weeks' gestation, the risk of spontaneous abortion ranges between only 2% and 2.3%[1,2]

The developmental changes of the embryo have been documented pathologically during the early period of embryonic life. These features can be identified and followed sonographically throughout the first trimester as evidence of normal or deviant development with advanced ultrasound equipment. Six principal factors are used for evaluation:

1. Gestational sac size and location
2. Yolk sac presence and integrity
3. Embryonic pole with or without pulsations
4. Embryo size
5. Visualization of embryonic heartbeats and movements
6. Fetal morphology

EMBRYOLOGY

First Week of Life

CONCEPTION. One male gamete (sperm) fuses with one female gamete (ovum).

CLEAVAGE. A rapid succession of mitotic divisions results in the production of a larger number of increasingly smaller cells called blastomeres. Cleavage occurs in the zygote as it makes its way through the fallopian tube to the uterine cavity. The mass of cells reaching the uterine cavity is now composed of 16 cells, the morula.

BLASTOCYST FORMATION. The morula enters the uterine cavity and forms a blastocyst, which soon develops an internal cavity called a blastocoele.

IMPLANTATION. The blastocyst attaches to and erodes through the epithelial lining of the uterus. With the appearance of the amniotic cavity the embryoblast becomes the embryonic disc.[3]

Second Week of Life

The blastocyst becomes embedded in the uterine endometrium; it then establishes communication with the maternal blood vessels for physiologic exchanges. Both the embryo and the extraembryonic membranes grow rapidly. Early in the second week the embryo is composed of two germ layers (bilaminar); by the end of the second week the primitive streak becomes evident. Also at the end of the second week, the bilaminar embryo becomes trilaminar, or composed of three germ layers: endoderm, mesoderm, and ectoderm.[3]

Third and Fourth Weeks of Life

The zygote has matured by day 20 into the blastocyst, a fluid-filled cyst lined with a trophoblast that contains a cluster of cells at one side called the inner cell mass. The blastocyst invades the endometrial stroma into the hyperplastic endometrium at the site of the inner cell mass on day 20 to begin implantation. This process is completed by day 23 as the endometrial membrane regenerates over the blastocyst. The endometrial cells adjacent to the blastocyst become modified to supply nourishment to the blastocyst; these cellular changes are referred to as the decidual reaction.

The primary (primitive) yolk sac forms at approximately 23 days menstrual age as the blastocyst cavity becomes lined by the exocoelomic membrane and hypoblast (primitive embryonic endoderm). As the extraembryonic coelom forms, the primary yolk sac is pinched off and extruded, resulting in the formation of the secondary yolk sac.[3] Standard embryology texts indicate that the secondary yolk sac actually forms at approximately 27 to 28 days menstrual age when the mean diameter of the gestational sac is approximately 3 mm. The secondary, rather than the primary yolk sac, is commonly identified by ultrasound. A portion of the secondary yolk sac becomes incorporated in the midgut; it is the extruded remnant of the secondary yolk sac that is seen on ultrasound. The former portion has been described as the provisceral yolk sac and the latter as the secondary yolk sac remnant. The provisceral yolk sac serves in the transfer of nutrition, blood development, primitive gut formation, and the cell and vessel generation of primordial germ cells. The remnant of the secondary yolk sac eventually lies between the amnion and chorion.

The embryonic disc is symmetric, with layers of ectoderm and endoderm in contact at the midline. The ectoderm develops into the neural plate and is transformed into the neural tube and the nervous system. The endoderm develops into the foregut, the hindgut, and the midgut. The three endodermal subdivisions represent the first appearance of the alimentary and respiratory systems. The mesoderm develops into the skeletal, muscular, urogenital, and cardiovascular systems. During the fourth week there is a rapid proliferation of the syncytiotrophoblast, forming primary chorionic villi by the end of the fourth week.[3]

Fifth Week of Life

During the fifth week the embryo is converted by the process of gastrulation from a bilaminar disc to a trilaminar disc composed of three primary cell layers: endoderm, mesoderm, and ectoderm. The primitive streak and *notochord* appear during gastrulation. The primitive streak forms the mesenchyme which gives rise to the connective tissue of the embryo and stromal components of all glands.

The formation of the neural plate and its closure to form the neural tube is known as the process of neurulation. This process begins in the fifth *menstrual* week in the thoracic region and extends caudally and cranially, resulting in complete closure by the end of the sixth *menstrual* week. Failure of closure of the neural tube results in neural tube defects, which occur at a rate of 1 to 2 per 1,000 live births.

Two tubes forming the primitive heart develop during the fifth week from splanchnic mesodermal cells. These tubes begin to pump into a primitive paired vascular system by the end of the fifth week, and a vascular network develops in the chorionic villi that connect through the umbilical vein to the primitive embryonic vascular network.[3] A systematic discussion of the development of each major area during this period follows.

Sixth Through Tenth Weeks of Life

Weeks 6 to 10 are referred to as the embryonic period during which essentially all of the adult internal and external structures form. Blood flow is unidirectional, by the end of the sixth week, and the heart attains its definitive form by the end of the eighth week. The peripheral vascular system develops slightly later and is completed by the end of the 10th week.

The primitive gut forms during the sixth week. The midgut herniates into the umbilical cord from the 5th week to the end of the 10th week. The rectum separates from the urogenital sinus by the end of the 8th week, and the anal membrane perforates by the end of the 10th week. The primitive kidneys ascend from the pelvis starting at approximately week 8 but do not reach the adult site until 11 weeks gestation. External genitalia are still in a nongender-specific state at the end of week 10. Limbs are formed with separate fingers and toes. Nearly all congenital malformations, except for abnormalities of the genitalia, originate before or during the embryonic period. The external genitalia do not reach mature fetal form until the end of the 14th week.[3]

SONOANATOMY

Gestational Sac

The embryo becomes completely imbedded within the decidua 9½ days after conception. This is about 24 days after menstruation in a normal 28-day cycle, or 3½ weeks' gestational age. As the exocoelomic cavity, or early gestational sac develops, a cystlike structure may be detectable on sonograms. Small gestational sacs, or focal echogenic thickenings of the endometrium at the site of implantation within the decidua, have been described.[4] This sonographic appearance is called the *intradecidual sign*.

This sign previously described[5] was based on the sonographic visualization of the three layers of decidua in early pregnancy. Nyberg et al[5] reported that the early gestational sac of the normal intrauterine pregnancy is characterized by a double echogenic ring appearance produced by the decidua capsularis and decidua parietalis. They suggested this may serve as a sign for an early intrauterine pregnancy, distinguishing it from ectopic pregnancy.

Gestational sac (Fig. 4–1) shape also has been used to predict normal pregnancy development. In the sagittal plane (Fig. 4–2), the gestational sac appears to be an ellipsoid; in the coronal plane it appears as a

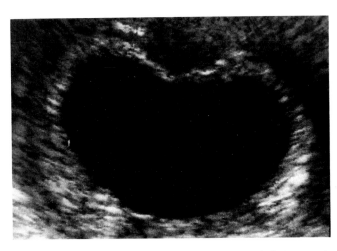

Figure 4–1. Gestational sac at 5½ weeks, observed via transvaginal ultrasonography. This transverse scan of the sac reveals an echogenic border representing the thickened decidua that outlines that entire gestational sac. Internally, the echolucent area represents the gestational sac fluid.

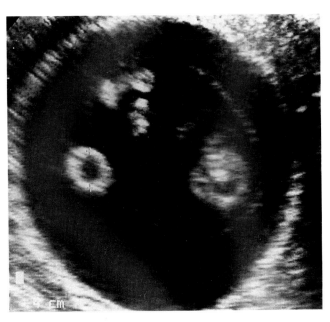

Figure 4–3. Cross-sectional view of an embryo and gestational sac observed via transvaginal ultrasonography. The decidua is clearly seen as an echodense margin within which is the echolucent gestational fluid. The lighter circumferential structure represents the amniotic membrane surrounding the embryo; the yolk sac with its echodense ring and an echolucent center can be observed separately. Note the calipers at the outer edges of the yolk sac(+'s).

circle (Fig. 4–3).[6] The presence, prominence, and continuity of the trophoblastic reaction surrounding the gestational sac have also been reported as sonographic markers to determine a normal pregnancy.[7]

The analysis of human chorionic gonadotropin (HCG) is the earliest biochemical test available for evaluation of pregnancy. Kadar et al[8] were the first to study and report on this subject. Using transabdominal sonography, they reported that a gestational sac should be visualized at a serum beta-HCG level greater than 6,500 mIU per mL in normal pregnancy. Nyberg et al[9] subsequently reported that a normal intrauterine gestational sac was always seen via vaginal sonography when the HCG level was greater than 1,800 mIU per mL (Fig. 4–4; Table 4–1; Table 4–2). In another study investigators reported that when the mean gestational sac diameter was equal to or greater

than 5 mm, the serum HCG level was equal to or greater than 1,800 mIU/mL in 70% of pregnancies studied.[10] They demonstrated a linear relationship between mean gestational sac growth and the maternal serum beta-HCG level in normal gestations.[10] In a study using transvaginal sonography Bateman et al[11] reported that the appearance of the gestational sac occurred at a total HCG level greater than 2,004 mIU per mL. In yet another transvaginal ultrasound study, the smallest gestational sac diameter detected was 2 mm. This occurred at a beta-HCG concentration of 141 mIU/mL.[12] The researchers concluded that in normal pregnancy a gestational sac should be consistently detectable via vaginal sonography at a beta-HCG level of 750 mIU per mL. This was the so-called safety margin or discriminatory zone.[12] Yeh et al[4] demonstrated the early sonographic appearance of the intrauterine gestational sac consistent with 3.5 weeks' gestation, about the same time the beta-HCG becomes positive.

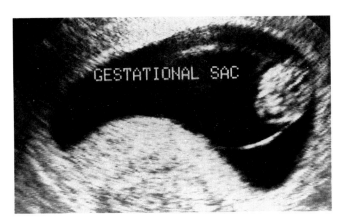

Figure 4–2. Transvaginal ultrasound of an embryo at 7 weeks' gestation, in a sagittal plane. The gestational sac fluid is seen, with the circumferential amnion suspended in the gestational sac and the embryo eccentrically located within the sac.

Embryo Growth

The embryo measures 8 to 14 mm in length in the sixth week, 14 to 20 mm in length in the seventh week, and 21 to 30 mm in length in the eighth week of gestation.

With advanced ultrasound equipment,[13–15] developmental anatomy of the embryo can be appreciated.

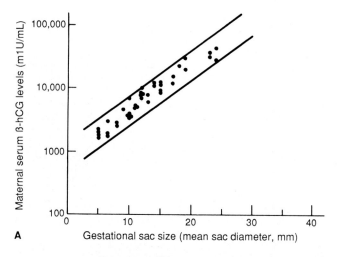
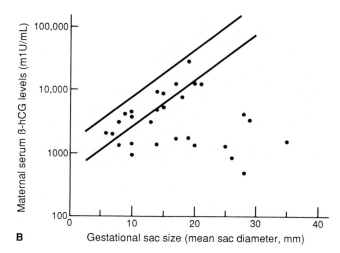

Figure 4–4. (A) Correlation of mean sac diameter with simultaneous serum hCG for 39 normal gestations. Solid lines represent the 95% confidence limits. **(B)** Mean sac diameter compared with serum hCG levels for 30 abnormal gestations. In 65% the hCG level was disproportionately low.

Sequential appearance of the embryonic organs during the first trimester can also be seen.

Yolk Sac

As previously noted, the extraembryonic coelom forms the primary yolk sac and eventually becomes pinched off and extruded, resulting in the formation of the secondary yolk sac at approximately 27 to 28 days menstrual age. The secondary yolk sac develops from the embryonic trilaminar disc and divides into two discrete portions. One portion becomes the definitive lining of the fetal gastrointestinal tract, whereas the other portion is extruded from the fetal body while maintaining contact with the fetal abdomen via the vitelline duct. The fetus itself is enclosed within the amniotic membrane, and the yolk sac and the vitelline duct are located in the fluid space outside the amnion. The secondary yolk sac forms when the mean gestational sac diameter is approximately 3 mm. It is the secondary rather than the primary yolk sac that is commonly identified by ultrasound. Later, owing to differential growth, the yolk sac lies between the amnion and the chorion.[3]

The yolk sac has a characteristic appearance of a bright ringlike structure with no internal echoes.[16,17] It can be visualized sonographically in the extra-amniotic cavity (Fig. 4–3). It can also be detected as early as the 5th week of gestation but disappears sonographically after the 12th week of gestation.[18,19]

TABLE 4–2. SAC SIZE VERSUS HCG LEVELS FOR NORMAL PREGNANCIES (n = 56)

Mean Sac Diameter (mm)	HCG Level (mIU/mL)		
		95% Confidence Limits	
	Predicted*	Lower	Upper
5	1,932	1,026	3,636
6	2,165	1,226	4,256
7	2,704	1,465	4,990
8	3,199	1,749	5,852
9	3,785	2,085	6,870
10	4,478	2,483	8,075
11	5,297	2,952	9,508
12	6,267	3,502	11,218
13	7,415	4,145	13,266
14	8,773	4,894	15,726
15	10,379	5,766	18,682
16	12,270	6,776	22,235
17	14,528	7,964	26,501
18	17,188	9,343	31,621
19	20,337	10,951	37,761
20	24,060	12,820	45,130
21	28,464	15,020	53,970
22	33,675	17,560	64,570
23	39,843	20,573	77,164
24	47,138	24,067	93,325

* Log (HCG) = 2.92 + 0.073 (MSD), R^2 = 0.93, $P < 0.001$.

Nyberg, DA, Filly, RA, Duarte Filho, DL, et al. Abnormal pregnancy: early diagnosis by US and serum chorionic gonadotropin levels. Radiology. 1986; 158:393–396.

TABLE 4–1. GESTATIONAL SAC DETECTION AND HCG LEVELS FOR NORMAL AND ABNORMAL GESTATIONS

HCG (mIU/mL)	Normal (n = 56)		Abnormal (n = 70)	
	No Sac	Sac	No Sac	Sac
< 1,800	17	0	35	12
> 1,800	0	39	4	19

Nyberg, DA, Filly, RA, Duarte Filho, DL, et al. Abnormal pregnancy: early diagnosis by US and serum chorionic gonadotropin levels. Radiology. 1986; 158:393–396.

BIOMETRY

Gestational Sac

It is possible to estimate gestational age on the basis of gestational sac size prior to visualization of the embryo. The gestational sac image in utero is recognized as a reliable marker of embryonic life.[6] A gestational sac appears as a hypoechogenic area usually located in the midline of the uterus, corresponding to the echodense line of the endometrium described earlier. The gestational sac can be visualized as early as 5 weeks of gestation.[6]

To quantify the sac size, the diameters in the sagittal (Fig. 4–2) and transverse planes (Fig. 4–3, Fig. 4–5) must be measured, obtaining the largest sac dimensions. The two sections should be perpendicular to each other.[6]

Nyberg et al[10] reported that the mean sac diameter of 5 mm was consistent with 35 menstrual days. Goldstein et al[6] reported that the normal rate of growth of the gestational sac throughout the first trimester occurs at an average rate of 0.1 cm per day,[14] with a range of 0.71 to 0.75[10] (Table 4–3). Goldstein et al[6] obtained a linear relationship between the measurements of the mean gestational sac growth and the crown–rump length growth. The earliest sonographic visualization of the embryo occurred when the mean gestational sac diameter reached 10 mm (Fig. 4–6). The embryonic heartbeat was visible when the mean gestational sac diameter measured 2 cm (Fig. 4–7), and embryo body movements were imaged when the mean gestational sac diameter reached 3 cm in size (Fig. 4–8).

TABLE 4–3. THE RELATIONSHIP AMONG GESTATIONAL AGE IN WEEKS, AND THE MEAN SAC SIZE, ± 2 SD, AND PERCENTILE DISTRIBUTION OF GESTATIONAL SAC IN MILLIMETERS

Gestational Age (weeks)	Gestational Means	Sac (mm) (± 2 SD)	Gestational Sac (mm)		
			10th	50th	90th
			percentile		
5	8	4	3	6	9
6	14	4	9	14	17
7	26	2	22	27	33
8	29	5	24	29	39

From Goldstein I, Zimmer EA, Tamir A, et al. Evaluation of normal gestational sac growth: appearance of embryonic heartbeat and embryo body movements using the transvaginal technique. Obstet Gynecol. 1991; 77:885–888; with permission.

Embryo and Fetal Growth

Ultrasound determination of the fetal crown–rump length (Fig. 4–9 and Fig. 4–10) in the first trimester of pregnancy was introduced by Robinson in 1973.[20] A normal curve of the fetal crown–rump length was derived between the 6th and 14th weeks of gestation, with an accuracy of within 3 days. Robinson and Fleming[21] showed that the fetal age could be estimated

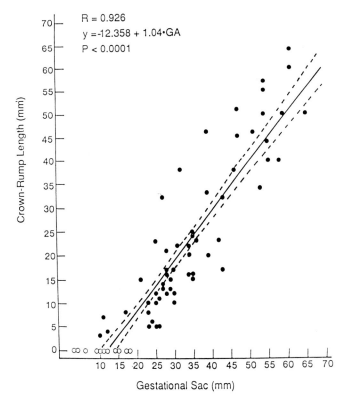

Figure 4–6. The linear relationship between crown–rump length in millimeters and mean gestational sac size in millimeters, with 95% confidence limits (dotted lines). The open circles represent gestational sacs that did not contain a detected measurable embryo (from Goldstein[6]).

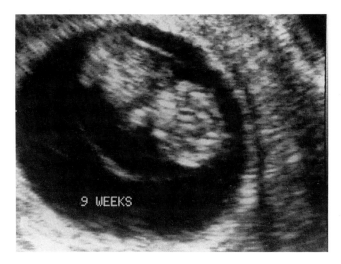

Figure 4–5. Transvaginal examination in a cross-sectional plane of a fetus at 9 weeks' gestation. The well-circumscribed gestational sac contains the amniotic sac, its fluid, and the fetus.

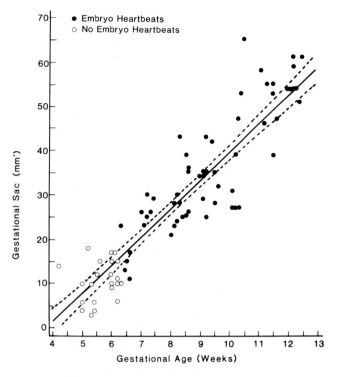

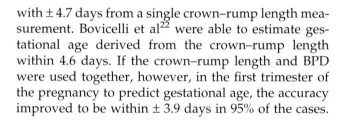

Figure 4–7. The relationship between mean gestational sac diameter in millimeters and gestational age in weeks. The closed dots represent embryo heartbeats; the open dots represent absence of embryo heartbeats (from Goldstein[6]).

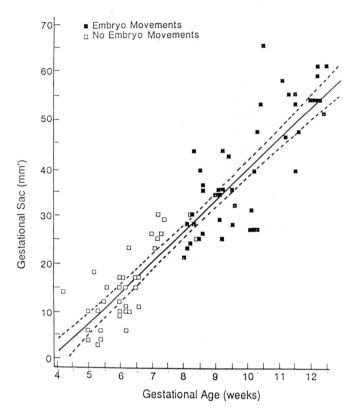

Figure 4–8. The linear relationship between mean gestational sac diameter in millimeters and gestational age in weeks with 95% confidence limits. The closed squares represent embryo movements; the open squares represent absence of embryo movements (from Goldstein[6]).

with ± 4.7 days from a single crown–rump length measurement. Bovicelli et al[22] were able to estimate gestational age derived from the crown–rump length within 4.6 days. If the crown–rump length and BPD were used together, however, in the first trimester of the pregnancy to predict gestational age, the accuracy improved to be within ± 3.9 days in 95% of the cases.

It appears that the crown–rump length is biologically stable and thus provides reproducible and reliable results. This finding suggests that the biologic variability of the crown–rump length is small. Drumm and coworkers[23] did not find any effect of maternal influences on the fetal crown–rump length. Other investigators have demonstrated that there are excep-

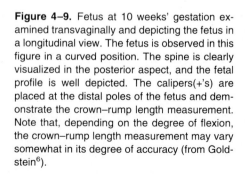

Figure 4–9. Fetus at 10 weeks' gestation examined transvaginally and depicting the fetus in a longitudinal view. The fetus is observed in this figure in a curved position. The spine is clearly visualized in the posterior aspect, and the fetal profile is well depicted. The calipers(+'s) are placed at the distal poles of the fetus and demonstrate the crown–rump length measurement. Note that, depending on the degree of flexion, the crown–rump length measurement may vary somewhat in its degree of accuracy (from Goldstein[6]).

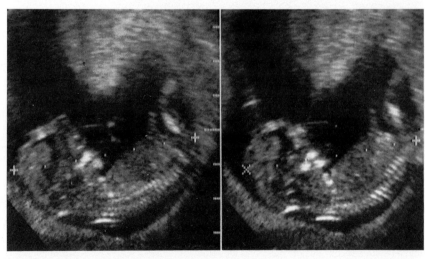

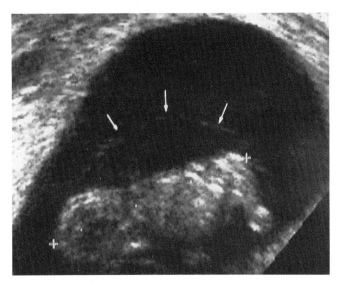

Figure 4–10 Transvaginal exam of a fetus at 10 weeks' gestation. A well-developed gestational sac, with an echogenic rim within representing the amniotic membrane (three arrows), is depicted. The fetus can be seen within the amniotic cavity. Note the fetal curvature, which represents a fetus in an extended position. The calipers(+'s) are depicted at either end of the fetus and measure the crown–rump length measurement (from Goldstein[6]).

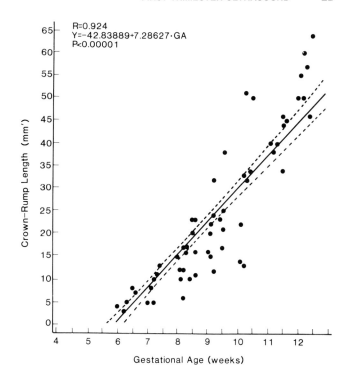

Figure 4–11. The linear relationship between crown–rump length in millimeters and gestational age in weeks with 95% confidence limits (from Goldstein[6]).

tions to that general rule. Female fetuses have a slightly smaller crown–rump length than that observed in male fetuses;[24] the fetus of early diabetic pregnancy has been reputed to be often smaller than the normal,[25,26] although this has been disputed by some. In some pregnancies complicated by threatened abortion, embryos are smaller than would be expected based on the last menstrual period.[27] Investigators also reported early growth retardation of the crown–rump length in the first trimester in fetuses with chromosomal abnormalities.[28]

A transvaginal ultrasound study[6] was recently conducted to determine the relationship between gestational age and crown–rump length growth (Fig. 4–9, Fig. 4–10, and Fig. 4–11), and between the crown–rump length growth and the mean gestational sac growth (Fig. 4–6).

Robinson[29] was the first to describe the presence of fetal heart movement using pulsed ultrasound. He detected the fetal heart movement from the 48th day of menstrual age by an abdominal approach. Investigators have determined embryonic heart motion at 6 weeks and 4 days in 94% and at 7 weeks' gestation in 100% of the cases using the transvaginal approach.[6] These authors determined that with an embryonic size of 5 mm or greater the embryonic heartbeat should be observed (Fig. 4–12), and with an embryonic size of 15 mm or greater, the fetal movements should be seen (Fig. 4–13). A well-performed crown–rump length measurement in the first trimester of the pregnancy is accurate within ± 5 days and is at least as accurate as

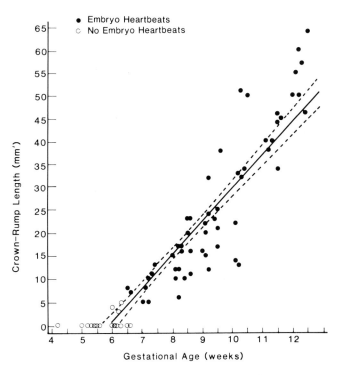

Figure 4–12. The relationship between crown–rump length in millimeters and gestation age in weeks. The closed circles represent embryo heartbeats; the open circles represent absence of embryo heartbeats (from Goldstein[6]).

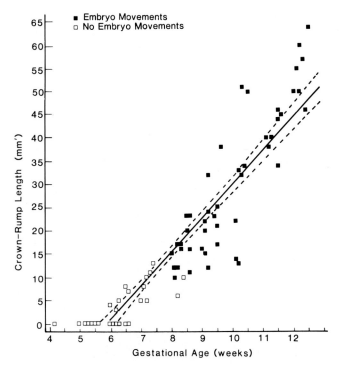

Figure 4–13. The linear relationship between crown–rump length in millimeters and gestational age in weeks, with 95% confidence limits. The closed squares represent embryo movements; the open squares represent absence of embryo movements (from Goldstein[6]).

the BPD measured early in the second trimester[30] (Table 4–4, Table 4–5, Table 4–6).

Yolk Sac

Measurements should be performed in the anteroposterior diameter and from the outer-to-outer margins to determine the yolk sac size (Fig. 4–3). The yolk sac diameter grows from a size of 2 mm in the fifth week of gestation to a maximum of 5 mm in the 11th week of gestation; then decreases in size. It is not usually detectable after the 12th week (Fig. 4–14). The yolk sac can be seen when the mean gestational sac diameter (average of the three gestational sac diameters: longitudinal, anteroposterior, and transverse) is 1 cm[18,31] (Table 4–7).

SONOPATHOLOGY OF FIRST-TRIMESTER PREGNANCY

Anembryonic Gestational Sac

Robinson[32] used the sac size alone as a criterion of abnormal pregnancy. The authors found a sac volume of 2.5 mL without evidence of embryonic echoes as a definitive sign of a blighted ovum even at the first sonographic exam. These investigators determined that if the sac was less than 2.5 ml in volume and failed

TABLE 4–4. ESTIMATION OF GESTATIONAL AGE (MENSTRUAL AGE) FROM CROWN–RUMP LENGTH (CRL) BASED ON 289 MEASUREMENTS IN 101 FETUSES

CRL (mm)	Gestational Age (Weeks + Days)
7	6+3
8	6+4
9	6+6
10	7+0
11	7+2
12	7+3
13	7+4
14	7+5
15	7+6
16	8+0
17	8+1
18	8+2
19	8+3
20	8+4
21	8+5
22	8+6
23	9+0
24	9+1
25	9+2
26	9+3
27	9+3
28	9+4
29	9+5
30	9+6
31	10+0
32	10+0
33	10+1
34	10+2
35	10+2
36	10+3
37	10+4
38	10+5
39	10+5
40	10+6
41	11+0
42	11+0
43	11+1
44	11+2
45	11+2
46	11+3
47	11+3
48	11+4
49	11+5
50	11+5
51	11+6
52	11+6
53	12+0
54	12+1
55	12+1
56	12+2
57	12+2
58	12+3
59	12+3
60	12+4

TABLE 4–4. (CONTINUED)

CRL (mm)	Gestational Age (Weeks + Days)
61	12+4
62	12+5
63	12+5
64	12+6
65	12+6
66	13+0
67	13+0
68	13+1
69	13+1
70	13+2
71	13+2
72	13+3
73	13+3
74	13+4
75	13+4
76	13+5
77	13+5
78	13+5
79	13+6
80	13+6
81	14+0
82	14+0
83	14+0
84	14+1
85	14+1

From Pedersen JF. Fetal crown–rump length measurement by ultrasound in normal pregnancy. Br J Obstet Gynecol. 1982; 89:926–930, with permission.

to increase by at least 75% in 1 week, this was also indicative of a blighted ovum (Fig. 4–15). Bernard and Cooperberg[7] concluded that if the gestational sac was larger than 2 cm in average diameter and lacking an embryonic echo, this represented nonviability of the pregnancy.

Nyberg et al[10] determined that gestational sacs were judged to be abnormal on the basis of specific sonographic criteria, including: 1) large mean size of the gestational sac (equal to or greater than 25 mm) without an embryo (Fig. 4–16), 2) distorted shape of

TABLE 4–5. THE RELATIONSHIP BETWEEN GESTATIONAL AGE IN WEEKS AND MEAN ± 2 SD OF THE CROWN–RUMP LENGTH IN MILLIMETERS

Gestational Age (weeks)	Crown–Rump Length (mm)	
	Mean	*± 2 SD*
6	3	2
7	8.5	3
8	14.5	5
9	21.5	7
10	29.0	7
11	41.0	4
12	54.0	6

TABLE 4–6. VARIATION IN GESTATIONAL AGE (MENSTRUAL AGE) ESTIMATES RELATIVE TO CROWN–RUMP LENGTH NOTED IN THREE REPORTS

Crown-rump length (cm)	Gestational age (weeks + days)		
	MacGregor et al	*Robinson and Fleming*	*Drumm et al*
1.0	7 + 5	7 + 0	6 + 6
1.1	7 + 6	7 + 1	7 + 1
1.2	8 + 0	7 + 3	7 + 2
1.3	8 + 1	7 + 4	7 + 3
1.4	8 + 1	7 + 5	7 + 4
1.5	8 + 2	7 + 6	7 + 5
1.6	8 + 3	8 + 0	7 + 6
1.7	8 + 4	8 + 1	8 + 0
1.8	8 + 5	8 + 2	8 + 1
1.9	8 + 5	8 + 3	8 + 2
2.0	8 + 6	8 + 4	8 + 3
2.1	9 + 0	8 + 5	8 + 4
2.2	9 + 1	8 + 6	8 + 5
2.3	9 + 1	8 + 6	8 + 6
2.4	9 + 2	9 + 0	9 + 0
2.5	9 + 3	9 + 1	9 + 1
2.6	9 + 4	9 + 2	9 + 2
2.7	9 + 4	9 + 3	9 + 3
2.8	9 + 5	9 + 3	9 + 3
2.9	9 + 6	9 + 4	9 + 4
3.0	9 + 6	9 + 5	9 + 5
3.1	10 + 0	9 + 6	9 + 6
3.2	10 + 1	9 + 6	10 + 0
3.3	10 + 2	10 + 0	10 + 0
3.4	10 + 2	10 + 1	10 + 1
3.5	10 + 3	10 + 1	10 + 2
3.6	10 + 4	10 + 2	10 + 3
3.7	10 + 4	10 + 3	10 + 3
3.8	10 + 5	10 + 3	10 + 4
3.9	10 + 6	10 + 4	10 + 5
4.0	10 + 6	10 + 5	10 + 5
4.1	11 + 0	10 + 5	10 + 6
4.2	11 + 1	10 + 6	11 + 0
4.3	11 + 1	11 + 0	11 + 0
4.4	11 + 2	11 + 0	11 + 1
4.5	11 + 3	11 + 1	11 + 2
4.6	11 + 3	11 + 1	11 + 2
4.7	11 + 4	11 + 2	11 + 3
4.8	11 + 5	11 + 3	11 + 4
4.9	11 + 5	11 + 3	11 + 4
5.0	11 + 6	11 + 4	11 + 5
5.1	12 + 0	11 + 4	11 + 5
5.2	12 + 0	11 + 5	11 + 6
5.3	12 + 1	11 + 5	12 + 0
5.4	12 + 1	11 + 6	12 + 0
5.5	12 + 2	11 + 6	12 + 1
5.6	12 + 3	12 + 0	12 + 2
5.7	12 + 3	12 + 1	12 + 2
5.8	12 + 4	12 + 1	12 + 3
5.9	12 + 4	12 + 2	12 + 3
6.0	12 + 5	12 + 2	12 + 4
6.1	12 + 6	12 + 3	12 + 5
6.2	12 + 6	12 + 3	12 + 5
6.3	13 + 0	12 + 4	12 + 6
6.4	13 + 0	12 + 4	12 + 6
6.5	13 + 1	12 + 5	13 + 0
6.6	13 + 2	12 + 5	13 + 0

From MacGregor SN, Tamura RK, Sabbagha RE, et al. Underestimation of gestational age by conventional crown–rump length dating curves. Obstet Gynecol. 1987; 70:344, with permission.

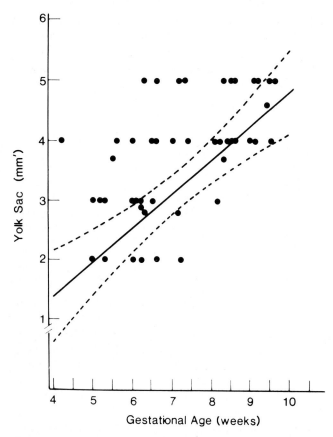

Figure 4–14. The relationship between yolk sac in millimeters and gestational age in weeks.

the gestational sac, 3) weak decidual reaction, 4) absence of a double decidual sac, and 5) low position. Two criteria, large sac and distorted shape, had 100% specificity and were called major criteria. The remaining criteria were less specific, although 100% specificity was achieved when three or more of these minor criteria were demonstrated. The authors concluded that experienced sonographers can reliably identify an abnormal gestational sac on a single examination in many cases (Fig. 4–17).

TABLE 4–7. THE RELATIONSHIP BETWEEN GESTATIONAL AGE IN WEEKS AND THE MEAN ± 2 SD OF YOLK SAC IN MILLIMETERS

Gestational Age (weeks)	Yolk Sac (mm)	
	Mean	*± 2 SD*
4	1.8	1
5	2.0	1
6	2.7	1
7	3.5	1
8	3.8	1
9	4.5	1
10	3.6	2
11	1.7	2
12	1.5	2

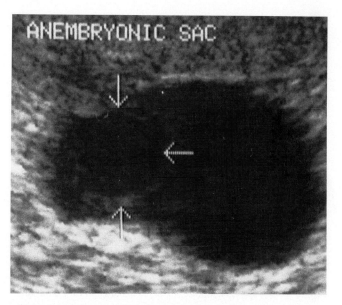

Figure 4–15. Transvaginal ultrasound exam of a pregnancy at 6½ weeks' gestation by last menstrual period with gestational sac borders not well defined. Internally, a small amniotic cavity can be recognized but no fetus or yolk sac is observed. These findings are typical of an anembryonic gestation.

The markers of abnormal pregnancy growth are: 1) mean gestational sac of greater than 2 cm, without embryonic heartbeat; 2) mean gestational sac greater than 3 cm, without embryonic body movements; 3) embryonic heartbeat not identifiable after 6 weeks and 4 days; 4) embryonic body movements not visualized after 8 weeks of gestation; 5) distorted shape of the gestational sac; 6) weak echogenic decidual reaction;

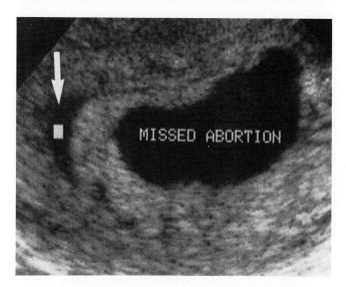

Figure 4–16. Pregnancy at 6 weeks' gestation examined transvaginally. There is a large gestational sac with well-defined borders and without embryo, yolk sac, or amniotic membrane within the gestational sac. An echolucent area (arrow) is outside the sac and represents a residual hemorrhage. These findings are indicative of a missed abortion.

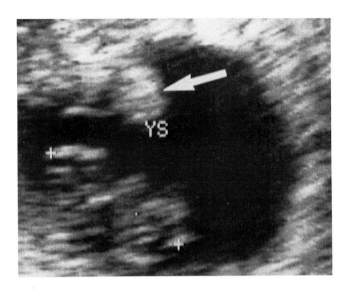

Figure 4–17. Transvaginal ultrasound examination of a pregnancy at 8 weeks' gestation. A gestational sac with fairly well-defined borders is seen with an embryo in the posterior aspect of the sac. The calipers(+'s) are seen at either end of the embryo and measure the crown–rump length. The yolk sac is seen in the upper portion of the gestational sac. Note that the yolk sac is highly echodense (arrow) and represents a sclerotic yolk sac. This pregnancy was not viable and resulted in a missed abortion.

7) absence of a double decidual sac; and 8) low position.[6, 10] Developmental events can be described using these sonographic markers.

Ectopic Pregnancy

The utility of ultrasound scanning for the diagnosis of tubal pregnancy is well established. The practical concept of the discriminatory zone HCG level, linked with sonographic findings, was proposed by Kadar et al[8] in 1981. They reported that an HCG level greater than 6,500 mIU per mL, in the absence of an intrauterine gestational sac on ultrasound, suggested a tubal pregnancy. Many tubal pregnancies were present, however, with HCG levels less than 6,500 mIU per mL. Transvaginal ultrasound imaging has significantly lowered the HCG discriminatory zone for the diagnosis of ectopic pregnancy.[11] Nyberg et al[33] reported that when the human chorionic gonadotropin level exceeded 1,800 mIU per mL, an intrauterine gestational sac is normally detected, and suggested that its absence is evidence for an ectopic pregnancy. Bateman et al[11] reported the doubling time for HCG in tubal pregnancies was 7.69 ± 9.8 days.

Investigators reported a lack of a visible embryo and a yolk sac in women with suspected ectopic pregnancies. They suggested that a yolk sac is reliable evidence for early intrauterine pregnancy and virtually excluded the possibility of an ectopic pregnancy.[34]

Some authors have suggested that blood within the uterine cavity cannot be distinguished from an abnormal intrauterine pregnancy.[9] Extrauterine findings, however, were of some value in predicting tubal pregnancy. The presence of a noncystic adnexal mass or fluid in the cul-de-sac were specific but not sensitive findings in detecting ectopic pregnancies. Transvaginal scanning was sensitive and specific in detecting cul-de-sac blood when the volume was greater than 100 mL. A typical adnexal mass may be present in some cases of extrauterine pregnancy.[35]

Investigators using transvaginal ultrasound reported the presence of fetal cardiac activity in the adnexa in 9% to 13% of ectopic pregnancies. These sonographic indices, the HCG titers, and the physical findings are all useful parameters for the diagnosis of extrauterine pregnancy.

Abnormal Yolk Sacs

The yolk sac, vascularized by means of the vitelline vessels, plays an integral role in hematopoiesis. Whether disturbances in yolk sac development should be considered as a primary cause of embryonic death or as a result of developmental anomalies of the embryo is unclear.

Although the yolk sac is a fetal structure, it is located outside the amnion and, in cases of spontaneous abortion (Fig. 4–17), the embryonic tissue may be evacuated, leaving the yolk sac behind.[36] Nyberg et al[19] found yolk sacs in only 16% of abnormal intrauterine pregnancies and in none of ectopic pregnancies.

Management of Abnormal Gestations

The following represent signs of inevitable abortion when termination of pregnancy may be considered: 1) the mean gestational sac is equal to or greater than 10 mm, with absence of an embryo; 2) the mean gestational sac is equal to or greater than 2 cm, with absence of fetal heart motion; 3) the mean gestational sac is equal to or greater than 3 cm, with absence of fetal motion; 4) the crown–rump length measurement is equal to or greater than 10 mm with absence of fetal heart motion; 5) the crown–rump length measurement is equal to or greater than 15 mm with absence of fetal movements.[13]

If the diagnosis is equivocal, then pregnancy management should be expectant with follow-up ultrasound and clinical examinations until a diagnosis can be made with certainty.

REFERENCES

1. Cashner KA, Christopher CR, Dysert GA. Spontaneous fetal loss after demonstrating of a live fetus in the first trimester. *Obstet Gynecol.* 1987;70:827–830.
2. Wilson RD, Kendrick V, Wittmann BK, et al. Sponta-

neous abortion and pregnancy outcome after normal first trimester ultrasound examination. *Obstet Gynecol.* 1986;67:352–355.

3. Moore KL, ed. *The Developing Human: Clinically Oriented Embryology,* 3rd ed. Philadelphia, Pa.: WB Saunders Co; 1982:14–139, 375–390.

4. Yeh HC, Goodman JD, Carr L, et al. Intradecidual sign: a US criterion of early intrauterine pregnancy. *Radiology.* 1986;161:463–467.

5. Nyberg DA, Laing FC, Filly RA, et al. Ultrasonographic differentiation of the gestational sac of early intrauterine pregnancy from the pseudogestational sac of ectopic pregnancy. *Radiology.* 1983;146:755–759.

6. Goldstein I, Zimmer EA, Tamir A, et al. Ultrasonographic evaluation of normal gestational sac growth: appearance of embryo heartbeat and embryo body movements using transvaginal technique. *Obstet Gynecol.* 1991;77:885–888.

7. Bernard KG, Cooperberg PL. Sonographic differentiation between blighted ovum and early viable pregnancy. *AJR.* 1985;144:597–602.

8. Kadar N, DeVore G, Romero R. Discriminatory hCG zone: its use in sonographic evaluation for ectopic pregnancy. *Obstet Gynecol.* 1981;58:156–160.

9. Nyberg DA, Filly RA, Duarte Filho DL, et al. Abnormal pregnancy: early diagnosis by US and serum chorionic gonadotropin levels. *Radiology.* 1986;158:393–396.

10. Nyberg DA, Laing FC, Filly RA. Threatened abortion: sonographic distinction of normal and abnormal gestational sac. *Radiology.* 1986;158:397–400.

11. Bateman BG, Nunley Jr WC, Kolp LA, et al. Vaginal sonography findings and hCG dynamics of early intrauterine and tubal pregnancies. *Obstet Gynecol.* 1990; 75:421–427.

12. Bernaschek G, Rudelstorfer R, Csaicsich P. Vaginal sonography versus serum human chorionic gonadotropin in early detection of pregnancy. *Am J Obstet Gynecol.* 1988;158:608–612.

13. Green JJ, Hobbins JC. Abdominal ultrasound examination of the first trimester fetus. *Am J Obstet Gynecol.* 1988;159:676–681.

14. Timor-Tritsch IE, Farine D, Rosen MG. A close look at early embryonic development with the high frequency transvaginal transducer. *Am J Obstet Gynecol.* 1988; 159:676–681.

15. Warren WB, Timor-Tritsch IE, Peisner DB. Dating the early pregnancy by sequential appearance of embryonic structures. *Am J Obstet Gynecol.* 1989;161:747–753.

16. Mantoni M, Peterson JF. Ultrasound visualization of the human yolk sac. *J Clin Ultrasound.* 1979;7:459–460.

17. Sauerbrei E, Cooperberg PL, Poland BJ. Ultrasound demonstration of the normal yolk sac. *J Clin Ultrasound.* 1980;8:217–220.

18. Goldstein I, Zimmer EA, Tamir A. The evaluation of normal yolk sac growth in normal and abnormal pregnancies using the transvaginal technique. (in preparation).

19. Nyberg DA, Mack LA, Harvey D, et al.: Value of the yolk sac in evaluating early pregnancies. *J Ultrasound Med.* 1988;7:129–135.

20. Robinson HP. Sonar measurement of fetal crown–rump length as means of assessing maturity in the first trimester of pregnancy. *Br Med. J.* 1973;4:28–31.

21. Robinson HP, Fleming JE. A critical evaluation of sonar "crown–rump" length measurements. *Br J Obstet Gynecol.* 1975;82:702–710.

22. Bovicelli L, Orsini LF, Rizzo N, et al. Estimation of gestational age during the first trimester by real time measurement of fetal crown–rump length and biparietal diameter. *J Clin Ultrasound.* 1981;9:71–75.

23. Drumm JE, Clinch J, MacKenzie G. The ultrasonic measurement of fetal crown–rump length as a method of assessing gestational age. *Br J Obstet Gynecol.* 1976; 83:417–421.

24. Peterson JF. Fetal crown–rump length measurement by ultrasound in normal pregnancy. *Br J Obstet Gynecol.* 1982;89:926–930.

25. Peterson JF, Peterson LM, Mortensen HB. Fetal growth delay and maternal hemoglobin A1c in early diabetic pregnancy. *Obstet Gynecol.* 1984;64:351–352.

26. Cousins L, Key TC, Schorzman L, et al. Ultrasonographic assessment of early fetal growth in insulin-treated diabetic pregnancies. 1988;159:1186–1190.

27. MacGregor SN, Tamura RK, Sabbagha RE, et al. Underestimation of gestational age by conventional crown–rump length dating curves. *Obstet Gynecol.* 1987;70:344.

28. Benacerraf BR. Intrauterine growth retardation in the first trimester associated with triploidy. *J Ultrasound Med.* 1988;7:153–154.

29. Robinson HP. Detection of fetal heart movement in the first trimester of pregnancy using pulsed ultrasound. *Br Med J.* 1972;4:466–468.

30. Kurtz AB, Needlman L. Ultrasound assessment of fetal age. In: Cullan PW, ed. *Ultrasonography in Obstetrics and Gynecology.* 2nd ed. Philadelphia, Pa.: WB Saunders Co; 1988:47–62.

31. Crooij MJ, Westhuis M, Schoemaker J, et al. Ultrasonographic measurement of the yolk sac. *Br J Obstet Gynecol.* 1982;89:931–934.

32. Robinson HP: The diagnosis of early pregnancy failure by sonar. *Br J Obstet Gynecol.* 1975:82:849–857.

33. Nyberg DA, Filly RA, Laing FC, et al. Ectopic pregnancy: diagnosis by sonography correlated with quantitative HCG levels. *J Ultrasound Med* 1987;6:145–150.

34. Nyberg DA, Mack LA, Harvey D, et al. Value of the yolk sac in evaluating early pregnancies. *J Ultrasound Med.* 1988;7:129–135.

35. Rottem S, Timor-Tritsch IE: Think ectopic. In: Timor-Tritsch, IE, Rottem S. eds., *Transvaginal Sonography,* 2nd ed. New York, NY: Elsevier; 1991:373–392.

36. Hurowitz SR. Yolk sac sign: sonographic appearance of the fetal yolk sac in missed abortion. *J Ultrasound Med.* 1986;5:435–438.

5

The Normal and Abnormal Fetal Head

The Normal Fetal Head

INTRODUCTION

The fetal head undergoes important developmental changes throughout gestation. These changes are not only quantitative modifications in the relative size of the intracranial structures or the compartments, but they also reflect quantitative growth. Ultrasound is highly effective in evaluating the fetal head. Cranial structures can be identified very early in gestation with the use of advanced, third-generation ultrasound machines. Ultrasound imaging provides a means of visualizing the sometimes subtle anatomic features of the fetal brain using an essentially simple technique. The normal biologic and mathematical growth of the fetal brain system is described in this chapter, and normative data on the overall morphology and changes in size of the fetal head throughout pregnancy is provided. The fetal head is regarded as a topographic map, divided into portions, with each described separately. Fetal head growth and development is assessed by the use of nomograms developed during the last two decades.

NORMAL INTRACRANIAL ANATOMY OF THE FETUS

The primary goals of examining the fetal head sonographically are to image and to depict a rather complex three-dimensional structure using a two-dimensional tool.[1-4] Therefore, a large number of scans taken in multiple planes are necessary.

The fetal brain undergoes important developmental changes during the first half of pregnancy. Such changes are not only related quantitatively to the modification in the ratio between the cerebral parenchyma and cerebrospinal fluid compartment, but they are also related to the shape of the ventricles and the parenchymal structure.[5-10] Some of these changes involve geometric modifications of the cerebral structures, as well as the sonographic appearance of the fetal brain. During early gestation the dominant fluid-filled lateral ventricles are easily recognized. This results in enhancement of the echogenicity, causing the distal cerebral cortex to appear more echogenic than later in gestation. In order to detect congenital anomalies of the fetal head and brain, it is necessary to become familiar with the normal sonographic appearance of these structures in different scanning planes and at different gestational ages.

Sonoanatomy

The axial, sagittal, and coronal planes are each used in the evaluation of the fetal head (Fig. 5–1, Fig. 5–2, and Fig. 5–3).[3] The latter two planes are difficult to obtain

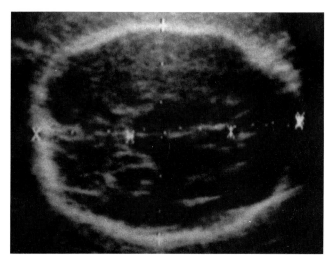

Figure 5–1. An axial scan of the fetal head at the level of the thalami. This plane is used for obtaining the biparietal diameter (BPD), which is shown by the verticle calipers(×'s).

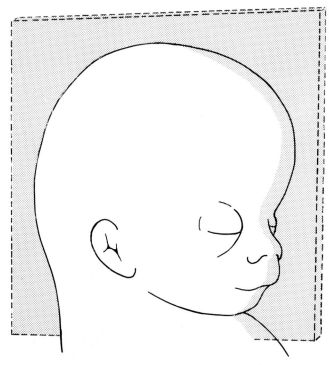

Figure 5–2. A sagittal scan of the fetal head shown schematically.

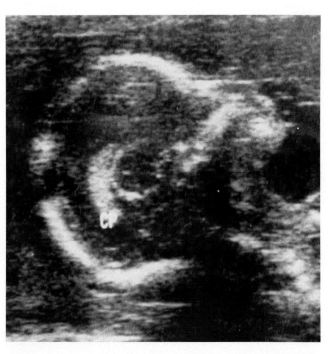

Figure 5–4. Transabdominal scan of a fetus at about 22 weeks' gestation showing the fetal head in profile. Most importantly, the choroid plexus (CP) is above the corpus callosum. Other normal craniofacial structures, such as the nasal area, the maxilla, the mandible, and the neck, are observed.

in transabdominal scanning but are often feasible via transvaginal sonography.

A scan of the fetal head along the anteroposterior axis will result in a sagittal view (Fig. 5–4, Fig. 5–5, and Fig. 5–6), while coronal views are obtained by scanning along the lateral axis (Fig. 5–7 and Fig. 5–8). Both require application of the transducer to the top of

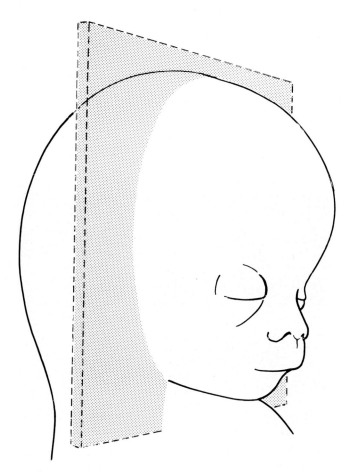

Figure 5–3. A coronal scan of the fetal head shown schematically.

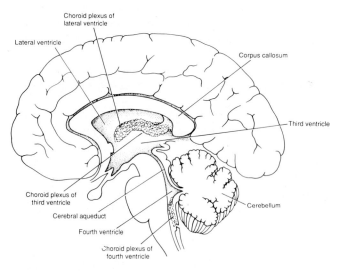

Figure 5–5. Schematic drawing of a fetal brain in a sagittal view demonstrating the ventricular system in relationship to other structures within the brain.

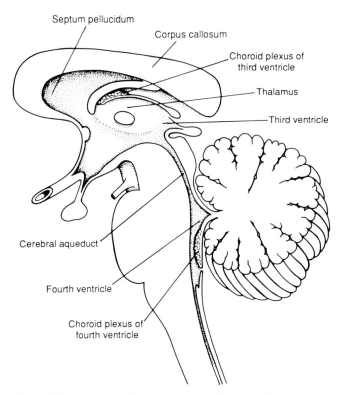

Figure 5–6. Schematic drawing of a sagittal section of the ventricular system. Note the lateral ventricle containing the choroid plexus; the third ventricle into which the cerebrospinal fluid will eventually flow; the cerebral aqueduct; and the fourth ventricle. Other structures identified include the corpus callosum and the cerebellum.

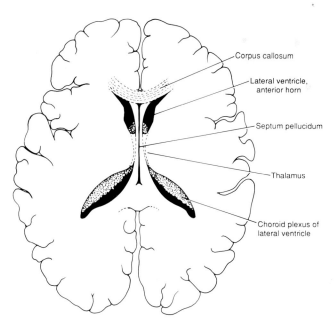

Figure 5–8. Schematic drawing of a coronal view of the fetal brain taken at midpoint in the midregion. Note the midline structures, including the corpus callosum, lateral ventricle, septum cavum pellucidum, thalamus, and choroid plexus of the lateral ventricle.

the fetal head, which is difficult to accomplish using a transabdominal technique.

The earliest identifiable structure in the lateral axial scan is the prominent choroid plexus, which almost entirely fills the lateral ventricle (Fig. 5–9). The considerable echogenicity of the choroid plexus early in

gestation is attributed to its high glycogen content, which enables it to serve as a principal energy source to the relatively hypovascular brain.[11] The cerebellar hemispheres, the cisterna magna, and the falx cerebri can be clearly identified by the beginning of the second trimester (Fig. 5–10 and Fig. 5–11).

This chapter emphasizes the axial planes and the

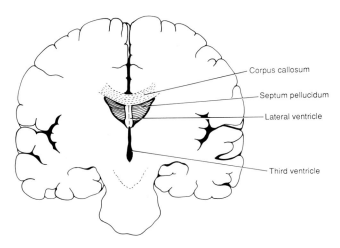

Figure 5–7. Schematic drawing of a coronal view of the fetal brain demonstrating the corpus callosum, the septum cavum pellucidum, the third and lateral ventricles. (Note: this coronal section was taken slightly anteriorly.)

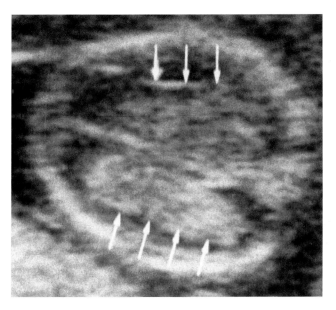

Figure 5–9. Transabdominal examination of the fetal head in an axial view at 13 weeks' gestation. The choroid plexuses are bilaterally located echodense masses which almost fill the entire fetal head. Arrows indicate the outer margin of the lateral ventricles.

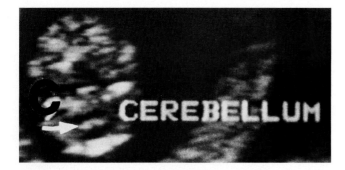

Figure 5–10. Transabdominal examination of a fetus at 10 weeks' gestation depicting the echodense structure of the cerebellum in the posterior fossa (arrow).

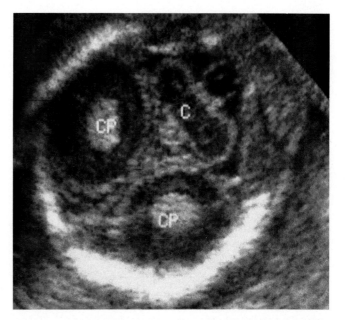

Figure 5–11. Transvaginal examination of a fetal head at approximately 15 weeks' gestation depicting the choroid plexuses (CP) surrounded by the echolucent lateral ventricles containing cerebrospinal fluid. The cerebellum is posterior (C) as is the echolucent cisterna magna. Note that the lateral ventricles appear semicircular in this view and are separated by the midline falx that lies between the cerebellum and the anterior skull table.

sonoanatomy of the fetal head at these planes, since the transabdominal exam is often used beyond the first trimester when the intracranial anatomy is best seen. An axial view is readily obtained with transabdominal scanning of the fetal head at a slight angle[12] (Fig. 5–12). For better fetal head evaluation a number of levels through the axial plane should be examined:

1. The highest axial zone goes through the bodies of the lateral ventricles (Fig. 5–13 and Fig. 5–14).
2. The next axial scanning zone passes through the frontal horns, atria, and occipital horn of the lateral ventricle (Fig. 5–15 and Fig. 5–16).
3. The third axial scanning zone is carried out at the level of the biparietal diameter (BPD) (Fig. 5–17).
4. The fourth axial zone passes through the midbrain and chiasmatic cistern.[3] At this level, the cerebral peduncles are seen as an echo-free, heart-shaped structure posterior to the active pulsation of the basilar artery, which is found in the interpeduncular cistern. A quadrangular echo-free area, corresponding to the chiasmatic cistern, can be observed anterior to

the interpeduncular cistern. Pulsation of the arteries of the circle of Willis are seen within this space, surrounding the echogenic optic chiasma.
5. The structure of the posterior fossa can be observed at a lower level.

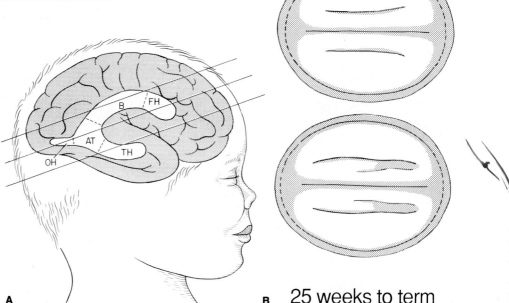

Figure 5–12. (A) Schematic diagram of a fetus in the sagittal view demonstrating the well-developed ventricular system from 25 weeks to term. Note the frontal horn (FH), the body (B), atrium (AT), occipital horn (OH), and the temporal horn (TH). **(B)** Schematic view of ventricular system resulting from axial plane through the most cephalad line in A.

A

B 25 weeks to term

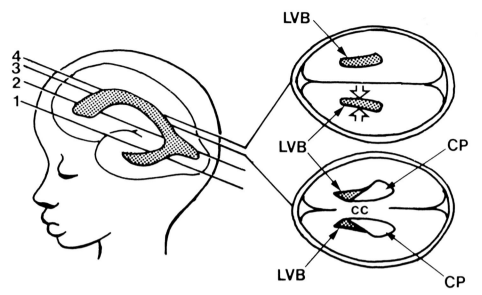

Figure 5-13. Schematic diagram of the fetal head with the horseshoe-shaped structure representing the fetal ventricular system. The lines drawn obliquely numbered 1, 2, 3, and 4 represent the various axial planes of sonographic examination possible. Numbers 3 and 4 represent levels at which the bodies of the lateral ventricle (LVB), and the corpus callosum (CC) can best be visualized, as shown schematically. Note the choroid plexus (CP) and lateral ventricular body (LVB) are both well-defined at level 3.

VENTRICULAR OR SUPERIOR LEVEL

Lateral Ventricles

There are two parallel lateral ventricles occupying the middle portion of the intracranial hemispheres (Fig. 5-18). The lateral ventricles are divided into five portions: anterior horn, body, atrium, posterior horn, and temporal horn.[3,5-8] Four periods of lateral ventricular growth are listed in the schematic illustration of the lateral ventricles:

1. The first period of growth is between 9 and 14 weeks' gestation, when the primitive lateral ventricle is seen with a prominent atrium (Fig. 5-19).
2. The second period of growth is between 15 and 16 weeks' gestation. The frontal horn (anterior horn), body, atrium, and temporal horn can be identified at this gestational age (Fig. 5-20).
3. The third period of growth is between 17 and 24 weeks' gestation, when the occipital horn (posterior horn) can be recognized (Fig. 5-21).

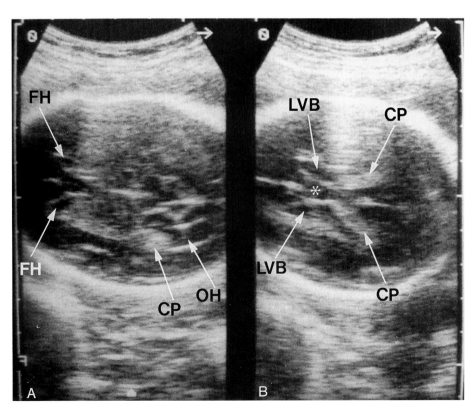

Figure 5-14. Ultrasound exam of the fetal head in the second trimester. **(A)** Axial view clearly identifying the frontal horns (FH), choroid plexus (CP), and occipital horn (OH). **(B)** Axial plane corresponding to level 3 in Figure 5-13. Note the choroid plexus (CP) in the body of the lateral ventricle (LVB). Asterisk shows echolucency representative of possible dilated third ventricle, in an otherwise normal fetus. (*Reprinted with permission from Reece EA, Hobbins JC, Mahoney J, et al. eds.* Medicine of the Fetus and Mother. *Philadelphia: JB Lippincott, 1992.*)

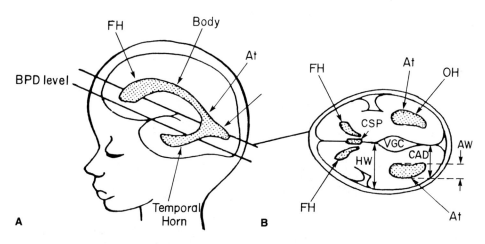

Figure 5–15. Schematic representation of ultrasound of fetal head at the level of the lateral ventricles. **(A)** Profile view showing horseshoe-shaped ventricular system. FH = frontal horn; At = atrium; temporal horn, body, and BPD level indicated. Anterior oblique line represents plane shown in B. **(B)** Representation of axial plane above the BPD level showing frontal horn (FH), occipital horn (OH), and portions of the atria (At). CAD = cerebroatrial distance; HW = hemispheric width; AW = atrial width; CSP = cavum septum pellucidum; VGC = vein of Galen.

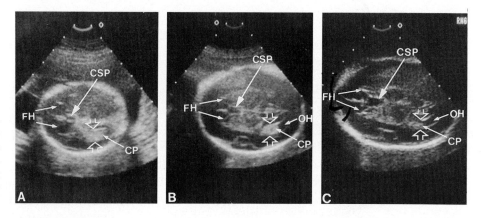

Figure 5–16. Axial scan of fetal head depicting the development of the occipital horn (OH) of the lateral ventricle. FH = frontal horn; CSP = cavum septum pellucidum; CP = choroid plexus. **(A)** Late first trimester. **(B)** Second trimester. **(C)** Early third trimester.

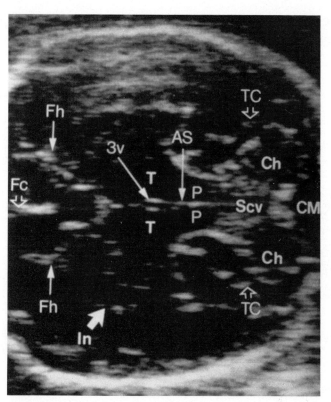

Figure 5–17. Transabdominal scan of a third-trimester fetus in a plane at the level of the biparietal diameter but slightly oblique. Several intracranial structures can be identified, including the midline falx cerebri (Fc), the frontal horns (Fh) of the lateral ventricles, and the insula (In). Midline structures, such as the third ventricle (3v), thalami (T), the aqueduct of Sylvius (AS), the cerebellar peduncles (P), the superior cerebellar vermis (Scv), cerebellar hemispheres (Ch), cisterna magna (CM), and the cerebellar tonsils (TC), are also easily visualized.

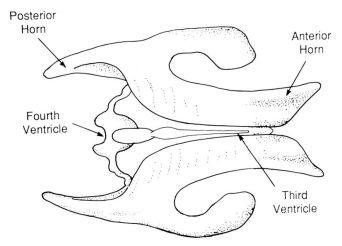

Figure 5–18. Diagrammatic representation of the ventricular system demonstrating the various portions of the ventricles: posterior horn, anterior horn, and third and fourth ventricles.

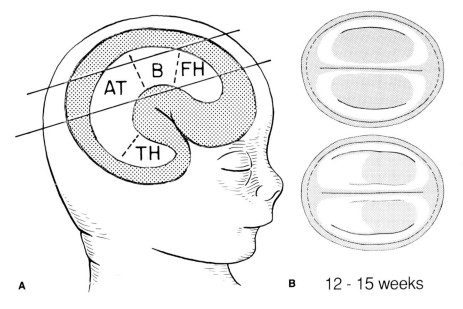

Figure 5–19. Diagrammatic representation of the fetal brain between 9 and 14 weeks' gestation specifically at the level of the lateral ventricles. **(A)** The line most cephalad represents the ultrasound beam in an axial plane. Note the frontal horn (FH), body (B), atrium (AT) and temporal horn (TH). **(B)** View of axial plane in A showing lateral ventricles filled almost entirely by the choroid plexus on either side of the midline. At this gestational age, the ventricle fills virtually the entire hemisphere.

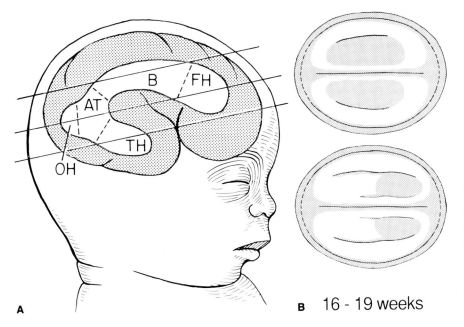

Figure 5–20. Schematic diagram showing the ventricular system in a midtrimester fetus. **(A)** Sagittal view illustrating the frontal horn (FH), the body (B), atrium (AT), occipital horn (OH), and the temporal horn (TH). **(B)** Schematic view of ventricular system resulting from axial plane through most cephalad line in part A. Note the ventricular size is similar to that in earlier gestation, but greater brain tissue is present.

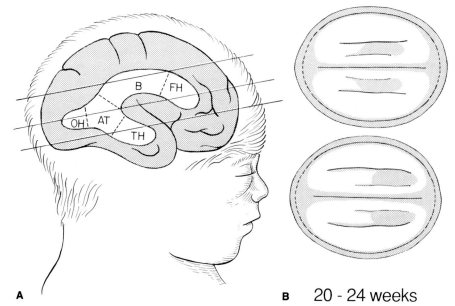

Figure 5–21. Schematic representation of fetal ventricular system at 20–24 weeks' gestation. **(A)** Sagittal view demonstrating the well-developed ventricular system. The line most cephalad represents the plane at which the ultrasound examination is done. **(B)** Schematic view of the well-defined ventricles seen in the axial plane described in A. There is significantly increased brain tissue compared with earlier gestation. The ventricular-width-to-hemispheric-width ratio decreases with advancing gestation.

A

B   20 - 24 weeks

4. The fourth period of lateral ventricular growth establishes the final shape of the lateral ventricle (Fig. 5–12).

Embryology

The lateral ventricles originate from the telocoele, the primitive neural cavity contained within the telencephalon and the primordium of the forebrain. Cleavage of the telencephalon along the sagittal plane results in a paired, symmetrical division of the internal telocoele, forming two distinct cavities. These cavities initially communicate with each other, with the inferior diacoele, and with the primitive third ventricle through the interventricular foramen.[5–8,13]

The rapidly growing hemispheres rotate in the following ways: bringing the rudimentary lateral ventricles to almost parallel planes and at the same time enfolding the thin membranous roof of the telocoele and the tela choroidea, deep in the brain. Throughout gestation, the lateral ventricles are stretched and molded by many developmental processes that occur within the forebrain, including the differential growth of the cerebral lobes, basal ganglia, and thalami, and the formation and deepening of cerebral sulci. Narrowing of the interventricular foramen by the developing thalamus and corpus striatum results in the formation of the foramen of Monro, which connect the lateral ventricles to the third ventricle and topographically divides the anterior end of the lateral ventricle or the frontal horn from the posterior body.

The definitive appearance of the frontal horn appears to be determined mainly by the growth of the basal ganglia of the corpus striatum and the genu of the corpus callosum, which results in a progressive reduction in size and molding of the internal lumen of the ventricle[13] (Fig. 5–6, Fig. 5–8, and Fig. 5–22).

Sonoanatomy

Early in gestation, the lateral ventricles are mostly occupied by relative space of the hemispheres and partially filled with the echogenic choroid plexuses. At midgestation, the size of the lateral ventricles remains fairly constant; the brain tissue increases in size, and thus gives the false impression of diminished size of the lateral ventricles.[5–7,14,15]

The frontal horn and the atrium appear prominent during early gestation.[5–8] The occipital horns do not develop prior to the 16th week of gestation. The atrium appears round and is pushed laterally owing to the increase of brain mass in between the midline and the medial wall of the lateral ventricles. The frontal horns, as well as the occipital horn, are occupied with fluid and are sonographically hypoechogenic in appearance. During pregnancy, therefore, the lateral ventricles diverge anteriorly and posteriorly.

The frontal horns are recognized as sonolucent areas resembling butterfly wings on both sides of the cavum septi pellucidae during the second and early third trimesters (Fig. 5–17). The frontal horns remain rounded until midpregnancy; later in gestation the edges appear straight. The lateral aspect of the frontal horns, occurring at right angles to the ultrasound beam, usually appears as a well-defined, straight echogenic line. It becomes difficult to visualize the lumen of the frontal horns after 30 weeks of gestation; it is easier, however, to recognize the lateral walls of the frontal horns of the lateral ventricles.

Biometry

The distance between the midline echo and the lateral wall of the lateral ventricle (internal ventricular width) measured in the second trimester is approximately one quarter of the distance of the hemisphere (hemispheric

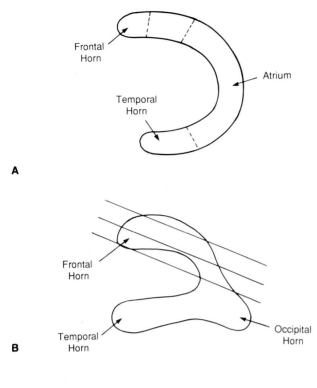

A

B

C

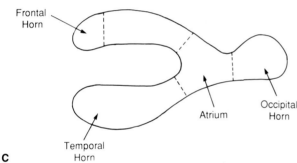

Figure 5–22. Diagrammatic representation of the developmental process of the lateral ventricles. **(A)** Note the half moon shape of the ventricle seen at about 12 weeks' gestation. Note the frontal horn, atrium, and temporal horn. **(B)** Development of the occipital horn, which is consistent with the ultrasound findings in a fetus of approximately 16–20 weeks' gestation. **(C)** Shape and contour of a mature ventricular system seen as early as midgestation. Note the development of the occipital horn.

distance); in the third trimester, it is approximately one third of the distance of the hemisphere.[14,16–21] Many nomograms are available to document the size of the lateral ventricles throughout gestation.

Only the lateral wall of the lateral ventricles could previously be clearly and consistently visualized during the third trimester. It is now possible to visualize both the lateral and the medial walls of the lateral ventricles throughout gestation with third-generation ultrasound equipment in many cases (Fig. 5–23, Fig. 5–24, and Fig. 5–25). Fewer nomograms are available for these varied determinations throughout pregnancy.[5–8]

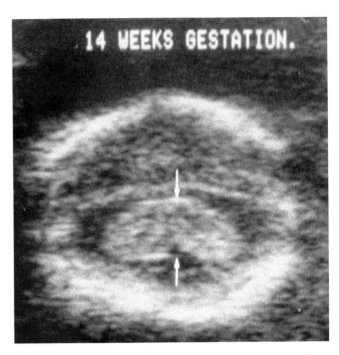

Figure 5–23. Transvaginal examination of the fetal head at about 14 weeks' gestation depicting the lateral ventricles and the choroid plexuses within these ventricles. In addition, both medial and lateral walls (arrows) of the lateral ventricles can be visualized.

Campbell[22] reported the normal values of the frontal horn and hemispheric width ratio from 14 to 21 weeks' gestation. The average ratio of the frontal horn distance and hemispheric width ratio at 14 weeks of gestation was about 60% and decreased to about 40% at 21 weeks' gestation. Other investigators[19] have re-

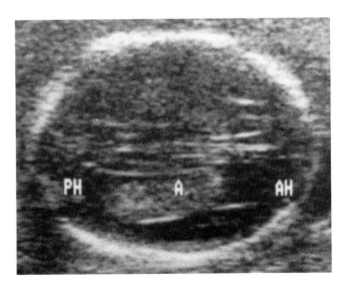

Figure 5–24. Transabdominal scan of a fetal head at about 16 weeks' gestation depicting the lateral ventricles. In this view, the lateral ventricle furthest from the transducer can be seen best, with the choroid plexus filling most of its body. The other visible aspects of the lateral ventricle include the posterior horn (PH), the atrial area (A) and the anterior, or frontal, horn (AH).

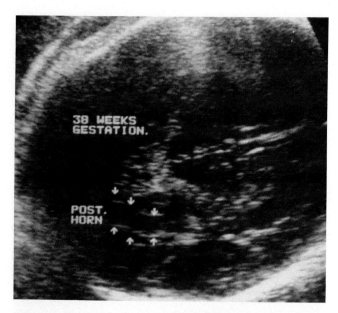

Figure 5–25. Axial view of the fetal head at about 38 weeks' gestation at a level above the biparietal diameter revealing the lateral ventricles. The medial and lateral walls of the posterior horn of the lateral ventricle are seen (arrows). The choroid plexuses are also seen as echodense structures within the ventricles.

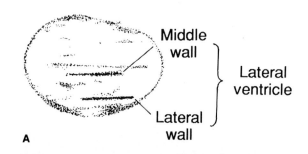

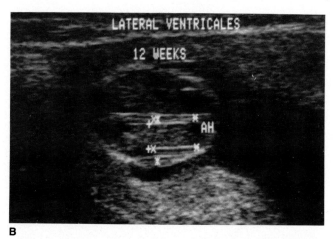

Figure 5–26. Representation of fetal brain at 12 weeks' gestation. **(A)** Schematic outline of the fetal brain. Note the horizontal midline representing the falx which divides the two hemispheres. Located inferiorly to the midline is the middle, or medial, wall of the lateral ventricle. Further lateral is the lateral wall of the lateral ventricle. **(B)** Ultrasound picture showing the features mentioned in part A (AH = anterior horn).

ported normal measurements of the bifrontal horn width distance between the lateral aspects of both frontal horns. They indicated that this distance increased with the gestation.

Goldstein et al[5] measured the cerebrofrontal horn distance (CFHD) of the lateral ventricles. The CFHD is measured between the falx cerebri and the lateral wall of the frontal horn of the lateral ventricles. The hemispheric width (HW) is obtained in the same plane: from the falx cerebri to the internal margin of the parietal bone. The authors[5] reported that despite an increase in absolute size throughout pregnancy of CFHD from a mean of 0.7 to 1.3 cm at term, the CFHD ratio and HW ratio steadily diminished throughout gestation, passing from a mean of 50% at 15 weeks' gestation to 28% at term. These data demonstrated that the HW increased from approximately 1.5 cm at 15 weeks' gestation to 4.5 cm at 40 weeks' gestation (Figs. 5–26 through 5–32).

The Bodies of the Lateral Ventricles

Sonoanatomy

The body is the portion of the lateral ventricle between the foramen of Monro and the atrium. It has been reported previously that the bodies of the lateral ventricles are narrow from midgestation and, therefore, are poorly visualized with sonography.[14,17,19] They can be seen, however, as two echogenic lines in the upper portion of the brain.[17,19]

Biometry

The internal diameter of the ventricular width of the body of the lateral ventricles between 15 and 22 weeks' gestation decreases from 6 mm to 3 mm, and between 22 weeks' gestation until term, a ventricular cavity of 3 mm or less is indicative of normality[7] (Fig. 5–13 and Fig. 5–14).

Atrium of the Lateral Ventricle

Sonoanatomy

The atrium, or trigone, is the triangular portion of the lateral ventricles that is connected anteriorly to the body, posteriorly to the occipital horn, and inferiorly to the temporal horn.[6] The middle and lateral walls of the posterior horn appear as echodense structures.

Biometry

The measurement of the atrial width (AW) is obtained by placing one electronic caliper at the medial wall

18 weeks

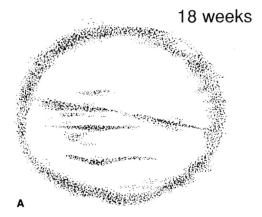

A

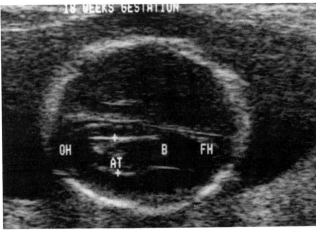

B

Figure 5–27. Representation of fetal brain at 18 weeks' gestation. **(A)** Schematic outline demonstrating the ventricular size approximately the same as at 12 weeks' gestation, although the hemispheric size is much larger. The ratio between ventricular width and hemispheric width, however, is smaller than at 12 weeks' gestation. **(B)** Ultrasound picture showing features similar to those described in part A. OH = occipital horn, AT = atrium, B = body, FH = frontal horn.

24 weeks

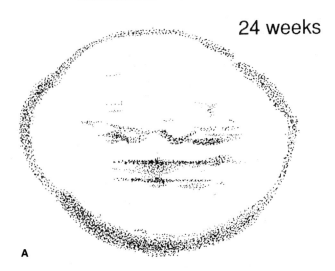

A

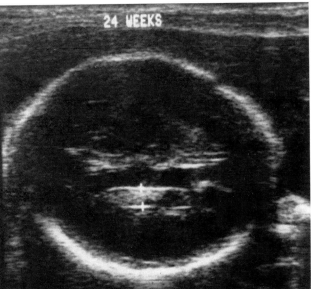

B

Figure 5–28. Representation of fetal brain at 24 weeks' gestation. **(A)** Schematic demonstrates that at 24 weeks ventricular size is similar to that of an earlier gestation, but brain parenchyma has significantly increased over the earlier gestation. As noted in Figure 5–29, the ratio between the ventricular width and the hemispheric width is thus much smaller, although the ventricular width remains approximately the same. **(B)** Sonographic appearance of the fetal brain at 24 weeks' gestation.

and the second caliper at the lateral wall of the atrial portion of the lateral ventricles. The cerebroatrial distance (CAD) is measured between the falx cerebri and the lateral wall of the atria. The HW is obtained in the same plane, from the falx cerebri to the internal margin of the parietal bone.[6] Hadlock and associates[15] reported normal values of the distance between the midline and the lateral wall of the atrium between 27 and 40 weeks of gestation. They found the *ratio* of the CAD to the HW to be fairly constant throughout gestation, ranging from 0.56 and 0.51. Campbell and Pearce[23] reported that the atrial width and hemispheric width ratio decreased from about 60% at 15 weeks' gestation to 30% at 24 weeks' gestation.

In contrast, Pilu et al[6] reported that the relative size of the AW of the lateral ventricles was found to be constant from 15 weeks of gestation until term and measured 0.7 ± 0.13 cm. The CAD, however, increased progressively from 1.1 cm at 15 weeks' gestation to 2.1 cm at 40 weeks' gestation, suggesting that it is the

brain parenchyma that increases with advancing gestational age (Fig. 5–15 and Fig. 5–33). Investigators agree, in any event, that an atrial width of 1 cm or less is considered normal and can be used to rule out the diagnosis of ventriculomegaly (hydrocephalus[24]).

Posterior Horn of the Lateral Ventricle

Sonoanatomy

The posterior, or occipital, horn of the lateral ventricles represents the posterior continuation of the atria of the lateral ventricles and appears sonographically

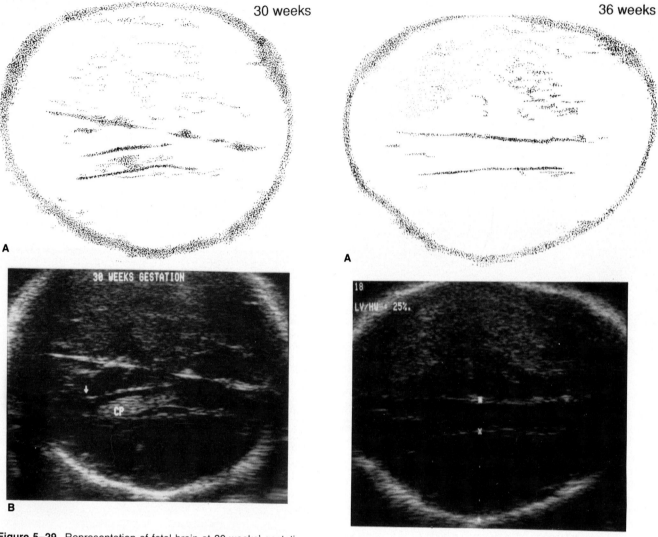

Figure 5–29. Representation of fetal brain at 30 weeks' gestation. **(A)** Schematic showing the relationship of the lateral ventricle to the brain parenchyma at this gestational age. **(B)** Ultrasound picture showing the relationship mentioned in part A.

Figure 5–30. Representation of fetal brain at 36 weeks' gestation. **(A)** Schematic demonstrating the fairly consistent ventricular width even at 36 weeks despite a significant increase in brain tissue. **(B)** Ultrasound picture showing the relationship between the lateral ventricle and the brain tissue at this gestational age.

as a sonolucent area in the posterior lobe in the fetal head[6] (Fig. 5–25).

Biometry

The measurements of the posterior horn of the lateral ventricles are obtained without including the brain tissue (Fig. 5–23). The posterior horn width (PHW) of the lateral ventricles is the distance between the medial and lateral walls of the posterior horn. The cerebroposterior horn distance (CPHD) is measured between the falx cerebri and the lateral wall of the posterior horn. The HW is obtained in the same plane, from the falx cerebri to the internal margins of the parietal bone. The PHW is found to be consistent throughout gestation, measuring between 5 mm and 9 mm.[6]

Third and Fourth Ventricles and Their Communications

The sonographic appearance of the third ventricle is a midline structure at the level of the thalami. The third ventricle is observed between the two lateral ventricles and anterior to the fourth ventricle on a coronal scan. The foramen of Monro connects this ventricle to the lateral ventricles at the roof of the third ventricle. Similarly, at the lower part of the third ventricle the aqueduct of Sylvius connects the third ventricle to the fourth ventricle.

The sonographic appearance of the fourth ventricle is below the level of the thalami, anterior to the

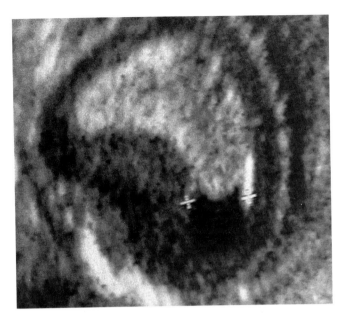

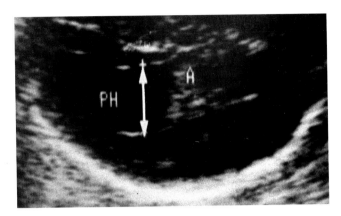

Figure 5–32. Ultrasound of fetal brain at 23 weeks' gestation. Sagittal view at the level of the lateral ventricle demonstrates its medial and lateral walls. The posterior horn (PH), the atrium (A), and the choroid plexus within the walls of the lateral ventricle are also visible. At this gestational age there is greater brain parenchyma present and thus a smaller ratio between ventricular and hemispheric width.

Figure 5–31. Ultrasound of fetal brain at 15 weeks' gestation demonstrating both the medial and lateral walls of the lateral ventricle as evidenced by the calipers(+'s). The choroid plexus is seen between the calipers(+'s) in the lateral ventricle.

cerebellar hemispheres, and can be identified in the midline. Small foramina of Magendie and Luschka serve as points of egress in the lower aspect of the fourth ventricle. These three very narrow pathways should be patent; otherwise, obstructive ventriculomegaly may result.

Biometry
The width of the third ventricle averages from 0.25 cm at 13 weeks' gestation to 0.82 cm at term.[16]

Choroid Plexus

Anatomic studies, using both animal models,[25] and sonographic investigations of the human fetus, have outlined the relatively large size of the choroid plexus.[12] The peculiar echogenicity of these structures in vivo has been attributed to a high glycogen content,

which is thought to represent a major energy supply for the rapidly growing cerebrum.[11]

Embryology
At 6 weeks' gestation the medial wall of the primitive lateral ventricles bulges within the cavity, forming a fold that is rapidly covered by pseudostratified epithelium and molded into a villous structure by the proliferation of underlying blood vessels. This structure develops into the choroid plexus, which is present in the lateral, third, and fourth ventricles. The choroid plexuses decrease in relative size with advancing gestation.[25]

Sonoanatomy
The choroid plexus is identified sonographically in the atrium of the lateral ventricles.[17] This organ appears hyperechogenic and fills the entire space of the atrium (Fig. 5–9 and Fig. 5–31). The choroid plexus is responsible for producing most of the cerebrospinal fluid. Modern sonographic ultrasound equipment shows choroid plexuses to contain many tiny hypoechogenic

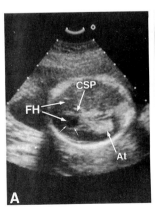
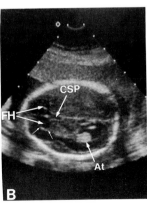
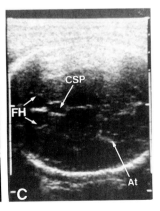

Figure 5–33. Ultrasound picture depicting axial scan of fetal head at the level of the atrium. Note choroid plexus within lumen of atrium (At). FH = frontal horn; CSP = cavum septum pellucidum. (A) View at late first trimester. (B) View at second trimester. (C) View at third trimester.

pockets, which represent fluid secretions from the plexus choroidea. Choroid plexuses are reduced in size and are no longer prominent sonographically after 20 weeks' gestation.

BPD OR MIDLEVEL

Thalami and Septum Cavum Pellucidum

The thalami appear, at the level of the basal ganglia, as a triangular echo-free area, divided in the midline by the third ventricle. It is possible to visualize the aqueduct of Sylvius posterior to the third ventricle. The cavum septum pellucidum normally fills the space between the frontal horns in the second trimester. The cavum septum pellucidum is decreased in size in the third trimester, and its "clover leaves" can be seen either as two symmetric lines or as a single line between the frontal horns. On the sides of the thalami, the hippocampal gyri appear as a circular area, lined on both sides by the cisterna magna and laterally by the atrium of the lateral ventricle. The frontal horn of the lateral ventricles can be visualized anteriorly to the thalami.[9]

Corpus Callosum

Embryology

The corpus callosum is a bundle of white-matter tracts of fibers that connect the two cerebral hemispheres, cross midline, and form the roof of the third ventricle. The corpus callosum is the largest of the median interhemispheric commissures. It is formed during the third and fourth months of fetal life from the lamina terminalis.[27]

Sonoanatomy

The corpus callosum is seen as a hypoechogenic band of tissue, superior to the third ventricle in the midline on the sagittal scan and forming the roof of the lateral ventricles on the coronal scan. A midsagittal scan demonstrates the corpus callosum.

Frontal Lobe

The landmarks of the thalami, cavum septum pellucidum, and the third ventricle are identified. The posterior landmark of the frontal lobe is established by the anterior edges of the medial wall of the frontal horn of the lateral ventricles and the anterior landmark of the frontal lobe as the middle hyperechogenic frontal bone[10] (Table 5–1, Table 5–2, and Table 5–3).

TABLE 5–1. MEASUREMENTS OF THALAMIC FRONTAL LOBE DISTANCE

Gestational Age (wk)	Percentile				
	10th	25th	50th	75th	90th
15	3.2	3.2	3.2	3.2	3.2
16	2.9	3.1	3.2	3.4	3.5
17	3.2	3.4	3.5	3.8	4.5
18	3.3	3.3	3.7	3.9	3.9
19	3.5	3.5	3.7	3.9	4.0
20	4.0	4.0	4.0	4.3	4.4
21	3.9	3.9	4.1	4.4	4.5
22	4.6	4.6	4.6	4.6	4.6
23	4.6	4.6	4.6	4.6	4.6
24	4.6	4.6	4.6	4.9	4.9
25	4.7	4.8	5.2	5.3	5.4
26	4.8	5.0	5.3	5.4	5.5
27	5.3	5.6	5.6	6.8	7.2
28	5.5	5.6	5.7	6.0	6.2
29	6.0	6.0	6.1	6.4	6.4
30	5.5	5.7	5.9	6.4	7.4
31	6.1	6.1	6.1	6.2	6.2
32	6.2	6.2	6.4	6.9	7.1
33	5.9	6.0	6.3	6.5	6.6
34	6.2	6.4	6.7	7.0	7.2
35	6.6	6.7	7.1	7.2	7.3
36	6.5	6.5	6.6	6.9	6.9
37	6.2	6.4	6.7	7.0	7.1
38	6.5	6.6	7.2	7.3	7.4
39	7.1	7.0	7.4	7.7	7.8
40	7.4	7.4	7.6	8.1	8.1

From Goldstein I, Reece EA, Pilu G, et al. Sonographic assessment of the fetal frontal lobe: a potential tool for prenatal diagnosis of microcephaly. Am J Obstet Gynecol. 1988;158:1057–1062, with permission.

TABLE 5–2. MEASUREMENTS OF THE FRONTAL LOBE DISTANCE (PERCENTILES)

Gestational Age (wk)	Percentile				
	10th	25th	50th	75th	90th
16	1.0	1.4	1.5	1.6	1.8
17	1.5	1.6	1.6	1.8	1.8
18	1.4	1.4	1.7	1.7	1.8
19	1.4	1.5	1.8	1.9	1.9
20	1.7	1.7	1.9	1.8	1.9
21	1.4	1.5	2.0	2.0	2.1
22	2.3	2.3	2.3	2.3	2.3
23	1.8	1.9	2.1	2.2	2.3
24	2.0	2.0	2.0	2.0	2.0
25	2.0	2.0	2.3	2.4	2.5
26	2.0	2.1	2.3	2.4	2.5
27	2.5	2.5	2.7	3.1	3.2
28	2.4	2.5	2.6	2.6	2.7
29	2.7	2.7	2.8	2.8	2.8
30	2.6	2.6	2.7	3.2	3.4
31	2.7	2.7	2.8	3.0	3.0
32	3.0	3.0	3.3	3.6	3.8
33	2.5	2.6	3.2	3.4	3.4
34	2.9	3.0	3.1	3.2	3.3
35	3.2	3.4	3.5	3.7	4.0
36	2.9	2.9	3.2	3.4	3.4
37	3.1	3.2	3.4	3.6	3.8
38	3.2	3.2	3.5	3.9	4.0
39	3.5	3.5	3.7	4.2	4.3
40	3.8	3.8	3.9	4.5	4.5

From Goldstein I, Reece EA, Pilu G, et al. Sonographic assessment of the fetal frontal lobe: a potential tool for prenatal diagnosis of microcephaly. Am J Obstet Gynecol. 1988;158:1057–1062, with permission.

TABLE 5–3. MEASUREMENTS OF THE MEAN ± 2 SD OF THE FRONTAL LOBE DISTANCE AND THALAMIC FRONTAL LOBE DISTANCE VERSUS GESTATIONAL AGE

Gestational Age (wk)	Frontal Lobe Distance (cm) (Mean ± 2 SD)	Thalamic Frontal Lobe Distance (cm) (Mean ± 2 SD)
15	1.4 ± 0.4	3.2 ± 0.4
16	1.4 ± 0.4	3.2 ± 0.4
17	1.6 ± 0.2	3.6 ± 0.6
18	1.6 ± 0.2	3.7 ± 0.6
19	1.7 ± 0.2	3.8 ± 0.4
20	1.7 ± 0.2	4.1 ± 0.4
21	1.8 ± 0.4	4.1 ± 0.4
22	1.8 ± 0.4	4.6 ± 0.4
23	1.8 ± 0.4	4.6 ± 0.4
24	1.9 ± 0.2	4.7 ± 0.4
25	2.2 ± 0.4	5.1 ± 0.6
26	2.3 ± 0.4	5.2 ± 0.6
27	2.5 ± 0.6	5.6 ± 0.8
28	2.8 ± 0.2	5.7 ± 0.4
29	2.7 ± 0.2	6.1 ± 0.4
30	2.8 ± 0.6	6.2 ± 1.2
31	2.9 ± 0.4	6.2 ± 0.8
32	3.0 ± 0.6	6.4 ± 0.8
33	3.1 ± 0.6	6.5 ± 0.6
34	3.2 ± 0.2	6.7 ± 0.6
35	3.2 ± 0.4	6.9 ± 0.6
36	3.2 ± 0.4	7.0 ± 0.4
37	3.4 ± 0.4	7.2 ± 0.6
38	3.5 ± 0.4	7.3 ± 0.8
39	3.7 ± 0.6	7.5 ± 0.8
40	4.0 ± 0.6	7.7 ± 0.8

From Goldstein I, Reece EA, Pilu G, et al. Sonographic assessment of the fetal frontal lobe: a potential tool for prenatal diagnosis of microcephaly. Am J Obstet Gynecol. 1988;158:1057–1062, with permission.

CEREBELLAR OR INFERIOR LEVEL

Posterior Fossa

The posterior fossa is easily identified by a suboccipito-bregmatic scan. The following organs are located in this part of the intracranial anatomy: the cerebellum (including the cerebellar hemispheres), the vermis, and the cisterna magna. At a slightly lower level the fourth ventricle is bordered posteriorly by the inferior vermis. The cerebellum can be identified by ultrasound as early as 10 weeks' gestation. It appears as two rounded, mildly echogenic areas corresponding to the cerebellar hemispheres. The cisterna magna lies between the cerebellum and occipital bone (sickle-shaped sonolucent area). The posterior fossa contents are large enough at 18 weeks' gestation and beyond to permit a detailed morphologic evaluation.

The transducer is first placed axial to the base of the skull and subsequently rotated posteriorly (Fig. 5–34) until the cerebellar hemispheres come into view. Continued movement of the transducer will allow demonstration of the cerebellar tonsils.[26]

The Cerebellum

Embryology

The cerebellum is formed from the dorsal part of the alar plates of the metencephalon. The cerebellar swelling appears initially at the end of the fourth week of gestation as a swelling overriding the fourth ventricle. By 6 weeks' gestation, the flocculonodular lobes develop, followed by the bilateral growth of the hemispheres, which eventually meet in the midline forming the vermis and the two lateral portions of the cerebellar lobes. The cerebellar swellings enlarge subsequently and become well-developed by the 12th week of gestation.[27,28]

Sonoanatomy

The cerebellum lies in the posterior fossa and is surrounded laterally by the dense petrous ridges and inferiorly by the occipital bone. Sonographic visualization of the cerebellum is possible as early as 10 to 11 weeks' gestation (Fig. 5–10). The characteristic image of the cerebellum by ultrasound appears as two lob-

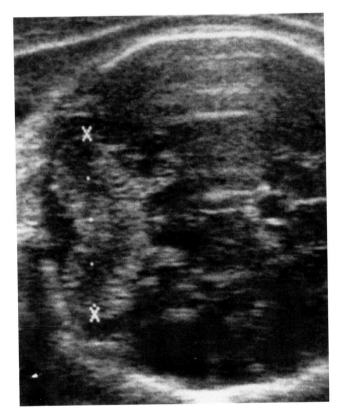

Figure 5–34. Sagittal scan of the fetal head at a level slightly below that used for the BPD and directed somewhat more inferiorly. The cerebellum is seen as a butterfly-shaped echodense structure in the posterior fossa; the calipers(x's) indicate the outer margins. Posterior to the cerebellum is the echolucent cisterna magna, and anterior to the cerebellum is a large echolucent area representing thalami divided by the midline falx. The cavum septum pellucidum is seen anteriorly as a small echolucent central area.

ules on either side of the midline located in the posterior cranial fossa (Fig. 5–11). The cerebellum is one structure of the fetal head easiest to detect sonographically, and it can be seen throughout gestation. The cerebellum is better visualized, however, before the third trimester.

The cerebellar hemispheres occupying the posterior portion of the intracranial fossa can be identified by the following landmarks: the thalami, cavum septum pellucidum, and the third ventricle. The characteristic butterfly-like appearance of the cerebellum is seen below the thalamic plane (Fig. 5–34).

Biometry

The transverse cerebellar diameters are obtained by identifying the aforementioned landmarks: the thalami, septum cavum pellucidum, and third ventricle, and then slightly rotating the transducer below the thalamic plane. The calipers are then placed at the outer-to-outer margins of the transverse cerebellar diameter. A nomogram comparing the transverse cerebellar diameter with gestational age is shown in Table 5–4 and Table 5–5). Sonographic evaluation of cerebellar growth reveals a linear relationship during the second trimester. The measurements in millimeters are

TABLE 5–4. CEREBELLAR MEASUREMENTS WITH ULTRASONOGRAPHY IN THE EVALUATION OF FETAL GROWTH AND DEVELOPMENT

Gestational age (wk)	Cerebellum (mm)				
	10	25	50	75	90
15	10	12	14	15	16
16	14	16	16	16	17
17	16	17	17	18	18
18	17	18	18	19	19
19	18	18	19	19	22
20	18	19	20	20	22
21	19	20	22	23	24
22	21	23	23	24	24
23	22	23	24	25	26
24	22	24	25	27	28
25	23	21	28	28	29
26	25	28	29	30	32
27	26	28	30	31	32
28	27	30	31	32	34
29	29	32	34	36	38
30	31	32	35	37	40
31	32	35	38	39	43
32	33	36	38	40	42
33	32	36	40	43	44
34	33	38	40	41	44
35	31	37	40	43	47
36	36	29	43	52	55
37	37	37	45	52	55
38	40	40	48	52	55
39	52	52	52	55	55

From Goldstein I, Reece EA, Pilu G, et al. Cerebellar measurements with ultrasonography in the evaluation of fetal growth and development. Am J Obstet Gynecol. 1987;156:1065–1069, with permission.

TABLE 5–5. A NOMOGRAM OF THE TRANSVERSE CEREBELLAR DIAMETER (mm)

Gestational Age (wk)	Percentile		
	10th	50th	90th
15	13	14	16
16	14	16	17
17	16	17	18
18	17	18	19
19	18	19	20
20	19	20	21
21	20	21	23
22	22	23	24
23	23	24	26
24	23	26	28
25	25	27	30
26	26	28	32
27	27	30	33
28	28	31	35
29	29	33	38
30	31	35	40
31	33	38	42
32	34	39	43
33	35	40	44
34	38	41	44
35	41	42	45
36	42	43	45
37	43	45	48
38	45	48	50
39	48	52	55
40	52	55	58

From Goldstein I, Reece EA, Pilu G, et al. Cerebellar measurements with ultrasonography in the evaluation of fetal growth and development. Am J Obstet Gynecol. 1987;156:1065–1069, with permission.

thus approximately equal to the gestational age in weeks during this period. A transverse cerebellar diameter of 17 mm, for example, is equal to a gestational age of 17 weeks. This statement is true between the gestational ages of 15 weeks and 22 weeks.[9] Later in gestation, however, the growth curve of the cerebellum does not permit this correlation.

Cisterna Magna

Sonoanatomy

The cisterna magna comprises a portion of the subarachnoid space that bathes the posterior fossa in the cerebrospinal fluid. It surrounds around the cerebellum posteriorly and is normally deepest in the midline, where invagination of this space occurs between the two cerebellar hemispheres. Although the cisterna magna usually occupies a small slitlike space in adults, it may be proportionally large in neonates, even in the absence of infratentorial pathology.[29] The cisterna magna appears as a hypoechogenic ellipsoid area, and the subarachnoid fluid in the cisterna magna delineates the cerebellum especially well.

TABLE 5–6. VISUALIZATION OF THE CISTERNA MAGNA IN 215 FETUSES WITHOUT EVIDENCE OF NEURAL TUBE DEFECTS

Menstrual Age (wk)	Cisterna Magna Depth (mm)					Cisterna Magna (Not Well Visualized)	Total
	1–2	3–4	5–6	7–8	9–10		
15–20	11	12	9	2	0	4	38
21–24	12	14	11	17	0	1	55
25–28	4	1	3	15	4	3	30
29–32	2	3	3	7	8	17	40
≥ 33	6	0	1	6	4	35	52
Total	35	30	27	47	16	60	215

From Mahony BS, Callen PW, and Tilly RA. The fetal cisterna magna. Radiology. *1984;153:773–776.*

Biometry

Standardized measurements for the midsagittal depth of the cisterna magna were prospectively obtained and measured 5 ± 3 mm[30] (Table 5–6).

Biometry of Fetal Skull

Biparietal Diameter

This measurement is obtained at the level of the thalami, the septum cavum pellucidum, and the third ventricle by placing the calipers at the outer echodense side of the proximal parietal bone to the inner echodense side of the distal parietal bone (Fig. 5–35). The thalami appear as two triangular echo-free areas. The slitlike third ventricle can be seen between the thalami. A cross-sectional view of the aqueduct of Sylvius can be seen inferior and posterior to the third ventricle. (Fig. 5–17, Table 5–7, and Table 5–8).

Occipitofrontal Diameter. This measurement is obtained at the level of the thalami, septum cavum pellucidum, and the third ventricle by placing the cali-

pers at the midechogenic line of the occipital and frontal bones (Table 5–9).

Head Circumference. Usually this is calculated using the measurements of the BPD and occipitofrontal diameter (OFD), or it can be measured directly.

$$HC = (BPD + OFD) \times 1.57$$

Cephalic Index. The cephalic index is calculated by the ratio between the BPD and OFD × 100. The normal range is 78.3% ± 4.4% (± 1 SD).[31]

$$CI = BPD/OFD \times 100 = 75\% \text{ to } 85\%$$

TABLE 5–7. RELATIONSHIP BETWEEN GESTATIONAL AGE AND BIPARIETAL DIAMETER

Gestational Age (wk)	Biparietal Diameter (mm)				
	10	25	50	75	90
15	30	31	33	34	35
16	34	34	35	36	38
17	36	37	38	40	43
18	38	40	42	43	44
19	42	43	45	46	48
20	45	46	47	48	53
21	48	49	50	52	57
22	50	51	53	54	55
23	53	54	56	58	60
24	56	59	60	61	64
25	61	61	63	66	68
26	63	64	65	66	67
27	64	67	68	69	70
28	68	69	70	71	72
29	71	72	74	76	79
30	72	74	75	75	79
31	75	78	76	81	84
32	75	78	80	81	83
33	80	80	81	82	87
34	81	82	84	86	91
35	78	83	87	89	93
36	84	85	88	89	91
37	87	87	89	92	92
38	87	87	90	93	94
39	92	92	92	92	92

From Goldstein I, Reece EA, Pilu G, et al. Cerebellar measurements with ultrasonography in the evaluation of fetal growth and development. Am J Obstet Gynecol. *1987;156:1065–1069, with permission.*

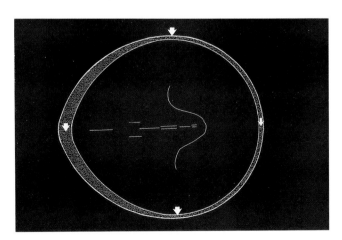

Figure 5–35. Schematic representation of fetal head at the level of the BPD. Measurement of the BPD is performed by placing calipers at the leading edges of the skull table as shown by arrows at the top and bottom of diagram. OFD is measured by placing calipers as shown by the laterally placed arrows.

TABLE 5–8. PREDICTED MENSTRUAL AGES FOR BPD VALUES FROM 2.0 TO 10.0 CM

BPD (cm)	Menstrual Age (wk)	BPD (cm)	Menstrual Age (wk)
2.0	12.2	6.1	25.0
2.1	12.5	6.2	25.3
2.2	12.8	6.3	25.7
2.3	13.1	6.4	26.1
2.4	13.3	6.5	26.4
2.5	13.6	6.6	26.8
2.6	13.9	6.7	27.2
2.7	14.2	6.8	27.6
2.8	14.5	6.9	28.0
2.9	14.7	7.0	28.3
3.0	15.0	7.1	28.7
3.1	15.3	7.2	29.1
3.2	15.6	7.3	29.5
3.3	15.9	7.4	29.9
3.4	16.2	7.5	30.4
3.5	16.5	7.6	30.8
3.6	16.8	7.7	31.2
3.7	17.1	7.8	31.6
3.8	17.4	7.9	32.0
3.9	17.7	8.0	32.5
4.0	18.0	8.1	32.9
4.1	18.3	8.2	33.3
4.2	18.6	8.3	33.8
4.3	18.9	8.4	34.2
4.4	19.2	8.5	34.7
4.5	19.5	8.6	35.1
4.6	19.9	8.7	35.6
4.7	20.2	8.8	36.1
4.8	20.5	8.9	36.5
4.9	20.8	9.0	37.0
5.0	21.2	9.1	37.5
5.1	21.5	9.2	38.0
5.2	21.8	9.3	38.5
5.3	22.2	9.4	38.9
5.4	22.5	9.5	39.4
5.5	22.8	9.6	39.9
5.6	23.2	9.7	40.5
5.7	23.5	9.8	41.0
5.8	23.9	9.9	41.5
5.9	24.2	10.0	42.0
6.0	24.6		

CALCULATED BPD VALUES (MEAN ± SD) AT MENSTRUAL AGES FROM 12 TO 40 WEEKS

Menstrual Age (wk)	Calculated BPD (cm)
12 (n = 2)	2.10 ± 0.13
13 (n = 3)	2.27 ± 0.06
14 (n = 4)	2.70 ± 0.14
15 (n = 12)	2.98 ± 0.16
16 (n = 32)	3.30 ± 0.13
17 (n = 36)	3.63 ± 0.18
18 (n = 24)	3.95 ± 0.15
19 (n = 23)	4.28 ± 0.24
20 (n = 19)	4.56 ± 0.24
21 (n = 27)	4.84 ± 0.21
22 (n = 27)	5.21 ± 0.22
23 (n = 21)	5.48 ± 0.27
24 (n = 24)	5.86 ± 0.21
25 (n = 16)	6.15 ± 0.17
26 (n = 22)	6.35 ± 0.25
27 (n = 17)	6.69 ± 0.19
28 (n = 17)	7.01 ± 0.16
29 (n = 11)	7.20 ± 0.17
30 (n = 17)	7.45 ± 0.25
31 (n = 20)	7.59 ± 0.19
32 (n = 10)	7.86 ± 0.26
33 (n = 22)	8.16 ± 0.23
34 (n = 22)	8.33 ± 0.16
35 (n = 7)	8.69 ± 0.21
36 (n = 19)	8.79 ± 0.17
37 (n = 8)	8.90 ± 0.24
38 (n = 15)	9.14 ± 0.27
39 (n = 36)	9.26 ± 0.43
40 (n = 20)	9.44 ± 0.30

* Menstrual age = $6.8954 + 2.6345 (BPD) + 0.008771 (BPD)^3$, [$r^2 = 98.7\%$]. From Hadlock FP, Deter RL, Harris RB, et al. Fetal biparietal diameter: a critical re-evaluation of the relation to menstrual age by means of real-time ultrasound. *J Ultrasound Med. 1982;1:97–104, with permission.*

The cephalic index should be used to verify that the size of the BPD is not affected by molding of the fetal head. Dolichocephaly is diagnosed by a cephalic index below 75%; brachycephaly is diagnosed by a cephalic index above 85%.

Lateral Ventricles. Measurement of the lateral ventricles is obtained superior to the level of the thalami by placing the calipers at the midechogenic line of the medial wall and at the lateral wall of the lateral ventricles (Fig. 5–36).

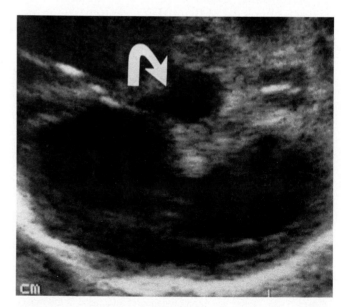

Figure 5–36. Transabdominal ultrasound examination of a fetus in the second trimester depicting triventricular hydrocephalus with dilation of the lateral ventricles and the third ventricle (arrowhead). This scan is taken in the axial view.

TABLE 5–9. NOMOGRAM OF THE GROWTH OF FETAL HEAD PARAMETER (in mm)

Week No.	Biparietal Percentile			Occipitofrontal Percentile			Head Perimeter Percentile		
	5th	50th	95th	5th	50th	95th	5th	50th	95th
10	9	14	18	7	14	21	26	50	74
11	13	17	22	11	18	25	38	63	87
12	16	21	25	16	23	30	51	75	100
13	20	24	29	20	27	34	64	88	112
14	23	28	32	24	31	38	76	101	125
15	27	31	36	29	36	43	89	113	138
16	30	35	39	33	40	47	101	126	150
17	34	38	43	37	44	51	114	138	163
18	37	42	46	41	48	55	126	151	175
19	40	45	49	46	53	60	138	163	187
20	44	48	53	50	57	64	150	175	199
21	47	51	56	54	61	68	162	187	211
22	50	55	59	58	65	72	174	198	223
23	53	58	62	62	69	76	185	210	234
24	56	61	65	65	72	79	196	221	245
25	59	64	68	69	76	83	207	232	256
26	62	67	71	73	80	87	218	242	266
27	65	70	74	76	83	90	228	252	277
28	68	72	77	80	87	94	238	262	286
29	70	75	79	83	90	97	247	271	296
30	73	77	82	86	93	100	256	281	305
31	75	79	84	89	96	103	265	289	313
32	77	82	86	92	99	106	273	297	322
33	79	84	88	95	102	108	281	305	329
34	81	86	90	97	104	111	288	312	336
35	83	87	92	99	106	113	294	319	343
36	84	89	93	102	109	116	300	325	349
37	86	90	95	104	111	118	306	330	355
38	87	91	96	105	112	119	311	335	359
39	88	93	97	107	114	121	315	339	364
40	89	93	98	108	115	122	319	343	367

From Jeanty P, Cousaert E, Hobbins JC, et al. A longitudinal study of fetal head biometry. Am J Perinatol. 1984;1:118–128, with permission.

Transverse Cerebellar Diameter. The sonographic evaluation of the cerebellar growth reveals a linear relationship during the second trimester. The pattern of growth of the cerebellum measured by transverse cerebellar diameter (TCD), however, follows the third-degree polynomial similar to the growth relationship between the TCD and BPD[9] (Table 5–2).

REFERENCES

1. McGahan JP, Phillips HE. Ultrasonic evaluation of the size of the trigone of the fetal ventricle. *J Ultrasound Med.* 1983;2:315–319.
2. Shepard M, Filly RA. A standardized plane for biparietal diameter measurement. *J Ultrasound Med.* 1982;1:145–150.
3. Romero R, Pilu G, Ghidini A, et al. The central nervous system: normal sonographic anatomy of the fetal central nervous system. In: *Prenatal Diagnosis of Congenital Anomalies.* Norwalk, Conn: Appleton-Century-Crofts; 1988:1–18.
4. Issacson G, Mintz MD, Cerlin ES. *Atlas of Fetal Sectional Anatomy.* New York, NY: Springer-Verlag; 1986.
5. Goldstein I, Reece EA, Pilu G, et al. Sonographic evaluation of the normal developmental anatomy of fetal cerebral ventricles. I: the frontal horn. *Obstet Gynecol.* 1988;72:588–592.
6. Pilu G, Reece EA, Goldstein I, et al. Sonographic evaluation of normal developmental anatomy of the fetal cerebral ventricles. II: the atria. *Obstet Gynecol.* 1989;73:250–256.
7. Siedler DE, Filly RA. Relative growth of the higher brain structures. *J Ultrasound Med.* 1987;6:573–576.
8. Goldstein I, Reece EA, Pilu G, et al. Sonographic evaluation of the normal developmental anatomy of the fetal cerebral ventricles. IV: the posterior horn. *Am J Perinatol.* 1990;7:79–83.
9. Goldstein I, Reece EA, Pilu G, et al. Cerebellar measurements with ultrasonography in the evaluation of fetal growth and development. *Am J Obstet Gynecol.* 1987;156:1065–1069.
10. Goldstein I, Reece EA, Pilu G, et al. Sonographic assessment of the fetal frontal lobe: a potential tool for prenatal diagnosis of microcephaly. *Am J Obstet Gynecol.* 1988;158:1057–1062.
11. Crade M, Patel J, McQuown D. Sonographic imaging of the glycogen stage of the fetal choroid plexus. *Am J Neuroradiol.* 1981;2:345–349.
12. Shepard M, Filly RA. A standardized plane for biparietal diameter measurement. *J Ultrasound Med.* 1982;1:145–149.
13. Kier EL. The cerebral ventricles: a phylogenetic and ontogenetic study. In: Newton TH, Potts DG, eds. *Radiology of the Skull and Brain: Anatomy and Pathology.* St. Louis, Mo: CV Mosby; 1977:2787–2914.
14. Pretorius D, Drose JA, Manco-Johnson ML. Fetal lateral ventricular ratio determination during the second trimester. *J Ultrasound Med.* 1986;5:121–124.
15. Hadlock FP, Deter RL, Park SK. Real-time sonography: ventricular and vascular anatomy of the fetal brain in utero. *AJR.* 1981;136:133–137.
16. Denkhaus H, Winsberg F. Ultrasonic measurement of the fetal ventricular system. *Radiology.* 1979;131:781–787.
17. Johnson ML, Dunne MG, Mack LA, et al. Evaluation of fetal intracranial anatomy by static and real-time ultrasound. *J Clin Ultrasound.* 1980;8:311–318.
18. Jeanty P, Dramaix-Wilmet M, Delbeke D, et al. Ultrasonic evaluation of fetal ventricular growth. *Neuroradiology.* 1981;21:127–133.
19. Fiske CE, Filly RA, Callen PW. Sonographic measurement of lateral ventricular width in early ventricular dilation. *J Clin Ultrasound.* 1981;9:303–309.
20. Chinn DC, Callen PW, Filly RA. The lateral cerebral ventricle in early second trimester. *Radiology.* 1983;148:529–531.
21. Chervenak FA, Berkowitz RL, Romero R, et al. The diagnosis of fetal hydrocephalus. *Am J Obstet Gynecol.* 1983;147:703–716.
22. Campbell S. Diagnosis of fetal abnormalities by ultrasound. In: Milunsky A, ed. *Genetic Disorders and the Fetus.* New York, NY: Plenum Press; 1979:431–467.

23. Campbell S, Pearce JM. Ultrasound visualization of congenital malformations. *Br Med Bull.* 1983;39:322–331.
24. Filly RA, Cardoza JD, Goldstein RB, et al. Detection of fetal CNS anomalies: A practical level of effort for a "routine" sonogram. *Radiology.* 1989;172:403–408.
25. Tennyson VM, Pappas GD. The fine structure of the developing telencephalic and myelencephalic choroid plexus in the rabbit. *J Compr Neurol.* 1964;123:379–383.
26. Pilu G, Romero R, Palma L, et al. Ultrasound investigation of the posterior fossa in the fetus. *Am J Perinatol.* 1987;4:155–159.
27. Moore K. The fetal period. In: *Clinically Oriented Embryology.* 1973; 3rd ed. Philadelphia, Pa: WB Saunders Co, 71–82.
28. Loeser JD, Lemire RJ, Alvord JR: The development of the folia in the human cerebellar vermis. *Anat Rec.* 1972;173:109–113.
29. Goodwin L, Quisling RG: The neonatal cisterna magna: ultrasonic evaluation. *Radiology.* 1983;149:691–695.
30. Mahony BS, Callen PW, Filly RA, et al. The fetal cisterna magna. *Radiology.* 1984;153:773–776.
31. Hadlock FP, Deter RL, Park SK. Real-time sonography: ventricular and vascular anatomy of the fetal brain in utero. *AJR.* 1981;136:133–137.

Abnormal Fetal Head Anatomy

HYDROCEPHALUS

Hydrocephalus is defined as a condition in which an excess of cerebrospinal fluid and intraventricular pressure is associated with ventricular enlargement. This increase in cerebrospinal fluid may result either from an increased production of fluid or obstruction of fluid egress from the ventricular system. Hydrocephalus occurs at an incidence of about 0.3 to 0.8 in 100 births and thus represents one of the commonest anomalies among live births.[1]

Etiopathology
Cerebrospinal fluid is formed at the level of the choroid plexus inside the lateral ventricles and flows into the third ventricle via the foramen of Monro down the aqueduct of Sylvius to the fourth ventricle. The fluid exits the fourth ventricle via the foramina of Luschka and Magendie into the subarachnoid space, where it bathes the cerebral structures, or via the foramen magnum into the spinal canal. Flowing along the subarachnoid cisterns, the fluid is then resorbed by the foram-

ina of Pacchioni, which are mainly distributed along the superior sagittal sinus. Congenital hydrocephalus results from an obstruction along the normal pathway of the cerebrospinal fluid in the vast majority of cases.

Hydrocephalus may be classified as follows:

1. Aqueductal stenosis
2. Communicating hydrocephalus
3. Dandy–Walker syndrome

Aqueductal Stenosis

Aqueductal stenosis is the most frequent cause of congenital hydrocephalus, accounting for more than 40% of reported cases.

Etiopathology
The aqueduct of Sylvius is the narrow channel connecting the third and the fourth ventricles through which cerebrospinal fluid traverses from the lateral ventricles to the subarachnoid space. An obstructive process or failure of the aqueduct to develop may be caused by various factors, including genetic, infectious, neoplastic, and developmental causes.

Genetic Causes. Genetic transmission may account for some cases of aqueductal stenosis; some of which may be caused by X-linked recessive transmission in about 25% of cases and affecting male infants.[2] Although X-linked recessive transmission does occur, multifactorial inheritance also has been suggested to account for other cases involving both males and females.[3,4]

Infectious Causes. Some of the TORCH viruses, along with mumps and influenza viruses have been implicated in aqueductal stenosis in animals.[5–7] In humans, however, there is evidence of inflammations in some cases and idiopathic causes in others. The precise mechanism associated with this maldevelopment is unknown.[8]

Neoplastic Causes. Tumors of various types may cause compression of the aqueduct and result in obstructive hydrocephalus.[9]

Spina bifida is most frequently associated with the communicating form of hydrocephalus, although aqueductal stenosis has been found in some cases. The mechanism for the hydrocephalus may be related to either extrinsic compression by the enlarged lateral ventricles or by downward traction of the tethered spinal cord.[10] Communicating hydrocephalus may lead to aqueductal stenosis, causing white matter edema and extrinsic compression.[10,11]

The natural history of congenital hydrocephalus is not completely understood. Information currently available results from biopsies made from those children undergoing shunt procedures. There is initial dis-

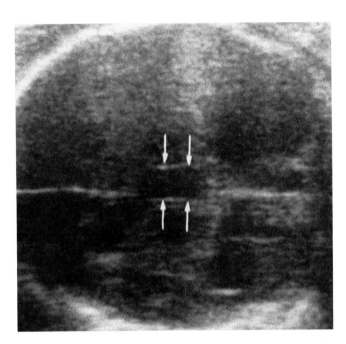

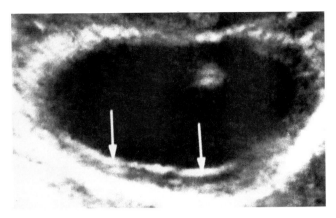

Figure 5–38. Transabdominal ultrasound examination of a fetus in the second trimester depicting severely dilated lateral ventricles bilaterally (arrows). The third and fourth ventricles are also dilated. These findings are most consistent with a diagnosis of communicating hydrocephalus.

Figure 5–37. Second-trimester examination of a fetus in the axial plane, using transabdominal ultrasound. Examination reveals lateral ventriculomegaly, as well as a third ventriculomegaly (four arrows). The finding of bilateral ventriculomegaly along with dilation of the third ventricle is diagnostic of obstruction of the aqueduct of Sylvius. This is sometimes referred to as triventricular hydrocephalus.

ruption in the ependymal lining, followed by edema of the white matter. This phase has been considered reversible. Later, the astrocytes proliferate, and the white matter undergoes fibrosis. The incidence of associated anomalies with aqueductal stenosis seems to be between 16% and 30%.[1]

Prenatal Diagnosis

The diagnosis of aqueductal stenosis is made by identifying dilation of the lateral ventricles (symmetric or asymmetric) and dilation of the third ventricle with the presence of a normal fourth ventricle (Fig. 5–36 and Fig. 5–37). Communicating hydrocephaly may present with the same appearance (Fig. 5–38), this is, when fourth ventricular dilation is mild. In this case distinction from aqueductal stenosis is not possible (Fig. 5–39 and Fig. 5–40). An effort should be made to scan the fetal spine to rule out open neural tube defects.[12]

Management and Outcome

Some parents may consider termination of pregnancy if the diagnosis is made before viability. Diagnosis after viability should lead to a management option based both on the severity of the hydrocephalus and fetal lung maturity. Neither cephalocentesis nor routine cesarean section are recommended in isolated aqueductal stenosis unless the cranium is very large. If there are other associated congenital anomalies, the manage-

ment, which might include cephalocentesis, depends on the most severe anomaly present.

The outcome for infants presenting with aqueductal stenosis is variable. Some of these fetuses will die in utero or in the neonatal period. The reported mortality ranges between 11% and 30%. The long-term prognosis has been examined: A mean IQ of 70 was reported in one study; in another the IQ was greater than 70 in one half of the treated cases. Normal intellectual development may also be possible.[13]

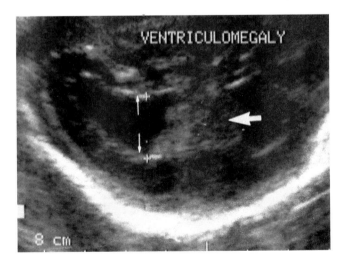

Figure 5–39. This is a sagittal scan of the lateral ventricles at a slightly oblique angle demonstrating the posterior horn of the lateral ventricles. The choroid plexus (large arrow) can be seen, with a dilation of the ventricular lumen (two small arrows). In addition, the calipers(+'s) measure the atrial width of the lateral ventricle. The dimension is in excess of the normal size of the normal atrial width of 1 cm. These findings suggest early ventriculomegaly without the characteristic alteration in the ratio of the ventricular width to hemispheric width.

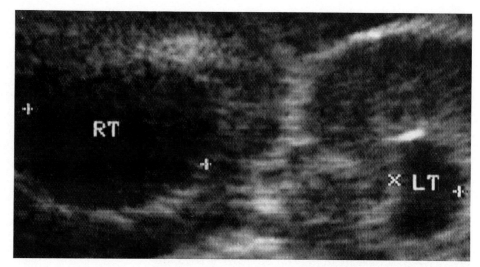

Figure 5–40. Transvaginal examination of a fetus in the second trimester depicting a right unilateral ventriculomegaly (RT). The calipers(+'s) outline the limits of the right ventriculomegaly. Calipers also depict the normal size of the left ventricle (LT). Etiology might include an obstructive process or unilateral fluid production from a choroid plexus papilloma.

REFERENCES

1. Williamson EM. Incidence and family aggregation of major congenital malformations of the central nervous system. *J Med Genet*. 1965;2:161–172.
2. Burton BK. Recurrence risk for congenital hydrocephalus. *Clin Genet*. 1979;16:47–53.
3. Price JR, Horne BM. Family history indicating hereditary factors in hydrocephalus. *Ment Retard*. 1968;6:40–41.
4. Carter CO, David PA, Laurence KM. A family study of major central nervous system malformations in South Wales. *J Med Genet*. 1968;5:81–106.
5. Johnson RT, Johnson KP, Edmonds CJ. Virus-induced hydrocephalus: development of aqueductal stenosis in hamsters after mumps infection. *Science*. 1967;157:1066–1067.
6. Margolis G, Kilham L. Hydrocephalus in hamsters, ferrets, rats and mice following inoculations with reovirus type I. *Clin Invest Med*. 1969;21:189–198.
7. Phillips PA, Alpers MP, Stanley NF. Hydrocephalus in mice inoculated by oronasal route with reovirus Type I. *Science*. 1970;168:858–859.
8. Drachman D, Richardson EP. Aqueductal narrowing, congenital and acquired: a critical review of histological criteria. *Arch Neurol*. 1961;5:552–556.
9. Russell DS. Observations on the pathology of hydrocephalus. *Special Report Series No. 265*. London. Her Majesty's Stationery Office; 1949.
10. Nugent GR, Al-Mefty O, Chou S. Communicating hydrocephalus as a cause of aqueductal stenosis. *J Neurosurg*. 1979;51:812–818.
11. Borit A, Sidman RL. New mutant mouse with communicating hydrocephalus and secondary aqueductal stenosis. *Acta Neuropathol*. 1972;21:316–331.
12. Romero R, Pilu G, Jeanty P, et al. The central nervous system. In: Romero R, Pilu G, Jeanty P, et al. *Prenatal Diagnosis of Congenital Anomalies*. Norwalk, Conn: Appleton & Lange; 1988:1–35.
13. McCullough DC, Balzer-Martin LA. Current prognosis in overt neonatal hydrocephalus. *J Neurosurg*. 1982;57:378–386.

Communicating Hydrocephaly

Communicating hydrocephaly may result from other mechanical obstruction outside the ventricular system, impairing resorption of the cerebrospinal fluid (CSF) and resulting in dilation of the subarachnoid space and ventricular system, or it may result from excessive production of CSF as in the case of a choroid plexus papilloma. The incidence of communicating hydrocephalus is about 40% of all cases of hydrocephalus.[1]

Etiopathology
Although the precise cause of communicating hydrocephalus is unknown, this maldevelopment has been associated with neural tube defects, subarachnoid hemorrhage—the most common cause, and obstructive lesions at the level of the superior sagital sinus resulting in impairment in fluid reabsorption. Choroid plexus papillomas may cause excess CSF formation also.[2–7]

The obstruction outside the ventricular system or the impaired resorption of the cerebrospinal fluid cause dilation of the subarachnoid space and eventually results in dilation of the lateral ventricles. The communicating hydrocephaly usually presents as tetraventriculomegaly, that is, dilation of the two lateral ventricles, the third ventricle, and the fourth ventricle.

Prenatal Diagnosis

Communicating hydrocephalus causes tetraventricular hydrocephaly; the dilation of the fourth ventricle, however, is minimal. The more specific sonographic image is the dilation of the subarachnoid cistern;[7] it is rarely detected, however. In the differential diagnosis of this anomaly, aqueductal stenosis must be excluded (Fig. 5–38, Fig. 5–39, and Fig. 5–40).

Management and Outcome

Termination of the pregnancy may be offered to parents if the diagnosis is made before viability. Cephalocentesis should not be used in third-trimester diagnoses of isolated communicating hydrocephalus, since this procedure is associated with high fetal morbidity and mortality. Cesarean section should be used for delivering fetuses with macrocephaly, fetal distress, or other usual obstetrical indications.

The outcome appears better, compared with other types of hydrocephaly. The mortality rate in isolated communicating hydrocephalus was 11% in one study, and in 84% of cases the IQ was greater than 70.[6]

REFERENCES

1. Burton BK. Recurrence risks for congenital hydrocephalus. *Clin Genet.* 1979;16:47–53.
2. Emery JL, Zachary RB. Hydrocephalus associated with obliteration of the longitudinal sinus. *Arch Dis Child.* 1956;31:651–655.
3. Ellington E, Margolis G. Block of arachnoid villus by subarachnoid hemorrhage. *J Neurosurg.* 1969;30:651–657.
4. Gutierrez Y, Friede RL, Kaliney WJ. Agenesis of arachnoid granulations and its relationship to communicating hydrocephalus. *J Neurosurg.* 1975;43:553–558.
5. Milhorat TH, Hammock MK, Davis DA, et al. Choroid plexus papilloma, I: proof of cerebrospinal fluid over production. *Child's Brain.* 1976;2:273–289.
6. Guthkelch AN, Riley NA. Influence of aetiology in prognosis in surgically treated infantile hydrocephalus. *Arch Dis Child.* 1969;44:29–35.
7. Pilu G, DePalma L, Romero R, et al. The fetal subarachnoid cisterns: an ultrasound study with report of a case of communicating hydrocephalus. *J Ultrasound Med.* (In press).

Dandy–Walker Syndrome

Dandy–Walker syndrome accounts for about 10% of all cases of hydrocephalus. This syndrome results from a posterior fossa cyst which usually creates a defect in the cerebellar vermis, enlargement of the transverse cerebellar diameter, and obstruction to the egress of cerebrospinal fluid from the ventricular system into the subarachnoid space. This obstructive process results in ventriculomegaly.

Etiopathology

Dandy–Walker malformation was originally believed to occur secondary to complete or partial obstruction or atresia of the foramina of Luschka and Magendie.[1] These foramina provide communication with the subarachnoid space, allowing the cerebrospinal fluid to flow from the upper ventricles into the subarachnoid space. The maldevelopment of the rhombencephalic midline structures, which derive from the primitive third cerebral vesicle, may also be responsible for this anomaly. Hypoplasia of the primary cerebellar vermis may be due to the early dilation or herniation of the rhombencephalic roof. Another theory suggests an imbalance in cerebrospinal fluid production among ventricles. Although the Dandy–Walker syndrome may not have a single etiology, when the condition was followed from early in pregnancy with ultrasound, a defect in the cerebellar vermis often seemed to be the first or only sign of the condition.[2]

The three main characteristics associated with Dandy–Walker syndrome are hydrocephalus, posterior fossa cyst, and cerebellar vermis defect. Although hydrocephalus may be essential in Dandy–Walker syndrome, such is not always the case, and it may be absent in the early prenatal period.

Dandy–Walker syndrome may be associated with agenesis of the corpus callosum or encephalocele.[3,4] Polycystic kidney and cardiovascular defects, particularly ventricular septal defect, have also been reported.[3–6]

Prenatal Diagnosis

Obstruction of the foramina of Luschka and Magendie leads to dilation of the ventricular system. Dilation of the fourth ventricle is the most prominent feature that distinguishes Dandy–Walker syndrome from the other types of hydrocephalus. Although hydrocephalus is often one of the signs leading to the diagnosis of Dandy–Walker syndrome, it may be absent in the prenatal period.[7,8] Therefore, the morphologic appearance of the posterior fossa and the biometric measurements of the TCD can be useful in the early prenatal diagnosis of this disorder. The diagnosis of Dandy–Walker syndrome should be considered whenever a cystic mass is visualized in the posterior fossa (Fig. 5–41 and Fig. 5–42).[4,9–12] Dilation of the cisterna magna and an arachnoid cyst, however, must be excluded.

Management and Outcome

Termination of pregnancy is considered by some parents if the diagnosis is made before viability. There is no consensus on management of the pregnancy if diagnosis is made after viability.

The survival rate of Dandy–Walker syndrome

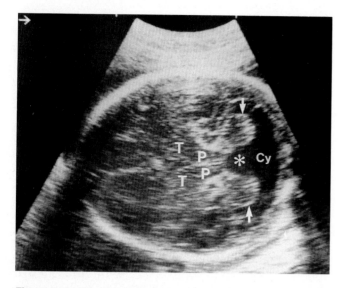

Figure 5–41. Transabdominal examination of a fetus in the second trimester. This axial plane depicts midline structures, such as the thalami (T), the cerebellar peduncles (P), and the cerebellar hemispheres (two small arrowheads). The cerebellar vemris is absent (*), and a cystic structure fills that area in the posterior fossa (Cy).

was reported to range between 70 and 90%. The IQ of the survivors is above 80 in almost 50% of the cases.[4,5]

REFERENCES

1. Dandy WE. The diagnosis and treatment of hydrocephalus due to occlusion of the foramen of Magendie and Luschka. *Surg Gynecol Obstet.* 1921;32:112–115.
2. Pilu G, Romero R, DePalma L, et al. Antenatal diagnosis and obstetrical management of Dandy–Walker syndrome. *J Reprod Med.* 1986;31:1017–1022.
3. Hart MN, Malamud N, Ellis WG. The Dandy–Walker syndrome: a clinico-pathological study based on 29 cases. *Neurology.* 1972;22:771–780.
4. Hirsch JF, Pierre KA, Renier D, et al. The Dandy–Walker malformation: a review of 40 cases. *J Neurosurg.* 1984; 61:515–522.
5. Sawaya R, McLaurin RL. Dandy–Walker syndrome: clinical analysis of 23 cases. *J Neurosurg.* 1981;55:89–98.
6. Olson GS, Halpe DC, Kaplan AM, et al. Dandy–Walker malformation and associated cardiac anomalies. *Child's Brain.* 1981;8:173–180.
7. Dempsey PJ, Koch HJ. In utero diagnosis of the Dandy–Walker syndrome: differentiation for extra-axial posterior fossa cyst. *J Clin Ultrasound.* 1981;9:403–405.

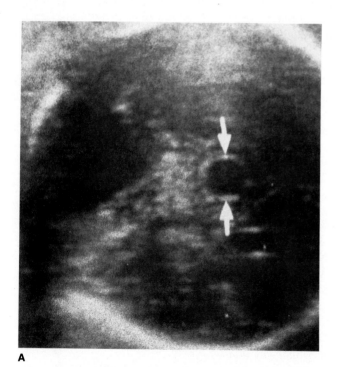

A

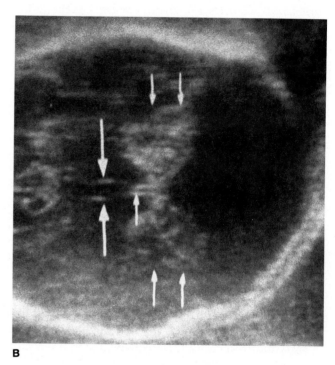

B

Figure 5–42. Variations on a prenatal diagnosis of posterior fossa cyst using ultrasound. **(A)** The cerebellum can be seen with expansion or splaying of the cerebellar hemispheres. There is also dilation of the fourth ventricle (arrows). This typically results from an obstructive process eventually leading to dilation of all ventricles, progressing from the fourth, third, and then to the lateral ventricles. **(B)** A large posterior fossa cyst with absent cerebellar vermis and splaying of the cerebellar hemispheres is shown (two smaller arrows bilaterally). The fourth and third ventricles are of relatively normal size. These findings indicate an earlier stage of the disorder, with relative normality of the ventricular system.

8. Fileni A, Colosimo C, Mirk P, et al. Dandy–Walker syndrome: diagnosis in utero by means of ultrasound and CT correlations. *Neuroradiology.* 1983;24:233–235.
9. Hatjis CG, Horbar JD, Anderson GG. The in utero diagnosis of a posterior fossa intracranial cyst (Dandy–Walker cyst). *Am J Obstet Gynecol.* 1981;140:473–475.
10. Kirkinen P, Jouppila P, Valkeakari T, et al. Ultrasonic evaluation of the Dandy–Walker syndrome. *Obstet Gynecol.* 1982;59(suppl):185–215.
11. Mahony BS, Callen PW, Filly RA, et al. The fetal cisterna magna. *Radiology.* 1984;153:773–776.
12. Taylor GA, Sanders RC. Dandy–Walker syndrome: recognition by sonography. *Am J Neuroradiol.* 1983;4:1203–1206.

MICROCEPHALY

Microcephaly is characterized by a head circumference below the normal range and is strongly associated with mental retardation in 30 to 60% of the cases.[1–3] Estimates of the incidence of microcephaly, based on observations made at birth, have varied from 1 in 6,250 to 1 in 8,500 live births.[4] A much higher incidence of 0.16% of live births was reported in the United States' Collaborative Perinatal Project in which infants through the first year of life were observed.[5]

Etiopathology
The causes of microcephaly are many; they may be divided into genetic mutations, chromosomal abnormalities, and environmental damage.

Genetic Mutations. Microcephaly may be inherited as an autosomal recessive trait, in association with consanguinity. Meckel syndrome is an example of an autosomal recessive genetic disorder with a constellation of abnormal features that may include microcephaly.[6]

Chromosomal Abnormalities. Structural chromosomal abnormalities, such as the 5p (or cri du chat) syndrome or trisomies, may cause microcephaly.[6]

Environmental Factors. The environmental causes of microcephaly may include intrauterine exposure to infectious agents (e.g., cytomegalovirus, toxoplasmosis, rubella); drugs (e.g., alcohol, certain anticonvulsives); maternal disease (e.g., phenylketonuria), or maternal radiation exposure.[6,7]

Sonoanatomy
Typical morphologic findings in the fetus with microcephaly involve changes in the shape of the head: a cone-shaped head, a large face, large ears, and narrowing, receding, and flattening of the forehead are features sometimes referred to collectively as a "pinhead" or "birdhead" (Fig. 5–43). Microcephaly is also

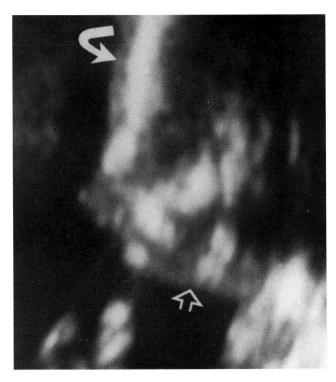

Figure 5–43. Profile of fetal face depicting the elongated forehead and its inclinations (curved arrow). The open arrow shows micrognathia.

associated with decreased size of the frontal lobe and flattening of the frontal bone, while other lobes of the fetal brain remain unchanged.[8,9]

Prenatal Diagnosis
True microcephaly can be diagnosed by serial measurements of fetal head growth. Some authors use a head circumference measuring 2 SD below the mean for gestational age,[3] while others use a head circumference measuring 3 SD below the mean for gestational age.[5,10] Some investigators use the biparietal diameter (BPD) as the key diagnostic parameter;[8] this criterion, however, can be modified by external pressure on the fetal head. Head circumference is thus considered more useful, since it would presumably be unaffected in these circumstances. The measurements of the growth of the fetal head circumference can be used appropriately during the second trimester as an indicator for gestational age estimation; there are great variations, however, in the head circumference in the third trimester. Romero and coworkers[3] suggested using the ratio of fetal head circumference to abdominal circumference as the parameter for the prenatal diagnosis of microcephaly. If a cutoff of 4 SD below the mean is used with traditional measurements, the false-positive rate would be reduced to 0% for femur length–head circumference, head–abdominal circumference, and occipital frontal diameter,[5] but the false negative rate would be increased.

The differential diagnosis of microcephaly includes symmetric fetal growth retardation. In cases of growth retardation, the head, abdomen, and occasionally long bones are below the normal range for the indicated gestational age. The abdominal circumference and long bone length are within normal limits, however, in cases of microcephaly. Reece et al[11] have shown recently that the measurements of the transverse cerebellar diameter (TCD) in growth-retarded fetuses remain relatively unchanged from normal.[11] It remains to be seen whether normal measurements of the TCD occur in microcephaly. The TCD tends to be smaller than normal in alcohol-related craniopathy.

Goldstein et al[9] demonstrated the pattern of growth of the frontal lobe, which is the organ most affected in microcephaly (Fig. 5–43). Measurements of the frontal lobe were obtained at the level of the thalami and the third ventricle. The posterior landmark of the frontal lobe was established by the anterior edge of the septum cavum pellucidum, and the anterior landmark by the hyperechogenic frontal bone. The thalami and the frontal lobe were measured by placing one caliper on the frontal bone (anterior edge) and another behind the thalami (posterior edge) (Table 5–7, Table 5–8, and Table 5–9).[9] The normal dimensions of the anterior cranial fossa and the frontal lobe of the fetal brain provided normative data against which fetuses suspected of having microcephaly or any other lesion affecting the anterior fossa could be evaluated. Preliminary findings indicate that the use of frontal lobe measurements may be more precise than conventional measurements for diagnosing microcephaly.[9]

Associated Anomalies

Microcephaly is often associated with other anomalies. Some have well-defined genetic or environmental causes, while in others, the precise etiology is not recognized. The heterogeneous nature of this disorder is also demonstrated by the variety of neuropathologic findings. Holoprosencephaly, agyria, absence of corpus callosum, or ventricular enlargement secondary to cortical atrophy may be present in some cases.

Management and Outcome

A detailed ultrasound evaluation and fetal karyotype should be performed. The pregnant patient is counseled on the basis of the most serious malformation if another malformation is found. If there is no associated abnormality, the patient is counseled on the degree of compromise of the head circumference. There is a *good chance* that the infant will be normal if the head circumference is between 2 to 3 SD below the mean. If the head perimeter is 4 SD below the mean,

however, the outcome is associated with mental retardation. The option of termination of pregnancy may be considered if the diagnosis is made before viability. Expectant management while awaiting spontaneous delivery is a reasonable approach if the diagnosis is made after viability. Since complicated delivery or fetal distress may occur, various obstetric options should be contemplated in advance, in consultation with patients.

Microcephaly is an untreatable condition. One study reported that when the head circumference was 3 SD below the mean, there was a 62% risk of moderate-to-severe mental retardation.[12] Pryor and Thelander[13] reported infants with head circumference measurements 4 to 7 SD below the mean to have a mean IQ of 35; those infants with measured head circumferences 7 SD below the mean, however, had a mean IQ of 20.

REFERENCES

1. Warkany JA, Dignan PJ. Mental retardation and developmental disabilities: an annual review. In: Warkany JA, ed. *Congenital Malformations: Microcephaly.* Chicago, Ill: Year Book; 1979;113–131.
2. Martin HP. Microcephaly and mental retardation. *Am J Dis Child.* 1970;119:128–131.
3. Romero R, Pilu G, Jeanty P, et al. *Prenatal Diagnosis of Congenital Anomalies.* Norwalk, Conn: Appleton & Lange; 1988:54–59.
4. Lemire RJ, Loeser JD, Leech RW, et al, Normal and abnormal development of human nervous system. In: Lemire RJ, Loeser JD, Leech RW, et al, eds: *Skull.* Hagerstown, Md: Harper & Row; 1975.
5. Chervenak FA, Jeanty P, Cantraine F, et al. The diagnosis of microcephaly. *Am J Obstet Gynecol.* 1984;149:512–517.
6. Warkany J, Dignan PSJ. Congenital malformations: microcephaly. *Mental Retard Rev.* 1973;5:113–120.
7. Warkany JA. *Congenital Malformations: Notes and Comments.* Chicago, Ill: Year Book; 1971;28:237–271.
8. Pescia G, Nguyen H, Deonna T. Prenatal diagnosis of genetic microcephaly. *Prenatal Diagn.* 1983;3:363–365.
9. Goldstein I, Reece EA, Pilu G, et al. Sonographic assessment of the fetal frontal lobe: a potential tool for prenatal diagnosis of microcephaly. *Am J Obstet Gynecol.* 1988; 158:1057–1062.
10. Kurtz AB, Wapner RJ, Rubin CS, et al. Ultrasound criteria for in-utero diagnosis of microcephaly. *J Clin Ultrasound.* 1980;8:11–16.
11. Reece EA, Goldstein I, Pilu G, et al. Fetal cerebellar growth unaffected by intrauterine growth retardation: a new parameter for prental diagnosis. *Am J Obstet Gynecol.* 1987;157:632–638.
12. Avery GB, Meneses L, Lodge A, et al. The clinical significance of "measurement microcephaly." *Am J Dis Child.* 1972;123:214–217.

13. Pryor HB, Thelander H. Abnormally small head size and intellect in children. *J Pediatr.* 1968;73:593–598.

ANENCEPHALY

Anencephaly is one of the most common neural tube defects characterized by absence of the cerebral hemispheres and the cranial vault.[1,2] Anencephaly occurs in approximately 1 in 1,000 births in the United States, and in 5 in 1,000 births in Ireland and Wales.[1–3]

Etiopathology

Anencephaly features an absence of the structures derived from the forebrain and skull; most of the cranial vault is absent. The forebrain and the midbrain are missing or replaced by rudimentary fibrovascular tissue, with scattered islands of neural elements. The facial bone and skull base are nearly normal in form, but the frontal bone, the parietal bones, and the occipital bone are absent or partially formed. The head itself is covered by a vascular membrane. Underneath the mass of fibrovascular tissue lie a few remnants of the cerebral hemispheres.[2,4,5]

The exact cause of anencephaly remains uncertain despite much speculation and research. Both family and epidemiologic studies suggest that anencephaly results from failure of closure of the anterior neuropore at approximately 24 days of fetal life, and that its etiology is multifactorial.[2]

Associated anomalies include spina bifida, cleft lip or palate, clubfoot, and omphalocele. Other characteristic features are a short neck, large tongue, and bulging eyes.[3]

Prenatal Diagnosis

The sonographic diagnosis of anencephaly is based on the findings of abnormal intracranial anatomy, abnormal or absent frontal bones, and prominent orbital structures. This conspicuous abnormality, often detected when the biparietal diameter (BPD) measurements of the fetus are attempted, is shown best on coronal views of the fetal face, where a typical "froglike" appearance may be observed. The diagnosis can be made as early as the 10th week of gestation. (Fig. 5–44 and Fig. 5–45).[6]

The intracranial anatomy can be easily identified by the end of the first trimester, when the choroid plexuses are prominent structures in the lateral ventricles; even the cerebellum can be identified.

The BPD and the occipitofrontal diameter (OFD) can be obtained in the 12th week of gestation. In cases in which these parameters cannot be visualized, a strong suspicion of anencephaly should be entertained. The diagnosis is sometimes made in the second or in the third trimesters, often in association with an

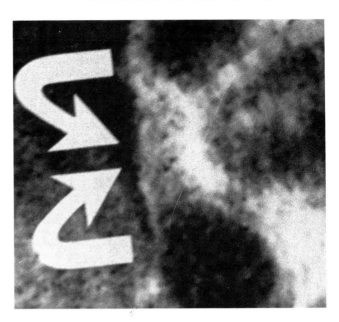

Figure 5–44. Transvaginal scan of a fetus at approximately 12 weeks' gestation. The fetal orbits are prominent and eyes are prominent and often described as froglike in appearance; the nasal area is also observed, but the calvarium is absent (curved arrows).

abnormal position of the fetus—breech or transverse. Occasionally when the fetus is in the vertex presentation, there may be difficulty in establishing the diagnosis because the base of the skull is deep in the maternal pelvis. Under these circumstances, transvaginal sonography is recommended.

Polyhydramnios is frequently associated with anencephaly, but its incidence varies from 30% to 98%.[3,6] The mechanism is unclear; it has been suggested that the polyhydramnios results from failure to swallow amniotic fluid secondary to central neurologic damage.[7]

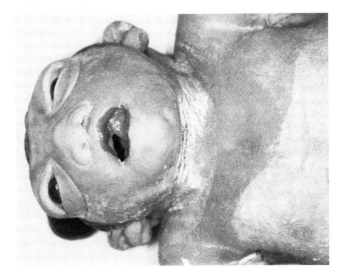

Figure 5–45. An anencephalic fetus with prominent eyes and absent calvarium. These findings are similar to those described in the sonographic picture.

Management and Outcome

Termination of pregnancy should be offered to patients carrying anencephalic fetuses. Some investigators have suggested that termination is justified even if this diagnosis is made in the third trimester.[3] Admittedly, such a position is controversial and not always an option because of local laws prohibiting abortion in the third trimester. The proponents of this position argue, however, that this condition is unequivocally incompatible with life, and death occurs within a few hours or days after birth. Premature delivery occurs in 50% of cases, while postterm pregnancies occur in 15% and livebirths in about 30%.

REFERENCES

1. Leench RW, Shuman RM. *Congenital Malformation in Neuropathy.* Philadelphia, Pa: Harper & Row; 1982;199.
2. Lemire RJ, Beckwith JB, Warkany J. *Anencephaly.* New York, NY: Raven; 1978.
3. Romero R, Pilu G, Jeanty P, et al. The central nervous system. In: Romero R, Pilu G, Jeanty P, et al. *Prenatal Diagnosis of Congenital Anomalies.* Norwalk, Conn: Appleton & Lange; 1988.
4. Campbell S, Johnstone FD, Holt EM, et al. Anencephaly: early ultrasonic diagnosis and active management. *Lancet.* 1972;2:1226–1227.
5. Fraser JE. Report on an anencephalic embryo. *J Anat.* 1921;56:12.
6. Goldstein RB, Filly RA. Prenatal diagnosis of anencephaly: spectrum of sonographic appearance and distinction from the amniotic band syndrome. *AJR.* 1988;151:547–550.
7. Giroud J. Anencephaly. In: Vinken GW, Bruyn FW, eds. *Handbook of Clinical Neurology.* vol. 32. Amsterdam: Elsevier/North Holland; 1978:175–208.

CEPHALOCELE

Cephalocele is an anomaly of the neural tube characterized by herniation of the intracranial contents through a bony defect in the skull. Meningocele describes protrusion of meninges only, at any site along the neural axis, while encephalocele is herniation of brain tissue.[1,2] Cephalocele is a rare anomaly. The frequency of occipital cephalocele is estimated at 0.3 to 0.8 in 1,000 births.[3]

Etiopathology

Like other neural tube defects, cephaloceles have a familial tendency.[1,2] Cephaloceles are frequent in Meckel syndrome and Warburg syndrome (genetic disorders with autosomal recessive inheritance), as well as in nongenetic diseases such as amniotic band syndrome.[4] They may also occur in cases of maternal diseases, for example, rubella, diabetes, and hyperthermia.[5]

Most cephaloceles are midline and result from either the overgrowth of the rostral portion of the neural tube, which may interfere with the closure of the skull, or failure of closure of the mesoderm.[1] Cephaloceles can be occipital (posterior) (Fig. 5–46), parietal (lateral), or frontal (anterior). The most common is the occipital cephalocele. The lesion varies in size and may or may not contain brain tissue. Frontal cephaloceles occur more frequently between the frontal and the ethmoidal bones (frontonasal cephaloceles). Some cephaloceles may not be obvious when located at the base of the skull or protruding inside the orbits, nasopharynx, or oropharynx. A frontal cephalocele is much more obvious, and almost always contains brain tissue.[6–9]

Associated anomalies may include polycystic kidney (Meckel syndrome), other neural tube defects (hydrocephaly) or primary microcephaly.[1,10] A posterior cephalocele with herniation of the cerebellum is termed Chiari type III deformity, which, together with aqueductal stenosis, is the major cause of hydrocephaly in these cases.[7] Frontal cephaloceles are often associated with the median cleft face syndrome (also known as the frontonasal dysplasia sequence) characterized by median cleft lip, cleft palate, or hypertelorism.[10]

Prenatal Diagnosis

The diagnosis is made by identifying an extracranial mass connected in some way to the fetal head.[6,11–16] The differential diagnosis includes cystic hygroma, teratoma, bronchiogenic cyst, hemangioma, and scalp edema. Efforts should also be made to identify the skull defect. This may not be easy, because the bony

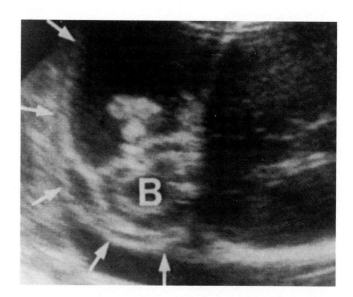

Figure 5–46. Ultrasound picture of fetal head depicting posterior herniation of brain tissue (B) at the base of skull and superior aspect of spine (arrows). This is consistent with an occipital cephalocele.

defect is usually smaller in proportion to the herniated brain mass. Cross-sectional scans should thus be taken carefully, especially in those cases when the intracranial anatomy is not clear. The examiner should always attempt to rule out cephalocele in cases of hydrocephaly, microcephaly, cystic hygroma, and scalp edema. A careful examination of the fetus is also indicated to exclude other associated anomalies when a diagnosis of cephalocele is made.

Management and Outcome

When the diagnosis of cephalocele is made before viability, termination of pregnancy should be offered. If the diagnosis is made after viability, however, the management depends on the amount of herniated brain tissue and the associated anomalies. A nonaggressive approach should be taken regarding medical management if these anomalies are incompatible with life. Parents should be included in all discussions and decisions regarding pregnancy management.

The prognosis of cephalocele is dependent on whether or not there is herniation of brain tissue. The presence or absence of hydrocephaly or microcephaly also plays a role in prognosis.

In a series of 68 patients with operatively corrected cephaloceles, Simpson et al[3] reported a 16% mortality rate. Of those remaining, 38 (56%) were normal or had slight disabilities; 14 (21%) had uncertain or significant mental defects; and 16 (23%) were severely disabled. There were no deaths, in contrast, to cases of simple meningocele. Mortality and intellectual development are both related to the size and site of the herniated lesion.

REFERENCES

1. Schulman K. Encephalocele. *Birth Defects Compendium.* 2nd ed. In: Bergsma D, ed, New York, NY: Alan R. Liss, Inc; 1979;390–391.
2. McLaurin RL. Cranium bifidum and cranial cephaloceles. In: Vinken SE, Bruyn FW, eds. *Handbook of Clinical Neurology.* vol. 32. Amsterdam: Elsevier/North Holland; 1978:209–218.
3. Simpson AD, David JD, White J. Cephaloceles: treatment, outcome, and antenatal diagnosis. *Neurosurgery.* 1984; 15:14–21.
4. Jones KL. *Smith's Recognizable Patterns of Human Malformation.* 4th ed. Philadelphia, Pa: W.B. Saunders Co.; 1988:710.
5. Cohen MM, Lemire RJ. Syndromes with cephaloceles. *Teratology.* 1982;25:161–172.
6. Graham D, Johnson TR, Winn K, et al. The role of sonography in the prenatal diagnosis and management of encephalocele. *J Ultrasound Med.* 1982;1:111–115.
7. Guthkelch AN: Occipital cranium bifidum. *Arch Dis Child.* 1970;45:104–109.
8. Carlan SJ, Angel JL, Leo J, et al. Cephalocele involving the oral cavity. *Obstet Gynecol.* 1990;75:494–496.
9. Fiske CE, Filly RA: Ultrasound evaluation of the normal and abnormal fetal neural axis. *Radiol Clin North Am.* 1982;20:285–288.
10. DeMyer W. The median cleft face syndrome. Differential diagnosis of cranium bifidum occultum, hypertelorism, and median cleft nose, lip, and palate. *Neurology.* 1967; 17:961–971.
11. Herzoa KA. The detection of fetal meningocele and meningoencephalocele by R-scan ultrasound: a case report. *J Clin Ultrasound.* 1975;3:307.
12. Sabbagha RE, Tamura RK, Dal Compo S, et al. Fetal cranial and craniocervical masses: ultrasound charateristics and differential diagnosis. *Am J Obstet Gynecol.* 1980;135:511–517.
13. Nicolini U, Ferrazzi E, Massa E, et al. Prenatal diagnosis of cranial masses by ultrasound: report of five cases. *J Clin Ultrasound.* 1982;11:170–174.
14. Chervenak FA, Issacson G, Mahoney MJ, et al. Diagnosis and management of fetal cephalocele. *Obstet Gynecol.* 1984;54:86–90.
15. Romero R, Pilu G, Jeanty P, et al. The central nervous system. In: Romero R, Pilu G, Jeanty P, et al. *Prenatal Diagnosis of Congenital Anomalies.* Norwalk, Conn: Appleton & Lange; 1988;46–49.
16. Cullen MT, Athanassiado AP, Romero R. Prenatal diagnosis of anterior parietal encephalocele with transvaginal sonography. *Obstet Gynecol.* 1990;75:489–491.

PORENCEPHALY

Porencephaly is a congenital anomaly with localized absence of cerebral mass resulting from intracerebral cystic cavities that contain cerebrospinal fluid. These cavities may communicate with the ventricular system sometimes causing ventriculomegaly.[1,2]

Etiopathology

True porencephaly is a developmental anomaly caused by failure in migration of cells destined to form the cerebral cortex.[3] This anomaly causes a local defect in both gray and white matter. In the absence of neural tissue the subarachnoid space expands to fill this void and therefore has the appearance of a cyst. Pseudoporencephaly may result from damage to the brain tissue occurring either before or after birth.[2,4,5] An example of traumatic pseudoporencephaly is a cyst, which develops after a cephalocentesis into the ventricular system of hydrocephalic infants.[1]

Sonoanatomy

True porencephaly is characterized by cystic cavities of variable sizes often located around the Sylvian fissure.[1-3] Many cavities are symmetric, with the corpus callosum either thin or absent.[3] It is frequently associated with microcephaly. Pseudoporencephaly is

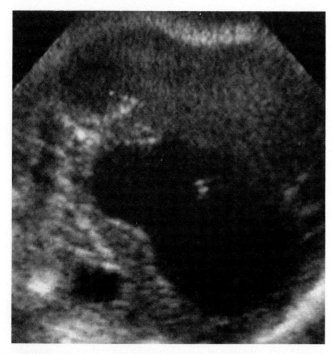

Figure 5–47. Intracerebral cystic cavity depicting the sonographic appearance of porencephaly.

almost always unilateral associated with histologic evidence of inflammation or ischemic injury.[4,5] Ventriculomegaly is seen in both porencephaly and pseudoporencephaly and is asymmetric.[6]

Prenatal Diagnosis
Porencephaly is diagnosed by the presence of multiple intracranial cystic structures (Fig. 5–47). They may be either bilateral or unilateral[3] and can be associated with complete distortion of the intracranial structures.[6]

Management and Outcome
Termination of pregnancy may be considered prior to viability, and cephalocentesis may be considered in cases of severe macrocephaly to avoid cesarean section. Infants with true porencephaly have a poor outcome, with severely impaired intellectual development and neurologic sequelae. Porencephaly is not treatable.

REFERENCES

1. Lorber J, Grainger RG. Cerebral cavities following ventricular punctures in the infants. *Clin Radiol.* 1963;14:98–100.
2. Sauerbrei EE, Cooperberg PL. Cystic tumors of the fetal and neonatal cerebrum: ultrasound and computed tomographic evaluation. *Radiology.* 1983;147:689–692.
3. Romero R, Pilu G, Jeanty P, et al. The central nervous system. In: Romero R, Pilu G, Jeanty P, et al. *Prenatal Diagnosis of Congenital Anomalies.* Norwalk, Conn: Appleton & Lange; 1988:50–52.
4. Benda CE. The late effects of cerebral birth injury. *Medicine.* 1945;24:71–75.
5. Cantu RC, LeMay M. Porencephaly caused by intracerebral hemorrhage. *Radiology.* 1967;88:526–530.
6. Chervenak FA, Berkowitz RL, Romero R, et al. The diagnosis of fetal hydrocephalus. *Am J Obstet Gynecol.* 1983; 147:703–716.

HYDRANENCEPHALY

Hydranencephaly is a variant of hydrocephaly characterized by the absence of most of the cerebral hemispheres and the replacement of brain tissue by cerebrospinal fluid.[1] It occurs in 0.2% of live births.[2,3]

Etiopathology
Hydranencephaly is a result of destructive intrauterine insult of vascular or infectious origin.[3] Myers[4] demonstrated in an animal model the induction of hydranencephaly by in utero occlusion of the carotid artery and jugular vein. This indicates that hydranencephaly may be caused by vascular occlusion and resulting tissue necrosis. Infection may also cause hydranencephaly, either by causing a necrotizing vasculitis or by local destruction of the brain tissue.[5] Dilation of the ventricular system results in either case, and cerebrospinal fluid fills the intracranial cavity.

There is variability in the extent of destruction of the cerebellar hemispheres. The destruction may be complete or partial, sparing portions of the temporal and occipital cortices.[1,6] The brain stem is usually present, although the thalami and the cerebellum may be smaller than normal. The head cavity is often filled with cerebrospinal fluid. Macrocrania does not occur in most cases. The falx cerebri may be absent or incomplete.

Prenatal Diagnosis
Hydranencephaly is diagnosed by the sonographic appearance of a large cystic mass filling the entire intracranial cavity along with the absence of midline structures and brain parenchyma. (Fig. 5–48). The most common diagnostic problems include the differentiation of hydranencephaly from severe hydrocephaly or porencephaly. There is evidence of cortical mantle in cases of porencephaly. The differential diagnosis may be almost impossible in cases of severe hydrocephaly. One way of differentiating hydranencephaly from severe hydrocephaly is that the former is usually associated with a normal biparietal[2,7–9] diameter (BPD).

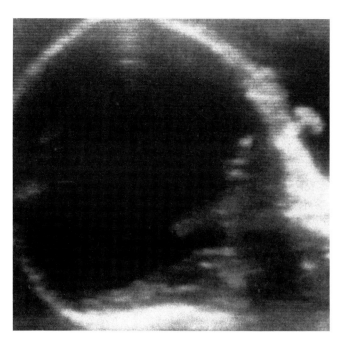

Figure 5–48. Transabdominal ultrasound examination of a fetus depicting hydranencephaly. Note the large cystic mass filling the intracranial cavity and the absence of midline structures and brain parenchyma.

Management and Outcome

The prognosis of hydranencephaly is poor, with severe neurologic sequelae at birth or resultant death. Termination of pregnancy should be considered prior to viability. If the diagnosis is clear, discussion with the parents should be entertained regarding not performing a cesarean section if fetal distress occurs in labor.

REFERENCES

1. Hamby WB, Krauss RF, Beswick WF. Hydranencephaly: clinical diagnosis. *Pediatrics.* 1950;6:371–376.
2. Romero R, Pilu G, Jeanty P, et al. The central nervous system. In: Romero R, Pilu G, Jeanty P, et al. *Prenatal Diagnosis of Congenital Abnormalities.* Norwalk, Conn: Appleton & Lange; 1988:52–54.
3. Sutton LN, Bruce DA, Schut L. Hydranencephaly versus hydrocephalus: an important distinction. *Neurosurgery.* 1980;6:34–38.
4. Myers R. Brain pathology following fetal vascular occlusion: an experimental study. *Invest Ophthalmol.* 1969;8:41–47.
5. Altshuler G. Toxoplasmosis as a cause of hydranencephaly. *Am J Dis Child.* 1973;125:251–252.
6. Johnson EE, Warner M, Simonds JP. Total absence of cerebral hemispheres. *J Pediatr.* 1951;38:69–72.
7. Fiske CE, Filly RA. Ultrasound evaluation of the normal and abnormal fetal neural axis. *Radiol Clin North Am.* 1982;20:285–296.
8. Lee TG, Warren BH. Antenatal diagnosis of hydranencephaly by ultrasound: correlation with ventriculomegaly and computed tomography. *J Clin Ultrasound.* 1977;5:271–273.
9. Pilu G, Rizzo N, Orsini LF, et al. Antenatal recognition of cerebral anomalies. *Ultrasound Med Biol.* 1986;12:319–326.

HOLOPROSENCEPHALY

Holoprosencephaly is a developmental malformation resulting from failure of cleavage of the prosencephalon. In its most severe form, cyclopia, has been reported to occur in 1 in 40,000 births. The true incidence of holoprosencephaly, however, is unknown because forms without facial defects may be unrecognized at birth.[1,2]

Etiopathology

The causes of holoprosencephaly include 1) chromosomal abnormalities (in particular trisomy 13, although it has also been reported in cases of trisomy 18 and other structural chromosomal defects);[3] 2) teratogenic agents, such as cytomegalovirus,[4] radiation,[5] or high dose salicylates;[6] 3) genetic factors including both autosomal dominant and autosomal recessive forms;[3,5,7] and 4) maternal disease states such as diabetes.[5]

The prosencephalon normally gives rise to the cerebral hemispheres and diencephalic structures, including thalami, third ventricle, and optic bulbs. This differentiation process is thought to be induced by precordial mesenchyme interposed between the roof of the mouth and the prosencephalon. This same tissue is responsible for the normal development of the median facial structures: forehead, nose, interorbital structure, and upper lip. Interference with the normal migration of the precordial mesenchyme thus leads to defects in both face and brain. The facial anomalies encompass a broad range of defects that are due to aplasia or varying degrees of hypoplasia of the facial structures.[5,8–10]

DeMyer[8] suggested the following classification for holoprosencephaly: 1) alobar, 2) semilobar, and 3) lobar. Alobar holoprosencephaly is characterized by absence of the interhemispheric fissure, a single primitive ventricle, fused thalami, and absence of the third ventricle, neurohypophysis, and olfactory bulbs. In semilobar holoprosencephaly, the cerebral hemispheres are partially separated posteriorly, but there is still a single ventricular cavity. Lobar holoprosencephaly is characterized by a well-developed interhemispheric fissure both anteriorly and posteriorly, with variable fusion of structures, such as the lateral ventricles or septum cavum pelucidae.

Prenatal Diagnosis

The characteristic feature of alobar and semilobar holoprosencephaly is the single ventricle and the undivided thalami.[11,12] The lobar form is characterized by nonseparated lateral ventricles, except for the frontal portion.[13,14] The contents of the posterior fossa are normal in all forms of holoprosencephaly (Fig. 5–49).

The most common facial defects include cleft lip or palate,[12] hypotelorism,[15,16] cyclopia,[11,17] absence of orbits and nose,[12] and identification of a proboscis.[11,18]

Management and Outcome

Termination of pregnancy is offered to patients if the diagnosis of holoprosencephaly is made before viability. Third-trimester diagnosis should lead to nonaggressive medical management and cephalocentesis in cases of macrocephaly.[12]

Infants with the alobar form usually die during the first year of life. Infants with the semilobar form may reach childhood but are severely handicapped.[5,10]

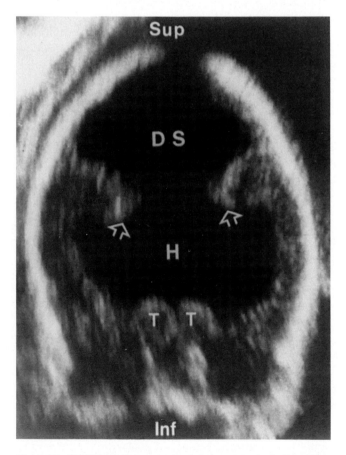

Figure 5–49. Midcoronal scan of a holoprosencephalic fetus. The cortex (arrows) is over the holoventricle (H), which amply communicates with the superior dorsal sac (DS). Note the fused thalami (T) on the floor of the ventricular cavity. Sup=superior; Inf=inferior. (*From Pilu G, Romero R, Jeanty P, et al. Criteria for the antenatal diagnosis of holoprosencephaly.* Am J Perinatal. *1987;4:41, with permission.*)

The lobar form may be compatible with a normal life span. The latter group is intellectually impaired, but some cases may be able to function independently in society.

REFERENCES

1. Blackwell DE, Spinnato JA, Hirsch G, et al. Antenatal ultrasound diagnosis of holoprosencephaly. *Am J Obstet Gynecol*. 1982;143:848–849.
2. Cayea FD, Balcar I, Alberti O, et al. Prenatal diagnosis of holoprosencephaly. *AJR*. 1984;142:401–402.
3. Roach E, DeMyer W, Conneally P, et al. Holoprosencephaly: birth data, genetic and demographic analysis of 30 families. *Birth Defects*. 1975;11:294–313.
4. Byrne PJ, Silver MM, Gilbert JM, et al. Cyclopia and congenital cytomegalovirus infection. *Am J Med Genet*. 1987;28:61–65.
5. DeMyer W. Holoprosencephaly. In: Vinken PJ, Bruyn GW, eds. *Handbook of Clinical Neurology*. vol. 32. Amsterdam: Elsevier/North Holland; 1978:431–478.
6. Benawra R, Manqurten HH, Duffell DR. Cyclopia and other anomalies following maternal ingestion of salicylates. *J Pediatr*. 1980;98:1069–1071.
7. Cohen MM. An update on the holoprosencephalic disorders. *J Pediatr*. 1982;101:865–869.
8. DeMyer W. Classification of cerebral malformations. *Birth Defects Original Article Series*. 1971;7:78–82.
9. DeMyer W, Zeman W, Palmer CG. The face predicts the brain: diagnostic significance of median facial anomalies for holoprosencephaly (arhinencephaly). *Pediatrics*. 1964;34:256–263.
10. DeMyer W, Zeman W. Alobar holoprosencephaly (iniencephaly) with median cleft lip and palate: clinical electroencephalographic and nosologic considerations. *Conf Neurol*. 1963;23:1–7.
11. Filly RA, Chinn DH, Callen FW. Alobar holoprosencephaly ultrasonographic prenatal diagnosis. *Radiology*. 1984;151:455–459.
12. Romero R, Pilu G, Jeanty P, et al. The central nervous system. In: Romero R, Pilu G, Jeanty P, et al. *Prenatal Diagnosis of Congenital Anomalies*. Norwalk, Conn: Appleton & Lange; 1988;59–65.
13. Fitz CR. Midline anomalies of the brain and spine. *Radiol Clin N Am*. 1982;20:95–104.
14. Fitz CR. Holoprosencephaly and related entities. *Neuroradiology*. 1983;25:225–238.
15. Chervenak FA, Isaacson G, Mahoney MJ, et al. The obstetric significance of holoprosencephaly. *Obstet Gynecol*. 1984;63:115–121.
16. Mayden KL, Tortoa M, Berkowitz RI, et al. Orbital diameters: a new parameter for prenatal diagnosis and dating. *Am J Obstet Gynecol*. 1982;144:289–297.
17. Benacerraf BR, Frigoletto FD, Bieber FR. The fetal face: ultrasound examination. *Radiology*. 1984;153:495–497.
18. Lev-Gur M, Maklad NF, Fatel S. Ultrasonic findings in fetal cyclopia: a case report. *J Reprod Med*. 1983;28:554–557.

AGENESIS OF THE CORPUS CALLOSUM

The corpus callosum is a white-matter structure that connects both cerebral hemisphers. It functions to coordinate information and exchange sensory stimuli between the two hemispheres. The incidence of agenesis of the corpus callosum at autopsy was reported to be 1 in 19,000.[1]

Etiopathology

Agenesis of the corpus callosum may be associated with chromosome disorders, including trisomy 18, and other structural defects.[2-4] A familial tendency has been reported.[5-8] Intrauterine infections, such as toxoplasmosis[9] and rubella,[10] are also associated with agenesis of the corpus callosum. Other possible etiologies include tuberous sclerosis,[11] mucopolysaccaridosis,[12] and median cleft face syndrome.[13]

The corpus callosum, a portion of the neural tube cephalic to the rostral neuropore, is derived from the lamina terminalis. The rostral part of the corpus callosum forms first, during the fourth month of gestation, while the caudal part develops only after the fifth month of gestation.[12,14] Thus, if an insult to this area occurs early in gestation, the resulting defect will consist of complete agenesis of the corpus callosum; an insult occurring during the fifth month of gestation, however, will result in only partial agenesis of the corpus callosum.[1]

Associated Anomalies

Dandy–Walker syndrome, microcephaly, macrocephaly, holoprosencephaly, and the median cleft syndrome, as well as cardiovascular, gastrointestinal, and genitourinary anomalies have been reported in association with agenesis of the corpus callosum.[15]

Prenatal Diagnosis

The diagnosis of agenesis of the corpus callosum can be made by sonography based on the following findings on axial imaging: 1) "flared" and modestly dilated occipital horns creating an appearance of a "butterfly;" 2) dilated frontal horns resulting in a "dumbbell" configuration; 3) dilated third ventricle in 50% of cases; and 4) absence of the cavum septum pellucidum. It is occasionally possible to obtain sagittal and coronal views through abdominal scanning. The same views can be beautifully obtained through transvaginal scanning in most cases when the fetus is in a vertex presentation. On coronal scan, the separated lateral ventricles, the absent cavum, and the absent corpus callosum are clearly appreciated. The cingulate sulcus has a "drooping" appearance, in addition.[16,17]

The differential diagnosis includes obstructive ventriculomegaly or brain atrophy resulting in hydrocephaly. Measurements of the cerebroatrial distance and the cerebroposterior horn distance of the lateral ventricles should be performed throughout gestation when agenesis of the corpus callosum is suspected. The orbital measurements should also be determined to rule out hypotelorism, and assessment of the fetal face should be made to rule out clefting.

Individuals with agenesis of the corpus callosum may have neurologic deficits, such as seizures, intellectual impairment, and psychosis.[1,12,14] These conditions, however, may be caused by cerebral anomalies that are often associated with agenesis of the corpus callosum.

Isolated agenesis of the corpus callosum may be asymptomatic or it may be manifested in some individuals by an inability to match stimuli in both hands, for example, to discriminate totally the sensation of different temperatures and weight.[1]

If the diagnosis of agenesis of the corpus callosum is entertained prenatally, it is important to look for other central nervous system anomalies.

Management and Outcome

No prenatal intervention is necessary, and obstetric care can continue essentially unaltered.

REFERENCES

1. Ettlinger G. Agenesis of the corpus callosum. In: Vinken GW, Bruyn PW, eds. *Handbook of Clinical Neurology.* vol. 32. Amsterdam: Elsevier/North Holland; 1978:285–297.
2. Grogono JL. Children with agenesis of the corpus callosum. *Dev Med Child Neurol.* 1968;10:613–616.
3. Warkany J, Passarge E, Smith LB. Congenital malformations in autosomal trisomy syndromes. *Am J Dis Child.* 1966;112:502–517.
4. Warkany J. *Congenital Malformations.* Chicago, Ill: Year Book Medical Publications; 1971.
5. Anderman E, Anderman F, Joubert M, et al. Three familial midline malformations of the central nervous system: agenesis of the corpus callosum and anterior horn cell disease, agenesis of the cerebellar vermis and atrophy of the cerebellar vermis. *Birth Defects, Original Article Series.* 1975;2:269–275.
6. Menkes JH, Philippart M, Clark DB. Hereditary partial agenesis of the corpus callosum. *Arch Neurol.* 1964; 11:198–202.
7. Naiman J, Fraser FC. Agenesis of the corpus callosum: a report of two cases of siblings. *AMA Arch Neurol Psychiatry.* 1955;74:182–184.
8. Shapira U, Cohen T. Agenesis of the corpus callosum in two sisters. *J Med Genet.* 1973;10:266–269.
9. Bartoleschi B, Cantore GP. Agenesia del corpo calloso in paziente affetto da toxoplasmosi. *Rev Neurol.* 1962;32: 79–84.
10. Friedman M, Cohen P. Agenesis of the corpus callosum

as possible sequal to maternal rubella during pregnancy. *Am J Dis Child.* 1947;73:178–182.

11. Elliott GB, Wollin DW. Defect of the corpus callosum and congenital occlusion of the fourth ventricle with tuberous sclerosis. *AJR.* 1961;85:101–109.

12. Loeser JD, Alvord EC. Agenesis of the corpus callosum. *Brain.* 1968;91:553–570.

13. DeMyer W. The median cleft face syndrome: differential diagnosis of cranium bifidum occultum, hypertelorism and median cleft nose, lip and palate. *Neurology.* 1967; 17:961–971.

14. Loeser JD, Alvord EC. Clinicopathological correlations in agenesis of the corpus callosum. *Arch Neurol.* 1968;18:745–756.

15. Parrish ML, Roessmann U, Levinsohn MW. Agenesis of the corpus callosum: a study of the frequency of associated malformations. *Ann Neurol.* 1979;6:349–354.

16. Babcock DS. The normal, absent and abnormal corpus callosum: sonographic findings. *Radiology.* 1984;151:449–453.

17. Gebarski SS, Gebarski KS, Bowerman RA, et al. Agenesis of the corpus callosum: sonographic features. *Radiology.* 1984;151:443–448.

INIENCEPHALY

Iniencephaly is a malformation consisting of a defect at the back of the skull, particularly at the level of the foramen magnum. It is often combined with severe lordosis or kyphoscoliosis of the fetal spine as well as rachischisis[1,2] (Fig. 5–50). The incidence of this anomaly is variable, 1 in 896 in England[3] and 1 in 65,000 in India.[4]

In approximately 85% of cases of iniencephaly other anomalies are found. These include cephalofacial, cardiovascular, abdominal, and limb defects.[2,5–7]

Prenatal Diagnosis
The sonographic diagnosis of an isolated iniencephaly is fairly difficult. A deformed short spine and hyperextension of the fetal head may lead to the diagnosis.[7]

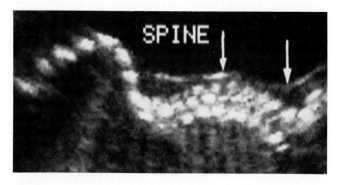

Figure 5–50. Picture of a spine depicting iniencephaly with kyphoscoliosis and rachischisis.

Management and Outcome
The prognosis of iniencephaly is poor, it is always fatal in the neonatal period.[8] Termination of pregnancy should be offered. Vaginal delivery may be complicated because of the hyperextended fetal head; cephalocentesis may thus be necessary to reduce the size of the head.[8,9]

REFERENCES

1. Abbott ME, Lochart FAL. Iniencephalus. *J Obstet Gynaecol Br Empire.* 1905;8:236–240.

2. Brodsky L. Four examples of iniencephalus with a statistical review of the literature. *Med J. Aust.* 1939;25:795–799.

3. Paterson SJ. Iniencephalus. *J Obstet Gynaecol Br Empire.* 1944;51:330.

4. Javant K, Mehta A, Sanghvi LD. A study of congenital malformations in Bombay. *J Obstet Gynaecol India.* 1960; 11:280–285.

5. David TJ, Illingworth CA. Diaphragmatic hernia in the southwest of England. *J Med Genet.* 1976;13:253–262.

6. David TJ, Nixon A. Congenital malformations associated with anencephaly and iniencephaly. *J Med Genet.* 1976; 13:263–265.

7. Romero R, Pilu G, Jeanty P, et al. The central nervous system. In: Romero R, Pilu G, Jeanty P, et al. *Prenatal Diagnosis of Congenital Anomalies.* Norwalk, Conn: Appleton & Lange; 1988;65–67.

8. Bluett D. Iniencephaly causing obstructed labor. *Proc R Soc Med.* 1968;61:1281–1282.

9. Cunningham L. Iniencephalus: a cause of dystocia. *J Obstet Gynaecol Br Cwlth.* 1965;72:299–303.

LISSENCEPHALY

Lissencephaly describes a developmental defect resulting in an absence of cerebral gyri. This condition often results from a deletion in the short arm of chromosome 17, or it may have an autosomal recessive etiology.[1,2]

Etiopathology
The gray matter of the cerebral cortex is formed by the prolongation of cells that migrate from the primitive neural tube. Lissencephaly is caused by the failure of these cells to migrate; therefore the gyri are not formed. Lissencephaly is associated with hydrocephaly, agenesis of the corpus callosum, and microcephaly.[3]

Sonoanatomy
There is almost complete absence of the cerebral gyri in lissencephaly, and the brain surface of the head appears smooth in the second half of gestation. The

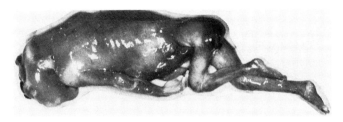

Figure 5–51. A 12-week anencephalic abortus.

thalami appear hypoplastic, and there is dilation of the lateral ventricles.[4,5]

Prenatal Diagnosis
The diagnosis may be made by the absence of cerebral gyri (Fig. 5–51). Effort should be made to identify the gyri in the second half of the pregnancy in all cases of microcephaly, hydrocephaly, and agenesis of the corpus callosum. This is best accomplished through transvaginal scanning. The thalami should also be carefully examined.

Management and Outcome
Although diagnosis of lissencephaly can be made prenatally, the diagnostic accuracy is unknown. Lissencephaly is associated with severe mental retardation and neurologic deficits of decerebration, including seizures, and spasticity. If the diagnosis is made before 24 weeks of pregnancy, termination should be offered. The clinician should discuss with the parents the possibility of nonintervention during the delivery, if the diagnosis is made late in pregnancy.

REFERENCES

1. Dobyns WB, Stratton RF, Parke JJ, et al. Miller–Diecker syndrome: lissencephaly and monosomy 17p. *J Pediatr.* 1983;102:552–558.
2. Dobyns WB, Kirkpatrick JB, Hittner, HM, et al. Syndromes with lissencephaly. *Am J Med Genet* 1984;18:509–526.
3. Dieker H, Edwards RH, Zurhein G, et al. The lissencephaly syndrome. *Birth Defects: Original Articles Series.* 1969;5:53–57.
4. Babcock DS. Sonographic demonstration of lissencephaly agyria. *J Ultrasound Med.* 1983;2:465–466.
5. Romero R, Pilu G, Jeanty P, et al. The central nervous system. In: Romero R, Pilu G, Jeanty P, et al. *Prenatal Diagnosis of Congenital Anomalies.* Norwalk, Conn: Appleton & Lange; 1988;70–71.

CRANIOSYNOSTOSIS

Craniosynostosis is characterized by early closure of the sutures of the skull. The incidence varies between 1 in 2,000 and 1 in 20,000 births.[1]

Etiopathology
Craniosynostosis is a feature of many heritable disorders, such as Crouzon syndrome or Apert syndrome. It can also result from a prenatal infection, for example, syphilis.[1]

Premature closure of the skull sutures results in alteration of the shape of the skull; this prohibits the normal growth of the brain mass. The result of this defect is brain dysfunction, visual impairment, and increased intracranial pressure.

Fibrous tissue can be found between the skull bones during normal intrauterine life. The possible mechanisms leading to craniosynostosis include hypoplasia of the fibrous tissue located between the skull bones, primary decrease in intracranial pressure, an abnormal ossification process, or obstruction in venous flow. The shape of the fetal head becomes dolichocephalic; the occipitofrontal diameter is dominant, or if brachycephalic, the biparietal diameter (BPD) is dominant.

Prenatal Diagnosis
Physiologic molding occurs during gestation and delivery, due to the fetal position. The calculated cephalic index is useful in the diagnosis of dolichocephaly or brachycephaly. The normal calculated cephalic index should be between 75 and 85%.

Dolichocephaly < 75%;   brachycephaly > 85%

Cephalic Index = BPD/OFD × 100 = 75 to 85%

If there is premature closure of the sagittal suture, the consequence is a larger OFD, with resulting dolichocephaly, or if there is early closure of the coronal suture, the result will be a larger BPD and resulting brachycephaly. This may give a cloverleaf skull type appearance; thanatophoric dysplasia should be ruled out. A smaller anterior fossa and hypertelorism will result from premature closure of the frontal suture. The prenatal diagnosis is easier in cases of a general closure of the head sutures.

Management and Outcome
The management should not be altered, since the outcome is generally good. The prognosis depends upon the severity of the defect and associated anomalies. Most infants do well, but cosmetic problems are reported. Ocular problems are associated with this anomaly, for example, exophthalmus, optic nerve at-

rophy, and effects due to an increase in intracranial pressure.[2]

REFERENCES

1. David DJ, Poswillo D, Simpson D. *The Craniosynostoses: Causes, Natural History and Management.* Berlin: Springer-Verlag, 1982.
2. Romero R, Pilu G, Jeanty P, et al. The central nervous system. In: Romero R, Pilu G, Jeanty P, et al. *Prenatal Diagnosis of Congenital Anomalies.* Norwalk, Conn: Appleton & Lange; 1988;1–79.

ACRANIA

Acrania is a complete or partial absence of the calvarium associated with an otherwise normal brain. The latter aspect distinguishes this anomaly from anencephaly in which the brain fails to develop completely.[1]

Sonoanatomy

The characteristic feature of acrania is the absence of the calvarium (Fig. 5–52). Differential diagnosis includes anencephaly and large encephalocele.[1,2]

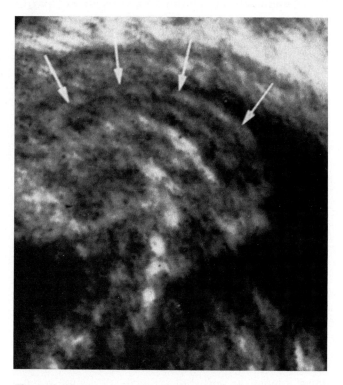

Figure 5–52. Transvaginal examination of a fetus at approximately 12 weeks' gestation with a diagnosis of acrania. In this figure, the brain tissue can be seen (arrows), but a calcified calvarium is absent.

Management and Outcome

This is a lethal abnormality; therefore termination of pregnancy or a nonaggressive approach is recommended.

REFERENCES

1. Mannes EJ, Crelin ES, Hobbins JC, et al. Sonographic demonstration of fetal acrania. *AJR.* 1982;139:181–182.
2. Romero R, Pilu G, Jeanty P, et al. The central nervous system. In: Romero R, Pilu G, Jeanty P, et al. *Prenatal Diagnosis of Congenital Anomalies.* Norwalk, Conn: Appleton & Lange; 1988;75–76.

CHOROID PLEXUS CYSTS

Choroid plexus cysts are believed to result from the accumulation of fluid and cellular debris in the folding neuroepithelium. These cysts have been observed in 0.6 to 2.3% of fetuses examined by ultrasound during the second trimester and are classified as bilateral in 67.6%, unilateral in 26.1%, and multiple in 6.3%.[1–3]

Prenatal Diagnosis

These choroid plexus cysts are fluid-filled structures of varying size that can be sonographically identified within the choroid plexus of the lateral ventricles and surrounded by normal tissue (Fig. 5–53). These cysts are round, with echodense margins. Papillomas of the

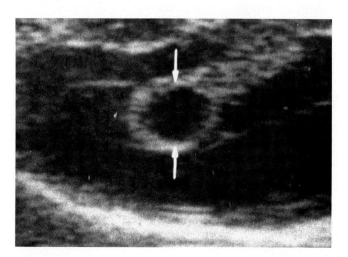

Figure 5–53. This is a saigttal scan of a fetus in the second trimester using transabdominal ultrasound. Both the medial and lateral walls along the ventricle can be seen in this plane, and the echodense structure of the choroid plexus is easily visualized within the lumen of the ventricle. An echolucent cystic structure within the substance of the choroid plexus is also readily observed (two arrows). The findings are consistent with choroid plexus cyst, without evidence of ventriculomegaly.

choroid plexus may also present in the same location, but a distinction can be made on the basis of the high hyperechogenicity of the solid papilloma. Most choroid plexus cysts are located within the atrium of the lateral ventricle, although some are located in the body of the lateral ventricle, giving the false impression of hydrocephaly.

Although the pediatric literature provides evidence that choroid plexus cysts may exist as asymptomatic findings in children, it appears that their detection in utero presents the risk of associated chromosomal anomalies (primarily trisomy 18), especially in the presence of other structural anomalies.[4-13] The overall incidence of chromosomal anomalies was 6.1% in a select referral group and 5.7% in a general population of patients.[14] Unfortunately, the incidence of aneuploidy associated with isolated choroid plexus cyst is unknown.

Management and Outcome

Once the choroid plexus cyst is identified, a complete and detailed sonographic survey of the fetal anatomy, including a fetal echocardiogram, should be undertaken. Chromosomal assessment should also be considered, especially in the presence of structural anomalies or persistence of the cyst, or in cases of large or multiple cysts.

REFERENCES

1. Benacerraf BR. Asymptomatic cysts of fetal choroid plexus in the second trimester. *J Ultrasound Med.* 1987; 6:475–478.
2. Chudleigh P, Pearce JM, Campbell S. The prenatal diagnosis of transient cysts of the fetal choroid plexus. *Prenat Diagn.* 1984;4:135–137.
3. Ostlere SJ, Irving HC, Lilfold RJ. Choroid plexus cysts in the fetus. *Lancet.* 1987;1:1491.
4. Ricketts NEM, Lowe EM, Patel NB. Prenatal diagnosis of choroid plexus cysts. *Lancet.* 1987;1:213–214.
5. Furness ME. Choroid plexus cysts and trisomy 18. *Lancet.* 1987;2:675–676.
6. Nicolaides KH, Rodeck CH, Gosden CM. Rapid karyotyping in non-lethal fetal malformations. *Lancet.* 1986; 1:283–287.
7. Baker GS, Gottlieb CM. Cyst of the choroid plexus of the lateral ventricle causing disabling headache unconsciousness: report of a case. *Mayo Clin Proc.* 1956;31:95–98.
8. De La Torre E, Alexander E, Courtland HD, et al. Tumors of the lateral ventricles of the brain. *J Neurosurg.* 1963;20:461–470.
9. Fakhry J, Schecter A, Tenner MS, et al. Cysts of the choroid plexus in neonate: documentation and review of the literature. *J Ultrasound Med.* 1985;4:561–563.
10. Benacerraf BR, Harlow B, Frigoletto FD. Are choroid plexus cysts an indication for second-trimester amniocentesis? *Am J Obstet Gynecol.* 1990;162:1001–1006.
11. Clark SL, DeVore GR, Sabey PL. Prenatal diagnosis of cysts of the fetal choroid plexus. *Obstet Gynecol.* 1988; 72:585–587.
12. Chitkara U, Cogswell C, Norton K, et al. Choroid plexus cysts in the fetus: a benign anatomic variant or pathologic entity?: report of 41 cases and review of the literature. *Obstet Gynecol.* 1988;72:185–189.
13. Fitzsimmons J, Wilson D, Mason JP, et al. Choroid plexus cysts in fetuses with trisomy 18. *Obstet Gynecol.* 1989; 73:257–260.
14. Gabrielli S, Reece EA, Pilu G, et al. The clinical significance of prenatally diagnosed choroid plexus cysts. *Am J Obstet Gynecol.* 1989;160:1207–1210.

CHOROID PLEXUS PAPILLOMA

The choroid plexus papilloma is an extremely rare intracranial neoplasm that accounts for 3% of all brain tumors in children. This tumor is usually unilateral and associated with hydrocephaly.[1]

Etiopathology

The choroid plexus is the main source of the cerebrospinal fluid (CSF) located in the ventricular system. A papilloma can occur in either the lateral, third, or fourth ventricles. The most common site of the choroid plexus papilloma, however, appears to be the atria of the lateral ventricles.[1] It appears to be unilateral in most cases, with only a few cases of bilateral choroid plexus papilloma reported.[2] This neoplasm can be either malignant or benign. Choroid plexus papilloma is associated with hydrocephaly. It can cause either the overproduction of cerebrospinal fluid, leading to communicating hydrocephalus, or obstruction to the flow of the cerebrospinal fluid, resulting in dilation of different portions of the ventricular system.[1,3-6]

Prenatal Diagnosis

Choroid plexus papilloma can mimic aqueductal stenosis, with the appearance of triventricular hydrocephalus, or it can appear as a tetraventricular hydrocephalus. These are the cases where the differential diagnosis seems to be difficult, and the echodense tumor needs to be demonstrated. The diagnosis of the choroid plexus papilloma appears easier in cases of unilateral hydrocephaly. The most significant parameters for the prenatal diagnosis are asymmetric size of the choroid plexus within the atria, appearance of the echodense tumor inside the choroid plexus, and hydrocephaly (Fig. 5–54).

Approximately 20% of choroid plexus papillomas

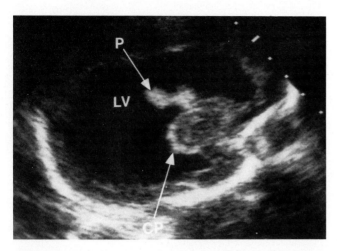

Fig. 5–54. Ultrasound exam of an early trimester fetus demonstrating hydrocephalus. Note the lateral ventricle (LV) that is massively dilated and the choroid plexus (P). In addition the echolucent structure is attached to the plexus, diagnostic of a choroid plexus papilloma being present and possibly causally related to the hydrocephalus.

become malignant. In benign cases, the operative outcome has shown good results. Mental retardation, however, is reported in 30% of the treated cases.[1]

Management and Outcome
There is no consensus on the optimum mode of delivery. Instrumental delivery, however, is contraindicated in cases of expanding hydrocephalus, since any trauma to the fetal head that may cause intracranial hemorrhage should be avoided.

REFERENCES

1. Matson DD, Crofton FDL. Papilloma of the choroid plexus in childhood. *J Neurosurg.* 1960;17:1002–1005.
2. Welch K, Strand R, Bresnan M, et al. Congenital hydrocephalus due to villous hypertrophy of the telencephalic choroid plexuses. *J Neurosurg.* 1983;59:172–175.
3. Eisenberg HM, McComb JG, Lorenzo AV. Cerebrospinal fluid overproduction and hydrocephalus associated with choroid plexus papilloma. *J Neurosurg.* 1974;40:381.
4. Turcotte JF, Copty M, Bedard F, et al. Lateral ventricle choroid plexus papilloma and communicating hydrocephalus. *Surg Neurol.* 1980;13:143–146.
5. Milhorat TH, Hammock MK, Davis DA, et al. Choroid plexus papilloma. *Child's Brain.* 1976;2:273–303.
6. Sahar A, Feinsod M, Beller AJ. Choroid plexus papilloma: cerebrospinal fluid dynamics. *Surg Neurol.* 1980;13:476–478.

6

The Fetal Face, Neck, and Thorax

Although sonographic examination of the fetal face, neck, and thorax is time-consuming, it can provide crucial diagnostic information. Structural abnormalities of the face, neck, and thorax are often seen in association with chromosomal aberrations and can provide the impetus for further genetic analysis. This chapter describes normal structural development and the sonographic approach to and evaluation of the fetal face, neck, and thorax. Clinical applications are discussed in relation to perinatal management.

The Fetal Face

INTRODUCTION

During the early stages of embryogenesis, genetic factors play the predominant role in development of the fetal face. In later stages, environmental influences increase in importance. Therefore, facial malformations may be the result of chromosomal aberrations as well as teratogenic factors.

Detailed ultrasonographic evaluation of the fetal face is useful in detecting the majority of facial anomalies. The fetal face can be visualized with ultrasound as early as late in the first trimester. Sagittal planes of the fetal face are the most useful in assessing the facial profile, including the forehead, nose, and jaw (Fig. 6–1). The ears can be visualized easily with this view, and can be recognized in greater detail (Fig. 6–2) as pregnancy advances. Next, a cross-sectional image of the fetal face should be completed to assess the integrity of the nose and lips (Figs. 6–3, 6–4 and 6–5). Mayden et al[1] recommended axial scans to measure the orbital diameters and to examine the upper lip and the anterior palate. If the examination is not completed successfully, the patient should be scheduled for a second evaluation.

In the coronal planes, one can visualize movements of the mouth, including protrusion of the tongue, "chewing" movements, and wide opening of the mouth (Fig. 6–6). The lens, iris, pupil, cornea, and extraocular structures, such as muscles, retro-orbital fat, and optic nerve also can be identified in this plane (Fig. 6–7).

Both orbits can be visualized using an axial scan slightly caudad to the one commonly used to determine the biparietal diameter. This view allows determination of the ocular biometry.[2,3] Nomograms of orbital diameters (Table 6–1) are available and can be used to date a pregnancy. By moving the transducer caudally, the anterior palate can be visualized, and a slight angulation permits visualization of the tongue within the oral cavity.

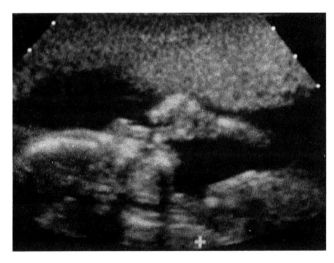

Figure 6–1. Profile of a fetus in the second trimester viewed by transabdominal ultrasonography. In this scan, a clear view of the fetal profile can be observed. The thumb is inserted directly into the fetal mouth.

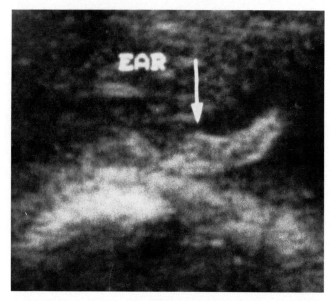

Figure 6–2. Second-trimester transabdominal ultrasound imaging of the fetal ear, which can be seen extending laterally from the fetal head (the "ear" is indicated by an arrow).

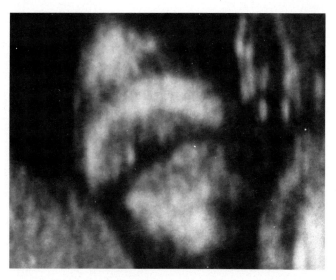

Figure 6–4. Second-trimester transabdominal ultrasound of the fetus demonstrating facial areas of the mouth and nose. The scan is taken in an inferior–superior plane and demonstrates the chin; the border of the lower lip; the semicircular, echodense, and intact upper lip; as well as the nose and nostrils.

ACCURACY OF ULTRASOUND DIAGNOSIS

Pilu et al[4] performed sonographic examinations between 18 and 40 weeks' gestation on 223 patients at risk for delivering fetuses with craniofacial malformations. The risk factors included a familial history of craniofacial malformations, extrafacial anomalies di-

agnosed on ultrasound, fetal chromosomal aberrations, and maternal drug intake (Table 6–2). Sonographic visualization of the face was possible in 151 of the patients (67.7%) on the first scan and in another 47 patients (21.1%) on the second scan; visualization was not possible in 25 patients (11.2%). Craniofacial malformations were detected in 14 (Table 6–3) of the 198 cases visualized antenatally, and all were confirmed

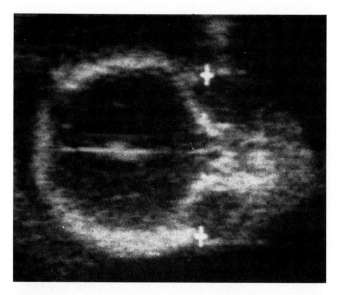

Figure 6–3. Sagittal scan of a fetus in the second trimester using transabdominal ultrasound. This is an oblique view showing both the head and portions of the fetal face; note the midline echoes in the head dividing the two cerebral hemispheres. The two orbits are clearly visualized with calipers (+'s) at either border demonstrating the method for measuring the outer orbital distances. The nasal area can be easily seen between the orbits.

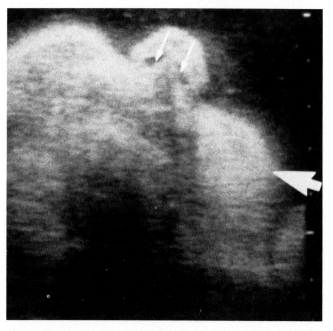

Figure 6–5. Transabdominal ultrasound of a fetus in the third trimester showing the nose, the nostrils (two small arrows) as well as the well-developed cheeks bilaterally (large arrowheads).

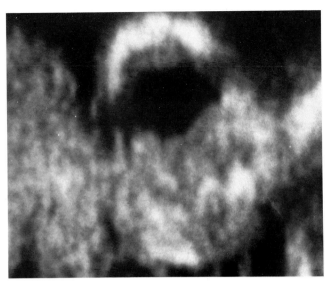

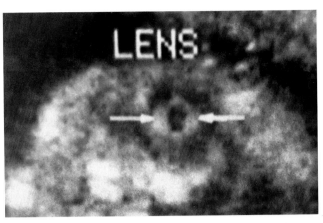

Figure 6–7. Transvaginal ultrasound in the early second trimester demonstrating a fetal orbit and the lens inside this orbit demarcated by two arrows.

Figure 6–6. Transabdominal scan of a second-trimester fetus in an oblique plane going inferior to superior. The open mouth shows the intact upper lip clearly defined as an echodense semicircle. The lower jaw and lip are less well defined.

TABLE 6–1. PREDICTED BIPARIETAL DIAMETER AND WEEKS' GESTATION FROM THE INNER AND OUTER ORBITAL DIAMETERS

Biparietal Diameter (cm)	Weeks' Gestation	Inner Orbital Diameter (cm)	Outer Orbital Diameter (cm)	Biparietal Diameter (cm)	Weeks' Gestation	Inner Orbital Diameter (cm)	Outer Orbital Diameter (cm)
1.9	11.6	0.5	1.3	5.8	24.3	1.6	4.1
2.0	11.6	0.5	1.4	5.9	24.3	1.6	4.2
2.1	12.1	0.6	1.5	6.0	24.7	1.6	4.3
2.2	12.6	0.6	1.6	6.1	25.2	1.6	4.3
2.3	12.6	0.6	1.7	6.2	25.2	1.6	4.4
2.4	13.1	0.7	1.7	6.3	25.7	1.7	4.4
2.5	13.6	0.7	1.8	6.4	26.2	1.7	4.5
2.6	13.6	0.7	1.9	6.5	26.2	1.7	4.5
2.7	14.1	0.8	2.0	6.6	26.7	1.7	4.6
2.8	14.6	0.8	2.1	6.7	27.2	1.7	4.6
2.9	14.6	0.8	2.1	6.8	27.6	1.7	4.7
3.0	15.0	0.9	2.2	6.9	28.1	1.7	4.7
3.1	15.5	0.9	2.3	7.0	28.6	1.8	4.8
3.2	15.5	0.9	2.4	7.1	29.1	1.8	4.8
3.3	16.0	1.0	2.5	7.3	29.6	1.8	4.9
3.4	16.5	1.0	2.5	7.4	30.0	1.8	5.0
3.5	16.5	1.0	2.6	7.5	30.6	1.8	5.0
3.6	17.0	1.0	2.7	7.6	31.0	1.8	5.1
3.7	17.5	1.1	2.7	7.7	31.5	1.8	5.1
3.8	17.9	1.1	2.8	7.8	32.0	1.8	5.2
4.0	18.4	1.2	3.0	7.9	32.5	1.9	5.2
4.2	18.9	1.2	3.1	8.0	33.0	1.9	5.3
4.3	19.4	1.2	3.2	8.2	33.5	1.9	5.4
4.4	19.4	1.3	3.2	8.3	34.0	1.9	5.4
4.5	19.9	1.3	3.3	8.4	34.4	1.9	5.4
4.6	20.4	1.3	3.4	8.5	35.0	1.9	5.5
4.7	20.4	1.3	3.4	8.6	35.4	1.9	5.5
4.8	20.9	1.4	3.5	8.8	35.9	1.9	5.6
4.9	21.3	1.4	3.6	8.9	36.4	1.9	5.6
5.0	21.3	1.4	3.6	9.0	36.9	1.9	5.7
5.1	21.8	1.4	3.7	9.1	37.3	1.9	5.7
5.2	22.3	1.4	3.8	9.2	37.8	1.9	5.8
5.3	22.3	1.5	3.8	9.3	38.3	1.9	5.8
5.4	22.8	1.5	3.9	9.4	38.8	1.9	5.8
5.5	23.3	1.5	4.0	9.6	39.3	1.9	5.8
5.6	23.3	1.5	4.0	9.7	39.8	1.9	5.9
5.7	23.8	1.5	4.1			1.9	5.9

Modified with permission from Mayden KL, Tortora M, Berkowitz RL, et al. Orbital diameters: a new parameter for prenatal diagnosis and dating. Am J Obstet Gynecol. 1982;144:289–297.

TABLE 6–2. INDICATIONS FOR ULTRASOUND EXAMINATION OF THE FETAL FACE

Indication	n	%
Other fetal anomalies detected by ultrasound	118	52.9
Familial history of craniofacial malformations	72	32.3
Maternal drug intake	25	11.2
Fetal chromosomal aberrations	8	3.6
TOTAL	223	

Reprinted with permission from Pilu G, Reece EA, Romero R, et al. Prenatal diagnosis of cranio-facial malformations with ultrasonography. Am J Obstet Gynecol. 1986;155:45–49.

postnatally. No false-positive diagnoses were made. Anomalies diagnosed sonographically included anopthalmia; anterior cleft lip (Fig. 6–8), cleft palate, or both, hypotelorism, and micrognathia. A negative diagnosis of craniofacial malformation was made in 184 cases with two false-negative results (1.0%). The fetal posterior palate is difficult to visualize sonographically because of the acoustic shadowing that arises from the surrounding bony structures; thus, defects in this area will generally escape identification. The results of the study by Pilu et al demonstrate that ultrasound is an accurate and reliable tool

for the prenatal diagnosis of craniofacial malformations.

Micrognathia was demonstrated in two fetuses in the series reported by Pilu et al[4] at 29 and 35 weeks of gestation. Because ultrasound performed in the second trimester in the latter case had revealed a seemingly normal jaw, some cases of micrognathia may evolve during the course of gestation, making an early diagnosis impossible.

Craniofacial malformations may be one feature of a number of syndromes with multisystemic involvement, and their recognition may have important clinical relevance. A classic example is represented by the holoprosencephalic malformations in which anomalies of the brain and face are closely correlated.[5] The list of congenital syndromes that may be suspected or recognized by the detection of a craniofacial malformation is extensive. Gorlin and coworkers,[6] completed an indepth review of the subject and identified approximately 150 syndromes involving craniofacial malformations with clinical implications.

Polyhydramnios has been reported to occur in 61.1% of cases of craniofacial malformations.[4] Increased amniotic fluid is often associated with severe cerebral anomalies, such as anencephaly or holo-

TABLE 6–3. CRANIOFACIAL MALFORMATIONS DIAGNOSED BY ULTRASONOGRAPHY

Case Number	Indication	Sonographic Findings	Weeks' Gestation	Postnatal Findings
1–7	Fetal holoprosencephaly	Hypotelorism Median cleft lip and palate Absent nasal bridge	22–30	Holoprosencephaly Median cleft lip and palate Absent nasal bridge
8	Fetal holoprosencephaly	Anophthalmia Median cleft lip and palate Absent nasal bridge	29	Holoprosencephaly Anophthalmia Median cleft lip and palate Absent nasal bridge
9	Fetal holoprosencephaly	Hypotelorism Proboscis	30	Holoprosencephaly Hypotelorism Proboscis (cebocephaly)
10*	History of Robin anomalad	Micrognathia	35	Micrognathia Posterior cleft palate (Robin anomalad)
11	Anencephaly	Micrognathia	29	Anencephaly Micrognathia
12†	Hydrocephalus	Hypotelorism Median cleft lip	31	Hydrocephalus Hypotelorism Median cleft lip (median cleft face)
13	Fetal holoprosencephaly	Hypotelorism	28	Holoprosencephaly Hypertelorism Median cleft lip and palate
14	Microcephaly	Micrognathia	33	Microcephaly Micrognathia 47,XY + 13

* Previously reported (see reference 6).
† Previously reported (see reference 12).
Reprinted with permission from Pilu G, Reece EA, Romero R, et al. Prenatal diagnosis of cranio-facial malformations with ultrasonography. Am J Obstet Gynecol. 1986;155:45–49.

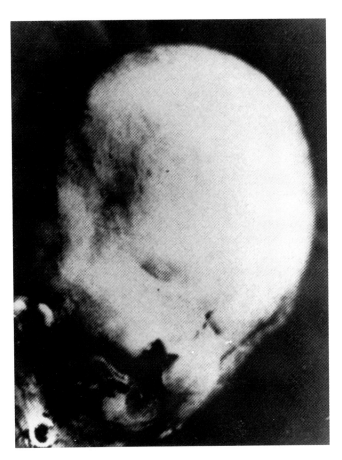

Figure 6–8. Second-trimester fetus viewed by transabdominal ultrasound. The scan is done in a direct on-face view and demonstrates the lower lip and the clefted upper lip, indicated by the small arrow. Directly above is the nasal area; the orbits can be seen on either side. Because this view is slightly oblique, the right orbit is better defined than the left.

prosencephaly, possibly because of a lack of fetal swallowing. In 17.6% of cases, however, no other anomalies were present. Because both micrognathia and cleft palate can interfere with fetal swallowing, we recommend including ultrasound examination of the fetal face as part of the clinical evaluation of pregnancies complicated by polyhydramnios.

PERINATAL OUTCOME AND MANAGEMENT

Craniofacial malformations can be identified as early as the second trimester of pregnancy. Many malformations, such as cleft lip and palate, can be treated postnatally with good cosmetic results. Although prenatal diagnosis will not alter obstetric management in such cases, it removes the "surprise factor," thereby allowing parents to prepare psychologically for the birth of a child with a craniofacial malformation. In more extreme cases, such as Robin's anomalad, where

a craniofacial malformation may jeopardize the newborn infant, a planned delivery with immediate neonatal assistance can be lifesaving.[7]

The Fetal Neck

INTRODUCTION

The intrauterine environment as well as congenital malformations can affect the prenatal development of the thorax and lungs. Recently, the use of high-resolution ultrasonography has improved our ability to visualize structures within the thorax and identify intrathoracic anomalies. A comprehensive sonographic examination of the fetal thorax should include identification of the position of the heart in the chest, the four-chamber view of the heart, and fetal lung growth. This section discusses the embryogenesis of normal lung development and the sonographic approach to the diagnosis of thoracic abnormalities.

SONOGRAPHIC APPROACH

Hata et al[8] studied the normal fetal neck via ultrasonography and found a linear relationship between fetal neck circumference and gestational age (Table 6–4). To measure neck circumference, they first assessed the fetal lie, then rotated the transducer into a cross-sectional plane. The fetal neck was then measured from outer-to-outer margins.

Sonographic evaluation and biometric measurement of the fetal neck can be useful in cases such as maternal diabetes, in which excess fetal adipose tissue may be deposited. There also have been reports of fetal neck masses (Table 6–5) that extrinsically obstruct the esophagus. These masses can be identified or diagnosed by careful examination of the fetal neck using ultrasonography.

TUMORS OF THE HEAD AND NECK

Cystic Hygroma

Etiopathology
Cystic hygroma, the most frequent fetal tumor of the head and neck, is found in 1 in 200 spontaneous abortuses.[9] These cysts present as sacs with or without

TABLE 6–4. ULTRASONOGRAPHIC MEASUREMENTS OF THE FETAL NECK CORRELATED WITH GESTATIONAL AGE

Gestational Age (Weeks)	Circumference of the Fetal Neck (mm) Percentile		
	5th	50th	95th
16	63	66	68
17	62	77	93
18	68	82	96
19	78	88	98
20	85	92	99
21	76	93	110
22	78	97	117
23	85	109	133
24	106	113	120
25	96	116	136
26	117	122	126
27	116	123	129
28	101	120	138
29	116	127	139
30	118	125	132
31	134	139	145
32	110	130	151
33	117	137	158
34	116	140	165
35	125	145	164
36	128	151	174
37	140	153	165
38	123	155	187
39	142	157	171
40	147	157	167

Reprinted with permission from Hata K, Hata T, et al. Ultrasonographic measurements of the neck correlated with gestational age. J Ultrasound Med. 1988;7:333–337.

multiple septations.[10] The lesions are the result of abnormalities of the lymphatic system in which the jugular lymphatic sacs fail to drain into the internal jugular vein, resulting in dilated lymphatic channels and a cystic appearance on ultrasound.

The lymphatic system is a complex network of thin-walled vessels that return tissue fluid to the jugular lymphatic sac, which in turn empties into the jugular vein. This system is established as early as the sixth week of gestation. Obstruction of these channels alters the development of the vessel systems, thereby causing dilation of the lymphatic channels with

TABLE 6–5. PRENATAL ULTRASOUND DIAGNOSIS OF FETAL TUMORS

Head and Neck Tumors
Cystic hygroma
Epignathus
Goiter
Hemangioma
Neuroblastoma
Proboscis
Thyroid teratoma

Modified with permission from Kurjak A, Zalud I, Jurkovic D, et al. Ultrasound diagnosis and evaluation of fetal tumors. J Perinat Med. 1989;17:173–193.

backup of tissue fluid.[10–12] When this obstructive process occurs at the level of the jugular lymphatic, it causes dilation of these vessels and leads to the characteristic cystic hygroma.[13] Chervenak and coworkers[13] suggested that more severe forms of obstruction with failure in communication can lead to progressive and severe lymphedema, nonimmune hydrops, or both. They also suggested that resorption of this fluid, or possibly the use of alternative channels for fluid drainage, sometimes results in the resolution of cystic hygromas.

Ultrasound Diagnosis

Prenatal diagnosis of cystic hygromas is not particularly difficult. Cystic hygromas have been successfully diagnosed prenatally as early as the first trimester of pregnancy and reported in the literature (Fig. 6–9 and Fig. 6–10).[11] Cystic hygromas are easily identified by the distorted appearance of the fetal neck. They are characterized by pericervical cystic structures located in the posterior-lateral area, some with septations, others without. The size of these lesions is variable; some may be small and confined to the neck region, whereas others may extend down to the back, trunk, or even pelvic area (Fig. 6–11). Most cystic hygromas are associated with fetal hydrops.

Because cystic hygroma is often associated with a number of other structural and chromosomal abnormalities, it is important to carry out a careful anatomic survey of the entire fetal anatomy when this diagnosis is suspected. Renal abnormalities, cardiac anomalies, single umbilical artery, and adrenal masses should be ruled out. Because this lesion is associated with Turner

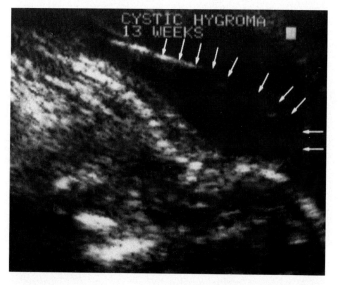

Figure 6–9. Transvaginal ultrasound examination of a fetus at 13 weeks' gestation demonstrating an echolucent cystic structure that extends from the level of the fetal head toward the thorax (small arrows). These findings are consistent with a cystic hygroma.

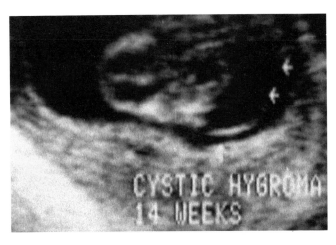

Figure 6–10. Transvaginal ultrasound of a fetus at 14 weeks' gestation demonstrating the echolucent cystic structure posterior to the fetal head. These findings are consistent with a cystic hygroma.

syndrome in about half the cases, fetal karyotyping also is recommended. In addition, other chromosomal abnormalities, such as trisomy 13, 18, and 21, have been reported.[9]

The differential diagnosis includes other cervical abnormalities, such as cephalocele, cystic teratoma of the neck, or cephalomeningocele. Cystic hygroma presents as an echolucent, fluid-filled, posterolateral sac originating in the pericervical area. Conversely, encephalocele, cystic teratoma, and cephalomeningocele all contain areas of echodensity consistent with herniation of brain tissue or neural elements.

Perinatal Outcome and Management
Obstetric management will vary, largely on the basis of karyotypic and sonographic findings. For example, if the diagnosis of cystic hygroma is made in the first trimester and if karyotypic analysis reveals trisomy 18, termination of the pregnancy can be offered to the patient. Similarly, if the diagnosis is made later in gestation, but before 24 weeks, and multiple congenital malformations or nonimmune hydrops are present, termination of the pregnancy may also be considered. Cystic hygroma with the presence of hydrops occurs in 50% to 90% of cases and is associated with a mortality rate of almost 100% (Fig. 6–12).[10,13] In approximately 25% of cases, neither a major congenital malformation nor nonimmune hydrops will be present, and the karyotype will be normal; these patients should be followed expectantly with serial ultrasound examinations.

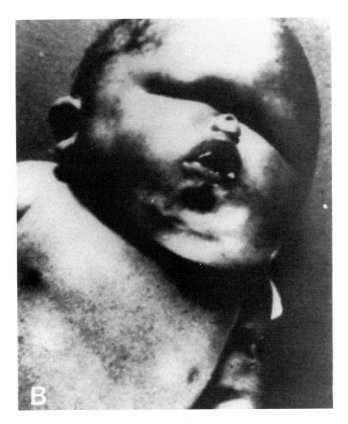

Figure 6–11. Second-trimester fetus examined by transabdominal ultrasonography revealing formation of edema of the skin over the thorax and the face as well as the scalp. In addition, pericardial effusion, best seen in the anterior border of the chest, as well as pleural effusion, best seen in the inferior and somewhat posterior aspect of the fetal heart, can be observed.

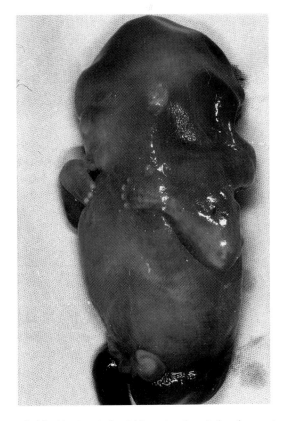

Figure 6–12. Abortus at about 14 weeks of gestation demonstrating a large multilocular cystic hygroma that extends from the neck down to the thoracic area and involves the scalp and facial areas as well.

Patients should be told that cystic hygromas can reabsorb spontaneously. If reabsorption does occur, they can expect a favorable neonatal outcome, although cosmetic surgery may be necessary postnatally.

Fetal Goiter

Etiopathology

Fetal goiter, enlargement of the thyroid gland, presents as a solid neck mass with some echolucent areas as observed by ultrasound. The most common cause is maternal ingestion of iodine preparations.[14] However, fetal goiter may also be the result of such maternal diseases as Grave's disease or the treatment of hyperthyroidism with iodine or, rarely, with propylthiouracil. In cases involving maternal Grave's disease, there is transplacental passage of a thyroid-stimulating substance, IgG immunoglobulin, which crosses the placenta and can cause hyperthyroidism of the fetus as well.

Fetal goiters resulting from maternal hypothyroidism may be the result of the mother's treatment, a deficiency of iodine, or a congenital metabolic disorder of thyroid synthesis. Congenital hypothyroidism, however, is rare.[15] Carswell and coworkers[14] reported the association of congenital hypothyroidism with maternal ingestion of as little as 12 mg per day of iodine preparations. It is therefore recommended that the physician should tailor the treatment to the mother's symptoms rather than attempt to achieve the nonpregnant, normal levels of thyroid hormones.

Ultrasound Diagnosis

The antenatal diagnosis of fetal goiter may be difficult and is based solely on the identification of a mass in the neck region that causes hyperextension of the fetal head (Fig. 6–13, Fig. 6–14, and Fig. 6–15). Few prenatal diagnoses of fetal goiter have been reported.[16,17] This mass may be solid, yet have a fairly homogeneous and echolucent consistency.[16,17] The mass may become so large that it actually precludes normal vaginal delivery because of the hyperextension of the fetal head.

When the mass compresses the fetal esophagus, polyhydramnios may result. Differential diagnosis of a neck mass in the fetus includes hemangiomas, cystic hygromas, teratomas, and bronchial cleft cysts. The accuracy of prenatal diagnosis is enhanced by the size of the lesion, its homogeneity, and the clinical setting.

Perinatal Outcome and Management

Medical management of the fetal goiter largely depends on its cause. Fetal goiter resulting from aggressive maternal therapy with propylthiouracil is best managed by significantly reducing the dose. Discon-

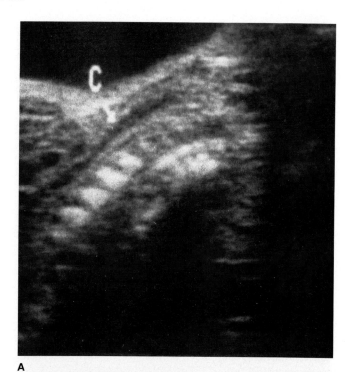

A

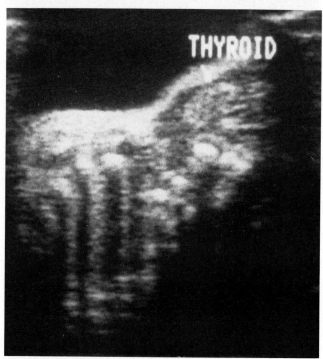

B

Figure 6–13. (A) Second-trimester transabdominal examination of a fetus depicting the fetal neck with the vertebral bodies shown as interrupted echodense nodular structures in the midline. Anteriorly is a narrow echolucent line (small arrow) representing the great vessel in the fetal neck (C). **(B)** This panel represents a fetus at approximately the same gestational age. The fetal chest and ribs are depicted by echolucent lines perpendicular to the horizontal and the fetal neck beyond the chest and to the right. In the neck, an enlarged thyroid gland and thyroid lobules can be clearly seen. These findings are diagnostic of fetal goiter. Such fetuses usually have a hyperextended head.

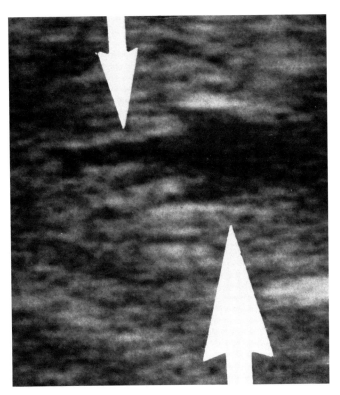

Figure 6–14. Ultrasound examination of the neck of a second-trimester fetus. In this scan, the upper arrow depicts the trachea, and the lower arrow depicts the laryngeal area.

tinuation of the drug is recommended for patients taking iodine. The fetal prognosis depends on the cause of the fetal goiter. Hypothyroidism diagnosed at birth requires aggressive supplemental treatment to prevent severe mental retardation.

If the goiter is large enough to cause hyperextension of the head, cesarean section is the optimum mode of delivery. On the other hand, if the mass is small and the head is not hyperextended, vaginal delivery can be attempted.

Other Neck Tumors

Other neck tumors include neuroblast of the neck with nodules within or on the surfaces of most of the abdominal organs and the heart. Hemangiomas and teratomas of the neck also can appear as a mixture of solid and cystic components. Like fetal goiter, these neck masses can compress the esophagus and, when extremely large, can lead to polyhydramnios.

The Fetal Thorax

INTRODUCTION

The American Institute of Ultrasound in Medicine recommends performance and documentation of a fetal cervical spine evaluation during the second and third trimesters of pregnancy. Because the majority of neck abnormalities will create a mass effect that distorts the normal anatomy and contours of the neck, such abnormalities are often associated with polyhydramnios. The location and characteristics of the mass, coupled with associated findings and a pertinent family history, are used for antenatal detection of neck abnormalities. Furthermore, if a neck mass is present, the sonographer should examine the fetus in detail because such masses are frequently seen in association with chromosomal abnormalities.

DEVELOPMENT OF THE LUNGS AND RESPIRATORY TRACT

The lung bud develops at the caudal end of the laryngotracheal tube and soon divides into two knoblike bronchial buds. In turn, each bronchial bud enlarges to form a primitive primary bronchus by the beginning of the fifth gestational week. The primary bronchi subdivide into secondary bronchi, and the latter continue to subdivide during the fifth week. Tertiary bronchi begin to form by the 7th week, and the respiratory bronchioles are present by the 24th week.

Lung development is divided into four stages: pseudoglandular, canalicular, terminal sac, and alveolar. The pseudoglandular period extends from the 5th to 17th week. During this period, the developing lung resembles a gland because the bronchial divisions are differentiating into the air-conducting system. All major elements of the lung have formed by the 17th week except those involved with gas exchange functions. Therefore, respiration is not possible during this time.

The canalicular period extends from the 16th to 25th week. This period overlaps the pseudoglandular period because cranial segments of the lungs mature faster than the caudal ones. During this period, the bronchi and bronchioles enlarge and the lung tissue becomes highly vascular. By 24 weeks, each terminal bronchiole has given rise to two or more respiratory bronchioles. Respiration is possible toward the end of this period because some thin-walled saccules called terminal sacs (primitive alveoli) have developed at the ends of the respiratory bronchioles and because these regions are well vascularized.

The terminal sac period lasts from the 24th week to birth. During this period, large numbers of terminal sacs develop, and the epithelium of the terminal sacs thins. Epithelial cells known as type I alveolar epithelial cells line the terminal sacs, and the capillaries begin to bulge into the sacs. By the 25th to 28th week of gestation, sufficient terminal sacs are present to permit survival of a prematurely born infant. Before this, the lungs are usually incapable of providing adequate gas exchange because the alveolar surface area is insufficient and the vasculature is underdeveloped.

The alveolar period begins in the late fetal period and ends in about the eighth year. Before birth, the immature alveoli appear as small bundles from the walls of the terminal sacs and the respiratory bronchioles.[18]

Development of the bronchial tree begins on about the 26th day after conception with the formation of the laryngotracheal groove. After the tracheoesophageal folds fuse, at about 16 weeks, the laryngotracheal bud is separated from the foregut. At the end of the pseudoglandular period, all the nonrespiratory airways exist to the level of the terminal bronchioles and are lined by thick columnar or cuboidal cells. At about 24 weeks, during the canalicular period, branching and differentiation of the respiratory airway begins. The epithelium is interrupted by ingrowth of capillaries. Progressive branching and differentiation of the respiratory airways occurs during the alveolar phase at about 32 weeks of gestation. Any alteration in the aforementioned sequence of events may result in a variety of malformations.

SONOGRAPHIC APPROACH

The circumference of the thorax is obtained after determining the position of the fetus. The fetal spine is visualized, and the transducer is then rotated until a cross-sectional view of the fetal thorax at the level of the four chambers of the heart is seen. A thoracic circumference measurement is then obtained either by direct measurement using electronic calipers along the perimeter of the view or by computation with the following formula:

$$\text{Thoracic circumference} = (T1 + T2) \times 1.57,$$

where T1 is the anteroposterior diameter of the fetal thorax and T2 is the maximum transverse diameter of the fetal thorax in a plane at a right angle to T1 (Tables 6–6 and 6–7).

Thoracic circumference/abdominal circumference, thoracic circumference/head circumference, thoracic circumference/humerus length, and thoracic circumference/femur length have been described as having a linear relationship with the thoracic circumference, the thoracic ratios, and gestational age be-

TABLE 6–6. EMBRYONIC TRUNK CIRCUMFERENCE AND ESTIMATION OF GESTATIONAL AGE

Trunk Circumference (mm)	Gestational Age ± 2 SD* (wk)
10	7.72 ± 0.5
12	7.99 ± 0.4
15	8.39 ± 0.3
17	8.64 ± 0.3
20	8.99 ± 0.2
22	9.22 ± 0.2
25	9.55 ± 0.2
27	9.75 ± 0.2
30	10.05 ± 0.2
32	10.23 ± 0.2
35	10.49 ± 0.2
37	10.65 ± 0.2
40	10.88 ± 0.2
42	11.02 ± 0.2
45	11.22 ± 0.2
47	11.33 ± 0.2
50	11.50 ± 0.2
55	11.72 ± 0.3
60	11.89 ± 0.5
65	12.01 ± 0.7
70	12.07 ± 0.9

* Overall, 2 SD = ± 3 days
Reproduced with permission from Reece EA, Scioscia AL, Green J, et al. Embryonic trunk circumference: a new biometric parameter for estimation of gestational age. Am J Obstet Gynecol. 1987;156:715.

tween 16 and 40 weeks' gestation (0.907 cm/week) (Table 6–8).[19]

A number of investigators have studied the ability of ultrasonographically derived chest circumference measurements to predict the existence of pulmonary hypoplasia (Figure 6–15).[20,21] Adequate fetal lung growth depends on a number of conditions. The necessary physical factors include adequate intrathoracic space, adequate intrauterine space, a sufficient amount of amniotic fluid, normal fetal breathing movements, and a normal balance of fluid volume and pressure within the trachea and potential airspaces.[22]

TABLE 6–8. MEAN VALUES WITH STANDARD DEVIATIONS FOR VARIOUS THORACIC RATIOS (N = 543)

Ratio	Mean Predictive Value	SD
Thoracic circumference: abdominal circumference*	0.89	0.06
Thoracic circumference: head circumference*	0.80	0.12
Thoracic circumference: humerus length	4.31	0.36
Thoracic circumference: femur length	4.03	0.33
Thoracic length: thoracic circumference	0.22	0.03
Thoracic length: humerus length*	0.93	0.13
Thoracic length: femur length	0.87	0.13

* Ratios did not vary significantly with gestational age
Reproduced with permission from Chitkara U, Rosenberg J, Chervenak FA, et al. Am J Obstet Gynecol. 1987,156:1069

TABLE 6–7. FETAL THORACIC CIRCUMFERENCE MEASUREMENTS*

Gestational Age (wk)	No.	Predictive Percentiles								
		2.5	5	10	25	50	75	90	95	97.5
16	6	5.9	6.4	7.0	8.0	9.1	10.3	11.3	11.9	12.4
17	22	6.8	7.3	7.9	8.9	10.0	11.2	12.2	12.8	13.3
18	31	7.7	8.2	8.8	9.8	11.0	12.1	13.1	13.7	14.2
19	21	8.6	9.1	9.7	10.7	11.9	13.0	14.0	14.6	15.1
20	20	9.5	10.0	10.6	11.7	12.8	13.9	15.0	15.5	16.0
21	30	10.4	11.0	11.6	12.6	13.7	14.8	15.8	16.4	16.9
22	18	11.3	11.9	12.5	13.5	14.6	15.7	16.7	17.3	17.8
23	21	12.2	12.8	13.4	14.4	15.5	16.6	17.6	18.2	18.8
24	27	13.2	13.7	14.3	15.3	16.4	17.5	18.5	19.1	19.7
25	20	14.1	14.6	15.2	16.2	17.3	18.4	19.4	20.0	20.6
26	25	15.0	15.5	16.1	17.1	18.2	19.3	20.3	21.0	21.5
27	24	15.9	16.4	17.0	18.0	19.1	20.2	21.3	21.9	22.4
28	24	16.8	17.3	17.9	18.9	20.0	21.2	22.2	22.8	23.3
29	24	17.7	18.2	18.8	19.8	21.0	22.1	23.1	23.7	24.2
30	27	18.6	19.1	19.7	20.7	21.9	23.0	24.0	24.6	25.1
31	24	19.5	20.0	20.6	21.6	22.8	23.9	24.9	25.5	26.0
32	28	20.4	20.9	21.5	22.6	23.7	24.8	25.8	26.4	26.9
33	27	21.3	21.8	22.5	23.5	24.6	25.7	26.7	27.3	27.8
34	25	22.2	22.8	23.4	24.4	25.5	26.6	27.6	28.2	28.7
35	20	23.1	23.7	24.3	25.3	26.4	27.5	28.5	29.1	29.6
36	23	24.0	24.6	25.2	26.2	27.3	28.4	29.4	30.0	30.6
37	22	24.9	25.5	26.1	27.1	28.2	29.3	30.3	30.9	31.5
38	21	25.9	26.4	27.0	28.0	29.1	30.2	31.2	31.9	32.4
39	7	26.8	27.3	27.9	28.9	30.0	31.1	32.2	32.8	33.3
40	6	27.7	28.2	28.8	29.8	30.9	32.1	33.1	33.7	34.2

* Measurements in centimeters.
Reproduced with permission from Chitkara U, Rosenberg J, Chervenak FA, et al. Am J Obstet Gynecol. *1987,156:1069*

The major space-occupying components of the intrathoracic space are the lung and the heart. Because the lungs fill almost the entire chest cavity, a decrease in lung mass secondary to pulmonary hypoplasia should be reflected by a decrease in the dimensions of the chest. When Nimrod and colleagues[20] compared their predictions of lung hypoplasia antenatally using sonographically determined chest circumference measurements with fetal outcomes and autopsy findings, their results demonstrated high sensitivity and speci-

ficity. This has led to the application of chest circumference measurements to cases of prolonged premature rupture of the membranes and oligohydramnios. Others have advocated the use of the ultrasonic ratio of fetal thoracic circumference to abdominal circumference as a better predictor of lung hypoplasia.[23]

In fact, Nimrod and colleagues[20] reported that 16 of 17 fetuses with chest circumference measurements below the fifth percentile for gestational age developed pulmonary hypoplasia; 15 of the 16 fetuses had

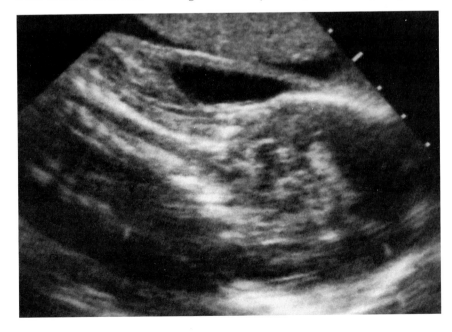

Figure 6–15. Second-trimester ultrasound examination of the fetal chest via transabdominal ultrasonography depicting a narrow chest and splaying of the articulations of the ribs as the chest forms a conical shape. In this case, there is severe oligohydramnios in the pregnancy with a diagnosis of renal agenesis. During real-time ultrasound examination, the heart is seen to involve almost the entire chest cavity.

a lethal form of the disease. In any event, the chest circumference, either alone or in combination with the abdominal circumference, clearly provides information that can be useful for determining lung development.

MALFORMATIONS OF THE THORAX

Congenital Chylothorax

Etiopathology

Chylothorax, the accumulation of chyle within the pleural cavity, is the most commonly encountered form of thoracic effusion seen in the prenatal period.[24-26] The chyle is clear, with abundant lymphocytes of about 60%.[24-26] The incidence of this disorder is 1 in 10,000, and males are affected twice as often as females.[23] Approximately 60% of effusions appear on the right, but fluid occasionally collects bilaterally.[24,27-30]

Although the etiology of chylothorax is unknown, some authors have postulated that the cause may be rupture or failed fusion of the thoracic lymphatic channels.[25,28,29] Chylothorax has also been reported in association with monosomy X, trisomy 21, and possible X-linked inheritance.[31]

Ultrasound Diagnosis

The most common sonographic findings include unilateral effusion; less common is bilateral effusion, with or without collapsed lungs (Fig. 6–16).[30,32] Because

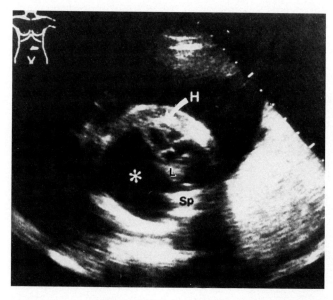

Figure 6–16. Chylothorax/hydrothorax. Transverse section of the fetal thorax demonstrating the fetal heart (H), lung (L), and spine (Sp). Fluid surrounding the heart (*) represents idiopathic hydrothorax or chylothorax. (*Reprinted with permission from Romero R, Pilu G, Ghidini A, et al. Prenatal Diagnosis of Congenital Anomalies. Norwalk, CT: Appleton & Lange, 1987:196*).

these sonographic findings of chylothorax are indistinguishable from other forms of pleural effusion, thoracentesis has been used for prenatal diagnosis of chylothorax. The use of hematologic indices remains controversial.[33,34] Findings include clear fluid with lymphocytosis.

Perinatal Outcome and Management

Brodman[35] studied 34 cases of chylothorax in infants and reported that the majority were symptomatic immediately after birth and that males predominated. Only three effusions were bilateral. Brodman found no correlation between the type of labor or mode of delivery, birth weight, onset of symptoms, site of infusion, or onset of respiratory distress.

The management of chylothorax depends on the severity of the disorder and the gestational age at which it is identified. Because chylothorax may be associated with chromosomal abnormalities, karyotypic analysis should be performed. The accumulation of fluid early in pregnancy can adversely affect lung development and therefore might lead to pulmonary hypoplasia and neonatal death, even in an otherwise normal fetus. Thoracentesis should be performed as fluid accumulation increases.[33-35] In our experience, such procedures might prevent the development of pulmonic hypoplasia.

The prognosis for fetuses affected by chylothorax is poor, especially when the condition occurs early in pregnancy. Spontaneous resolution of these effusions is rare; mortality rates range from 15% to 50%.[25,35] Neonates that survive the initial postnatal period are candidates for surgical ligation of the thoracic duct.[35,36,37]

Cystic Adenomatoid Malformation

Etiopathology

Cystic adenomatoid malformation is a unilateral hamartoma that usually presents in the immediate postnatal period as a serious respiratory emergency. Other clinical presentations include stillbirth, neonatal or perinatal death, progressive respiratory distress in the newborn, and acute or chronic pulmonary infection in the older infant and child.[38-40] Fetal hydrops and maternal polyhydramnios have been reported in association with this lesion.[41-43]

Cystic adenomatoid malformations result from abnormal induction of surrounding mesenchymal differentiation by the ramifying bronchial buds.[44,45] This leads to the overgrowth of bronchioles with adjacent but noncommunicating alveolar ducts and sacs. Two subtypes of cystic adenomatoid malformations have been identified. The macrocystic type contains single or multiple large cysts that are 5 mm or more in diameter. The microcystic type of cystic adenomatoid

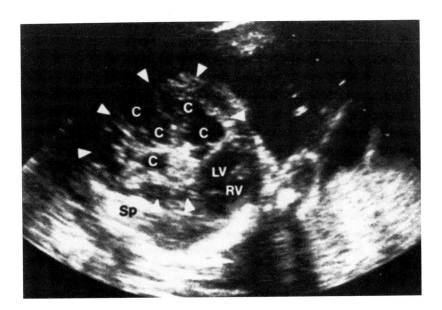

Figure 6–17. Macrocystic adenomatoid malformation. Transverse section through the fetal thorax demonstrating dextrorotation of the fetal heart (LV, left ventricle; RV, right ventricle) caused by a large multilocular cystic mass (C) (outlined by arrowheads). The spine (Sp) is located posteriorly. (*Reprinted with permission from* Journal of Ultrasound Medicine. *1;131:1982*).

malformation contains predominantly solid cysts that are generally smaller than 5 mm in diameter.[46] There is a slight predominance among males. However, all ethnic groups are affected equally. These lesions occur in both term and preterm infants and with equal frequency in both lungs. Single- and multiple-lobe involvement has been described.[44,45]

Three subtypes of cystic adenomatoid malforma-

tion have been described on the basis of pathologic features.[45,46] Type I lesions typically have one isolated large cystic cavity with trabeculations of the wall and smaller adjacent cavities with normal lung parenchyma. Type II is characterized by multiple small cysts up to 1 cm in diameter. Type III is a predominantly solid lesion. All three subtypes share the common histologic features of an increase in terminal bronchiolar structures, a polypoid configuration of the cuboidal-columnar epithelium lining the cystic structures, and an increase in elastic tissue in areas lined by cuboidal-columnar epithelium often associated with polypoid projections without inflammation.

Pleural effusion and hydrops are commonly seen in association with these lesions.[40,44,47] Increased accumulation of fluid enhances the likelihood of pulmonary hypoplasia.[22]

Polyhydramnios is also a commonly associated feature of cystic adenomatoid malformations; it is reported to occur in 30%[44] to 80% of cases.[43] Miller and colleagues[44] reported a 15% incidence of both hydrops and hydramnios, and nearly 50% of fetuses were stillborn. They postulated that increased amniotic fluid might be secondary to either excess secretion by the abnormal lung or decreased absorption by the malformed or hypoplastic adjacent lung. Fetal hydrops could also be caused by lymphatic obstruction of the mass or by direct compression of the heart by the expanding lesion, resulting in reduced cardiac output. It has been reported, however, that as much as 65% of cystic adenomatoid malformations remain asymptomatic during the perinatal period.[47]

Ultrasound Diagnosis

The finding of a solid space-occupying lung lesion with gross mediastinal shift in association with maternal polyhydramnios, fetal hydrops, or both, but with

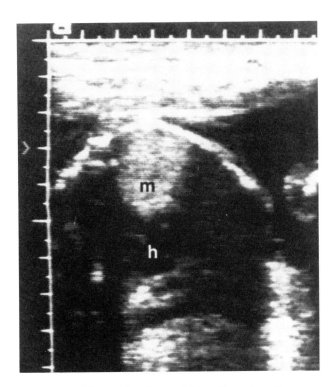

Figure 6–18. Microcystic adenomatoid malformation. Transverse section of the fetus demonstrating an echodense mass (m) filling the right hemithorax. The mediastinum and heart (h) are deviated to the left. (*Reprinted with permission from* Obstetrics and Gynecology. *70;631:1987*).

no other detectable anomalies should raise the possibility of congenital cystic adenomatoid malformation. A diagnosis of macrocystic tumors in a fetus depends on the presence of small peripheral cysts (Fig. 6–17). Identifying microcystic tumors is more difficult; this type is visualized as an echodense mass that replaces the lung (Fig. 6–18). Either type of tumor can result in significant displacement of the mediastinum and heart.[48-50]

Miller and colleagues[44] have described type III cystic adenomatoid malformations in a fetus who presented at 32 weeks' gestation with polyhydramnios and an abnormally thick hydropic placenta. The lung was described as voluminous, with the heart displaced to the right. The echogenicity was consistent with that of a solid organ. Autopsy and histologic examination confirmed type III congenital cystic adenomatoid malformation. Graham and associates[49] described the sonographic appearance of the type III lesion as extremely echogenic. The differential diagnosis of these lesions includes a solid tumor or other lung lesion, such as extralobar pulmonary sequestration.

Perinatal Outcome and Management

The most common initial signs seen in children born with cystic adenomatoid malformation are respiratory distress and cyanosis.[51] The respiratory distress is the result of displacement and compression of the normal pulmonary tissue. The pressure and concomitant pleural effusion early in pregnancy can lead to pulmonary hypoplasia.

Prenatal management depends on the gestational age at diagnosis as well as the presence or absence of hydrops and polyhydramnios. In the absence of hydrops and polyhydramnios, the outcome is relatively good. Repeated thoracentesis has been shown to improve the chance of survival in these cases.[41] Surgical correction is possible postnatally.[48] However, the fetus that is anomalous and has hydrops as well as polyhydramnios has an extremely poor prognosis.[41,42,51] Therefore, if the diagnosis is made before 24 weeks, termination of the pregnancy may be advised. Conversely, for diagnoses made after 24 weeks, a nonaggressive neonatal approach may be recommended.

The prognosis is better for infants with a macrocystic lesion: the overall survival rate is as high as 70%, compared with 20% for those with the microcystic lesion.[41] Again, fetuses without associated anomalies, hydrops, or pulmonary hypoplasia tend to have a better outcome.[31,41,51] The survival rate for the type I lesions is 69%, whereas the mortality rate for type III has been reported to be almost 100%. This high mortality rate appears to be related to the extreme mediastinal shift and associated circulatory and respiratory embarrassment.[52]

Almost all infants with congenital adenomatoid malformation have respiratory distress. Madewell and his associates[52] reported that approximately 66% of affected infants have onset of respiratory distress immediately after birth; however, as many as 25% of infants remain asymptomatic for a week or longer. Respiratory dysfunction secondary to pulmonary hypoplasia or compression of the thoracic viscera can result in heart failure.[53]

This cystic mass tends to expand progressively after birth, leading to air trapping.[37,39] Immediate surgical decompression, the treatment of choice, has been shown to be well tolerated by infants.[47] Survival depends on both the extent of the hypoplasia and the state of lung maturation.[53]

Ueda and colleagues[54] reported a case of asymptomatic congenital cystic adenomatoid malformation in which a small embryonal rhabdomyosarcoma was subsequently diagnosed. This represents one of the rare cases in which a malignant tumor arises within a congenital malformation.

Bronchopulmonary Sequestration

Etiopathology

Bronchopulmonary sequestration is a rare congenital thoracic defect. An accessory or dysplastic segment of lung exists that is supplied by a systemic artery but may be anatomically distinct from the remainder of the lobe (extralobar) or may be included in the substance of the lung. In the latter case, the segment may or may not have bronchial communication with the remaining bronchial tree.[55-57]

The sequestration of pulmonary tissue has been defined as masses of pulmonary tissue that have no communication with the bronchial tree.[55,56] Three types of bronchopulmonary sequestration are described: 1) intralobar, part of the lobe of a lung, 2) extralobar, a separate lobe still attached to the main pulmonary mass, and 3) complete sequestration, entirely independent of the lungs.

Intralobar bronchopulmonary sequestrations are confined to the visceral pleura. There is adjacent normal lung tissue and venous drainage into the left atrium.[18] This form is generally located basally and vertebrally, and both sides of the lung are involved with equal frequency. The lower lobes are affected in about 98% of cases. The arterial supply is generally from the thoracic aorta, whereas the pulmonary veins almost always drain this lesion.[36,39] In the extralobar type, the most common type observed in newborns, the lesions are enclosed within their own pleura and drain into the right atrium.[58] Approximately 90% of extralobar lesions reside in the posterior left costophrenic sulcus.[58] The arterial supply and venous drainage are primarily from the systemic vessels.[58,59] In contrast to the intralobar variety, which can be either cystic or solid in appearance, the extralobar type tends to resemble normal lung tissue.[59,60] Rarely do

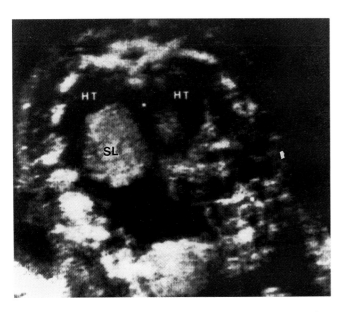

Figure 6–19. Bronchopulmonary sequestration. Transverse section through the fetal thorax demonstrating sequestered extralobar lung segment (SL) and hydrothorax (HT). (*Reprinted with permission from* Journal of Ultrasound Medicine. *1;131:1982*).

sequestrations of both types coexist, involving an entire lung, or occurring bilaterally.[55,56]

Although the pathogenesis of these lesions remains obscure, a number of anatomic variables may be associated with this lesion:

The arterial supply may be from a systemic or a pulmonary artery or both.
Communication with the gastrointestinal tract may or may not be present.
The venous drainage may be to a systemic or a pulmonary vein or both.
A sequestered mass of pulmonary parenchyma may exist within or outside the visceral pleura of the ipsilateral normal lung.
The diaphragm may or may not be defective.[54,60]

Some investigators call attention to the aberrant systemic artery and the developing bronchial bud that sequesters this from the rest of the respiratory tract.[18,55,61,62] There also appears to be a slight preponderance in males, and the left lung field is more commonly involved.[41,42,50,55,58,63]

Ultrasound Diagnosis

Although it is possible to diagnose the intralobar and extralobar forms of bronchopulmonary sequestration before birth, doing so can be difficult and requires expertise.[64] As is shown in Figure 6–19, the extralobar lesion may appear on ultrasound as a discrete echodense lesion in the left costophrenic sulcus.

Perinatal Outcome and Management

As we have described in previous sections, lung masses of significant size, with or without pleural effusion, tend to have a poor fetal outcome. Therefore, termination of the pregnancy may be offered when the diagnosis is made before 24 weeks of gestation. Other prognostic predictors include the presence of polyhydramnios, pleural effusion, fetal hydrops, or a mediastinal shift. Fetal outcome in the presence of the above complications is uniformly poor: mortality rates are as high as 100%.[65]

Bronchogenic Cysts

Etiopathology

Bronchogenic cysts result from abnormal budding of the laryngotracheal tube. These cysts often remain attached to the tracheobronchial tree and may be found in the area of the trachea, mediastinum, or pulmonary lung tissue (Fig. 6–20).[66] In approximately 30% of cases, aberrant budding will occur early in bronchial

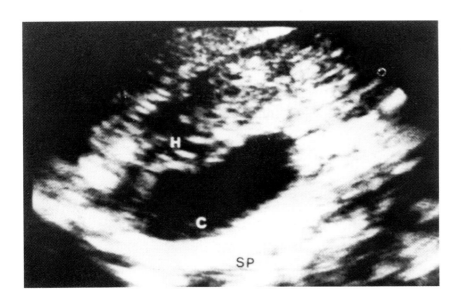

Figure 6–20. Bronchogenic cyst. Longitudinal section of the fetal chest demonstrating a large unilocular cyst (C) posterior to the heart (H). The spine (Sp) is located posterior to the cyst. (*Reprinted with permission from* Obstetrics and Gynecology. *70;628:1987*).

development; therefore, these cysts will assume a periesophageal or mediastinal location. In 70% of cases, the cysts occur as intraparenchymal lesions and are observed later in development.[67] These cysts can be single or multiple, contain mucoid fluid, and are lined by pseudostratified columnar epithelium. The lower lobes are involved more often than the upper lobes; however, right and left lung fields and male and female fetuses are equally affected.[66]

Ultrasound Diagnosis

Prenatal sonographic diagnosis of intraparenchymal lesions requires identification of thin-walled sonolucent cysts without an associated diaphragmatic defect or echodense septae.[67,68] When these lesions are suspected, other potential defects, such as diaphragmatic hernia or macrocystic adenomatoid malformations, should be excluded. If the lesion is mediastinal, other differential diagnoses include midline lesions, such as goiters, teratomas, and vascular malformations.[69]

Perinatal Outcome and Management

Following prenatal diagnosis of intrathoracic cysts, no special antenatal management is required. Serial ultrasound examinations are advised to screen for evidence of fetal hydrops or polyhydramnios. Most importantly, however, these infants must be evaluated immediately after birth so that respiratory assistance can be initiated if needed and appropriate medical and/or surgical management can be instituted promptly.

Although bronchogenic cysts may be well tolerated, especially if they appear as isolated lesions, they can cause postnatal obstruction of bronchioles, leading to recurrent infection in the respiratory tract or compression of the airway.[70] Most infants do well after surgical excision of these lesions.[69,71]

REFERENCES

1. Mayden KL, Tortora M, Berkowitz RL, et al. Orbital diameters: a new parameter for prenatal diagnosis and dating. *Am J Obstet Gynecol.* 1982;144:289–297.
2. Steward RE. Craniofacial malformations: clinical and genetic considerations. *Pediatr Clin North Am.* 1978;25:485–515.
3. Slavkin HC. Congenital craniofacial malformations: issues and perspectives. *J Pros Dent.* 1984;51:109–118.
4. Pilu G, Reece EA, Romero R, et al. Prenatal diagnosis of craniofacial malformations with ultrasonography. *Am J Obstet Gynecol.* 1986;155:45–50.
5. Saunders RC, James AE. *The Principles and Practice of Ultrasonography in Obstetrics and Gynecology.* 3rd ed. Norwalk, Conn: Appleton-Century-Crofts; 1985.
6. Gorlin RJ, Pindborg JJ, Cohen MM. Syndromes of the head and neck. 2nd ed. New York: McGraw-Hill; 1976.
7. Pilu G, Romero R, Reece EA, et al. The prenatal diagnosis of Robin anomalad. *Am J Obstet Gynecol.* 1986;154:630–632.
8. Hata K, Hata T, Takamiya O, et al. Ultrasonographic measurements of the neck correlated with gestational age. *J Ultrasound Med.* 1988;7:333–337.
9. Smith DW, Jones KL. *Recognizable Patterns of Human Malformation: Genetic Embryologic and Clinical Aspects.* 3rd ed., Philadelphia, Pa: WB Saunders, Co; 1982, p. 472.
10. Byrne J, Blanc WA, Warburten O, et al. The significance of cystic hygroma in fetuses. *Hum Pathol.* 1984;15:61–67.
11. Gustavii B, Edval H. First trimester diagnosis of cystic nuchal hygroma. *Acta Obstet Gynecol Scand.* 1984;63:377–378.
12. Kurjak A, Zalud I, Jerkovic D, et al. Ultrasound diagnosis and evaluation of fetal tumors. *J Perinat Med.* 1989;17:173–193.
13. Chervenak FA, Isaacson G, Blakemore KJ, et al. Fetal cystic hygroma: cause and natural history. *N Engl J Med.* 1983;309:822–825.
14. Carswell F, Kurr MM, Hutchinson JH. Congenital goiter and hypothyroidism produced by maternal injection of iodides. *Lancet.* 1970;1:1241–1243.
15. Fisher DA, Dussault JH, Fole TP Jr, et al. Screening for congenital hypothyroidism: results of screening one million North American infants. *J Pediatr.* 1979;94:700–705.
16. Weiner S, Scarf JI, Bolognesi RJ, et al. Antenatal diagnosis and treatment of fetal goiter. *J Reprod Med.* 1980;24:39–42.
17. Barone CM, Van Natta FC, Kourides IA, et al. Sonographic detection of fetal goiter and unusual causes of hydramnios. *J Ultrasound Med.* 1985;4:625–627.
18. Moore KL. *The Developing Human: Clinically Oriented Embryology.* 3rd ed. Philadelphia, Pa: WB Saunders, Co; 1982:219–223.
19. Chitkara U, Rosenberg J, Chervenak FA, et al. Prenatal sonographic assessment of the fetal thorax: Normal values. *Am J Obstet Gynecol.* 1987;156:1069–1074.
20. Nimrod C, Davies D, Iwanicki S, et al. Ultrasound prediction of pulmonary hypoplasia. *Obstet Gynecol.* 1986;68:495–497.
21. Nimrod C, Nicholson S, Davies D, et al. Pulmonary hypoplasia testing in clinical obstetrics. *Am J Obstet Gynecol.* 1988;158:277–280.
22. Kitterman JA. Fetal lung development. *J Dev Physiol.* 1984;6:67–82.
23. Johnson A, Callan NA, Bhutan: VK, et al. Ultrasonic ratio of fetal thoracic to abdominal circumference: an association with fetal pulmonary hypoplasia. *Am J Obstet Gynecol.* 1987;157:764–769.
24. Randolph JG, Gross RE. Congenital chylothorax. *Arch Surg.* 1957;74:405–419.
25. Van Aerde J, Campbell AN, Smith JA, et al. Spontaneous chylothorax in newborns. *Am J Dis Child.* 1984;138:961–964.
26. Chernick V, Reed MH. Pneumothorax and chylothorax in the neonatal period. *J Pediatr.* 1970;76:624–632.
27. Lange IR, Manning FA. Antenatal diagnosis of congenital pleural effusions. *Am J Obstet Gynecol.* 1981;140:839–840.
28. Perry RE, Hodgman J, Cass AB. Pleural effusion in the neonatal period. *J Pediatr.* 1963;62:838–842.

29. Yancy WS, Spock A. Spontaneous neonatal pleural effusion. *J Pediatr Surg.* 1967;2:313–319.

30. Thomas DB, Anderson JC. Antenatal detection of fetal pleural effusion and neonatal management. *Med J Aust.* 1979;2:435–441.

31. Yoss BS, Lipsitz PJ. Chylothorax in two mongoloid infants. *Genetics.* 1977;12:357–360.

32. Defoort P, Thiery M. Antenatal diagnosis of congenital chylothorax by gray scale sonography. *J Clin Ultrasound.* 1978;6:47–48.

33. Benacerraf BR, Frigoletto FD. Mid-trimester fetal thoracentesis. *J Clin Ultrasound.* 1985;13:202–204.

34. Benacerraf BR, Frigoletto FD, Wilson M. Successful midtrimester thoracentesis with analysis of the lymphocyte population in the pleural effusion. *Am J Obstet Gynecol.* 1986;155:398–399.

35. Brodman RF. Congenital chylothorax: recommendations for treatment. *NY J Med.* 1975;75:553–557.

36. Petres RE, Redwine FO, Cruikshank DP. Congenital bilateral chylothorax: antepartum diagnosis and successful intrauterine surgical management. *JAMA.* 1982;248:1360–1361.

37. Andersen EA, Hertel J, Pedersen SA, et al. Congenital chylothorax: management by ligature of the thoracic duct. *Scand J Thorac Cardiovasc Surg.* 1984;18:193–195.

38. Moncrieff MW, Cameron AH, Astley R, et al. Congenital cystic adenomatoid malformation of the lung. *Thorax.* 1969;24:476–487.

39. Fisher JE, Nelson ST, Allen JE, et al. Congenital cystic adenomatoid malformation of the lung: a unique variant. *Am J Dis Child.* 1982;136:1071–1074.

40. Adzick NS, Harrison MR, Glick PL, et al. Fetal cystic adenomatoid malformation: prenatal diagnosis and natural history. *J Pediatr Surg.* 1985;20:483–488.

41. Kohler HG, Rymer BA. Congenital cystic malformation of the lung and its relation to hydramnios. *J Obstet Gynaecol Br Commonwealth.* 1973;80:130–134.

42. Aslam PA, Korones SB, Richardson RL, et al. Congenital cystic adenomatoid malformation with anasarca. *JAMA.* 1970;212:622–624.

43. Glaves J, Baker JL. Spontaneous resolution of maternal hydramnios in congenital cystic adenomatoid malformation of the lung: antenatal ultrasound features: case report. *Br J Obstet Gynaecol.* 1983;90:1065–1068.

44. Miller RK, Sieber WK, Unis EJ. Congenital adenomatoid malformation of the lung. *Pathol Annu.* 1980(pt 1);387–407.

45. Oestoer AG, Fortune DW. Congenital cystic adenomatoid malformation of the lung. *Am J Clin Pathol.* 1978;70:595–604.

46. Stocker JT, Madewell JE, Drake RM. Congenital cystic adenomatoid malformation of the lung: classification and morphologic spectrum. *Hum Pathol.* 1977;8:155–171.

47. Wolfe SA, Hertzler JH, Philippart AO. Cystic adenomatoid display of the lung. *J Pediatr Surg.* 1980;15:925–927.

48. Halloran LG, Silverberg SG, Salzber AM. Congenital cystic adenomatoid malformation of the lung. *Arch Surg.* 1972;104:715–717.

49. Graham D, Winn K, Dex W, et al. Prenatal diagnosis of cystic adenomatoid malformation of the lung. *J Ultrasound Med.* 1982;1:9–12.

50. Stauffer UG, Salvoldelli G, Mieth D. Antenatal ultrasound diagnosis in cystic adenomatoid malformation of the lung: case report. *J Pediatr Surg.* 1984;19:141–142.

51. Sawyer DR, Mosadomi A. A case of congenital cystic adenomatoid malformation of the lung with associated anomalies. *Afr J Med.* 1980;26:220–222.

52. Madewell JE, Stocker JT, Korsower JM. Cystic adenomatoid malformation of the lung. *AJR.* 1975;124:436–438.

53. Frenckner B, Freyschuss U. Pulmonary function after lobectomy for congenital lobar emphysema and congenital cystic adenomatoid malformation: a follow-up study. *Scand J Thorac Cardiovasc Surg.* 1982;16:293–298.

54. Ueda K, Gruppo R, Unger F, et al. Rhabdomyosarcoma of lung arising in congenital cystic adenomatoid malformation. *Cancer.* 1977;40:383–388.

55. Khalil KG, Kilman JW. Pulmonary sequestration. *J Thorac Cardiovasc Surg.* 1975;70:928–937.

56. Sade RM, Clouse M, Ellis FH Jr. The spectrum of pulmonary sequestration. *Ann Thorac Surg.* 1974;18:644–658.

57. Choplin RH, Sieell MJ. Pulmonary sequestration: six unusual presentations. *AJR.* 1980;134:695–700.

58. Horowitz RN. Extralobar sequestration of lung in newborn infant. *Am J Dis Child.* 1965;110:195–197.

59. Stocker JT, Kagan-Hallet K. Extralobar pulmonary sequestration: analysis of 15 cases. *Am J Clin Pathol.* 1979;72:917–925.

60. Romero R, Chervenak FA, Kotzen J, et al. Findings of extralobar pulmonary sequestration. *J Clin Ultrasound.* 1986; 5:283–299.

61. Savic B, Birtell FJ, Tholen W, et al. Lung sequestration: Report of seven cases and review of 540 published cases. *Thorax.* 1979:34:96–101.

62. Kilman JW, Battersby JS, Taybi H, et al. Pulmonary sequestration. *Arch Surg.* 1965;90:648–649.

63. Carter R. Pulmonary sequestration. *Ann Thorac Surg.* 1969;7:68–88.

64. Demos NJ, Teresi A. Congenital lung malformations. A unified concept and a case report. *J Thorac Cardiovasc Surg.* 1975;70:260–264.

65. Buntain WL, Woolley MM, Mahour GH, et al. Pulmonary sequestration in children: a twenty-five year experience. *Surgery.* 1977;81:413–420.

66. Rogers LF, Osmer JC. Bronchogenic cyst. A review of 46 cases. *AJR.* 1964;91:273–275.

67. Lebrun D, Avni EF, Goolaaerts JP, et al. Prenatal diagnosis of a pulmonary cyst by ultrasonography. *Eur J Pediatr.* 1985;144:399–402.

68. Mayden KL, Tortora M, Chervenak FA, et al. The antenatal sonographic detection of lung masses. *Am J Obstet Gynecol.* 1984;148:349–352.

69. Bower RJ, Kiesewetter WB. Mediastinal masses in infants and children. *Arch Surg.* 1977;112:1003–1009.

70. Eraklis AJ, Griscom NT, McGovern JB. Bronchogenic cysts of the mediastinum in infancy. *N Engl J Med.* 1969;281:1150–1155.

71. Ramenofsky ML, Leape LL, McCauley RGK. Bronchogenic cyst. *J Pediatr Surg.* 1979;14:219–224.

7

The Heart and Fetal Echocardiography

INTRODUCTION

Cardiac malformations are among the most common forms of congenital malformations observed, and occur in about 8 of 1,000 live births[1-3] and even more frequently in lost pregnancies.[4] Congenital heart disease (CHD) does not result from a mendelian pattern of genetic inheritance but from multifactorial causes, with chromosomal aberrations accounting for 4% to 5% of cases. Mendelian transmission and environmental factors contribute to only a fraction of known cases even though a high frequency of cardiac anomalies occurs in children of mothers with CHD.[1,5,6]

Congenital heart disease can be diagnosed prenatally, and increasing numbers of fetuses are being evaluated for possible cardiovascular defects.[7-10] Although detailed cardiac scanning cannot be recommended in all pregnancies, the use of the four-chamber view during routine sonography is a prudent approach for screening the entire obstetric population.[10]

A formal fetal echocardiogram is best done at about 20 to 22 weeks, when the four-chamber view is easy to visualize and the outflow tracts can be imaged and scrutinized. Although examination of the fetal heart becomes more difficult as pregnancy progresses, a complete examination is feasible even in late pregnancy. Table 7-1 lists the normal dimensions of the heart throughout fetal life.

In fetal echocardiography, a systematic approach is used to evaluate the cardiac anatomy. The left and right sides of the fetal heart are evaluated by first determining the position of the fetal head and spine. In this position, certain internal organs, such as the stomach, hepatic vessels, abdominal aorta, and inferior vena cava, can be assessed (Fig. 7-1). A transverse section of the fetal chest allows one to demonstrate the four-chamber view (Fig. 7-2) and to examine 1) the position of the heart, 2) the apex of the heart, which points to the left, 3) the integrity of the atrial and ventricular septae, and 4) the relative sizes of the atria and ventricles. As Pilu[1] pointed out, real-time imaging

of the leaflets can be used to determine the patency of the mitral and tricuspid valves and the more apical insertion of the latter valve. It also can distinguish the structural features of the right and left ventricles and determine the presence of the moderator band of the trabecula septomarginalis at the apical end of the right ventricle.

The left and right outflow tracts can be visualized by tilting the transducer cephalad. With some added angulation, the main pulmonary artery, the ductus arteriosus, and the aortic arch can be observed (Fig. 7-3). Nomograms of normal ventricles and great vessels derived from M-mode imaging (Fig. 7-3) can be useful for comparing ventricles and great vessels suspected of being abnormal. M-mode ultrasound also can be

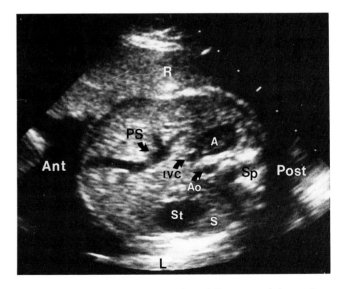

Figure 7-1. Transverse cross section of the upper abdomen in a second-trimester fetus demonstrating visceral situs. The portal situs (PS), the anatomic landmark of the hilus of the liver, can be clearly recognized. The stomach (St), spleen (S), inferior vena cava (IVC), and abdominal aorta (Ao) are demonstrated. (Ant = anterior, Post = posterior, R = right, L = left, A = right adrenal gland.) (*Reprinted with permission from Reece EA, Hobbins JC, Mahoney J, et al, eds. Medicine of the Fetus and Mother. Philadelphia: JB Lippincott, 1992.*)

TABLE 7–1. NORMAL CARDIAC DIMENSIONS

Week	Transverse Diameter (mm)			Longitudinal Diameter (mm)			Volume (cm³)		
	5th Percentile	50th Percentile	95th Percentile	5th Percentile	50th Percentile	95th Percentile	5th Percentile	50th Percentile	95th Percentile
12	4	5	6	5	6	7	0.038	0.067	0.096
13	5	6	7	6	7	9	0.072	0.127	0.182
14	6	7	8	8	9	10	0.128	0.225	0.322
15	7	8	10	9	10	12	0.213	0.374	0.535
16	8	10	11	10	12	14	0.336	0.588	0.840
17	9	11	13	12	14	16	0.504	0.883	1.262
18	10	12	15	13	15	18	0.726	1.271	1.816
19	11	14	16	14	17	20	1.008	1.764	2.520
20	13	15	18	16	19	22	1.356	2.373	3.390
21	14	17	20	18	21	24	1.776	3.106	4.436
22	15	18	21	19	23	26	2.273	3.975	5.677
23	16	20	23	21	24	28	2.851	4.987	7.123
24	18	21	25	22	26	30	3.519	6.155	8.791
25	19	23	27	24	28	32	4.282	7.490	10.698
26	20	24	28	25	30	34	5.150	9.008	12.866
27	22	26	30	27	32	36	6.130	10.723	15.316
28	23	27	32	28	33	38	7.232	12.649	18.066
29	24	29	34	30	35	40	8.458	14.795	21.132
30	25	30	35	31	37	42	9.812	17.163	24.514
31	26	32	37	32	38	44	11.284	19.743	28.202
32	28	33	38	33	40	46	12.857	22.505	32.153
33	29	34	40	34	41	47	14.498	25.388	36.278
34	30	35	41	35	42	49	16.155	28.301	40.447
35	30	37	43	36	43	50	17.750	31.107	44.464
36	31	38	44	37	44	51	19.180	33.626	48.072
37	32	39	45	37	45	52	20.308	35.642	50.976
38	33	39	46	38	46	53	20.966	36.913	52.860
39	33	40	47	38	46	54	20.903	37.156	53.409
40	33	41	48	38	46	55	19.478	35.580	51.682

Reprinted with permission from Jeanty P, Romero R, Cantraine, et al. Fetal cardiac dimensions: a potential tool for the diagnosis of congenital heart defects. Journal of Ultrasound in Medicine. *1984;3:359–364.*

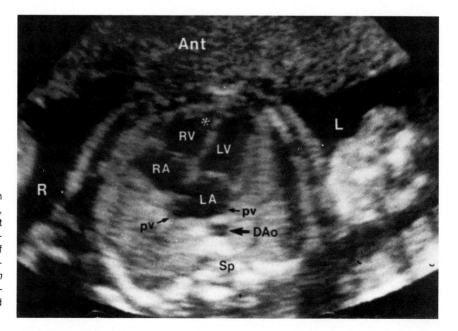

Figure 7–2. Four-chamber view of the heart in a second-trimester fetus. (RV = right ventricle, LV = left ventricle, RA = right atrium, LA = left atrium, pv = pulmonary veins, DAo = descending aorta, SP = spine, * = the moderator band of the trabecula septomarginalis. Other abbreviations are identified in Fig. 7–1.) (*Reprinted with permission from Reece EA, Hobbins JC, Mahoney J, et al, eds.* Medicine of the Fetus and Mother. *Philadelphia: JB Lippincott, 1992.*)

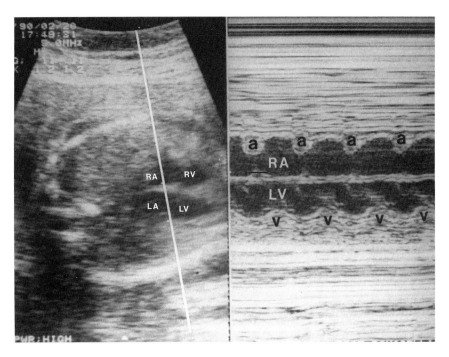

Figure 7–3. TM-mode evaluation of cardiac chambers. The M line is directed across the right atrium (RA) and left ventricle (LV). Undulations of the walls of the cardiac chambers indicate atrial and ventricular contractions. This sonogram allows precise calculation of atrial and ventricular frequency. The atrioventricular sequence of excitation can be inferred as well. (*Reprinted with permission from Reece EA, Hobbins JC, Mahoney J, et al, eds.* Medicine of the Fetus and Mother. *Philadelphia: JB Lippincott, 1992.*)

used in the identification and differential diagnosis of fetal dysrhythmias.[1,11–14]

A number of researchers[15–23] have found that, in most cases, pulsed Doppler recordings of blood flow through the mitral and tricuspid valves, the great vessels, and the inferior vena cava are adequate between the 18th and 20th weeks (Fig. 7–4). Consequently, such recordings also can be used to substantiate insuf-

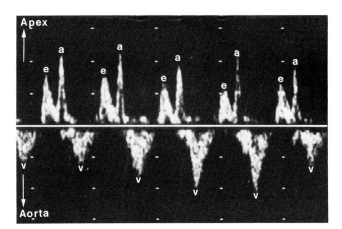

Figure 7–4. Doppler sonogram of the left ventricle in a 20-week-old fetus obtained by positioning a 4-mm large sampling gate below the mitral valve. Blood flow coursing along both the inflow and outflow tracts is registered. During diastole, blood moves away from the atrioventricular valve toward the cardiac apex. Two distinct velocity peaks can be recognized: the e peak, corresponding to passive venous filling, and the a peak, corresponding to atrial systole. During ventricular systole, blood flows in the opposite direction (v), moving toward the aortic valves. This sonogram allows us to infer the atrioventricular sequence of excitation. (*Reprinted with permission from Reece EA, Hobbins JC, Mahoney J, et al. eds.* Medicine of the Fetus and Mother. *Philadelphia: JB Lippincott, 1992.*)

ficiency of the atrioventricular valves (Fig. 7–5), especially when used in combination with two-dimensional and M-mode ultrasound. The prognosis is likely to be poor when structural heart disease is associated with hydrops and valvular insufficiency.[17]

Fetal echocardiography can be used effectively in the prenatal identification of CHD. Some defects are easy to identify, whereas others are more difficult to recognize. Anomalies more easily diagnosed include intracardiac defects, such as the ones involving the ventricular septum and those associated with hypoplasia or enlargement of the cardiac chambers. Greater expertise and sophistication are required to diagnose abnormal connections between the ventricles and the great arteries, such as transposition of the great vessels and coarctation of the aorta.

ABNORMAL RHYTHMS

Fetal Dysrhythmias

The transient dysrhythmias involving tachycardia, bradycardia, or ectopic beats that are common in fetuses are usually clinically insignificant. As Allan et al[24] pointed out, however, symptoms such as the following are abnormal and need further evaluation: a sustained bradycardia of less than 100 beats per minute (bpm), a sustained tachycardia of more than 200 bpm, and irregular beats detected in more than 1 in 10 beats. These dysrhythmias can be evaluated by 1) simultaneously imaging the mitral and tricuspid valves and the motion of the ventricular walls, 2) imaging the aortic valve and motion of the atrial walls,

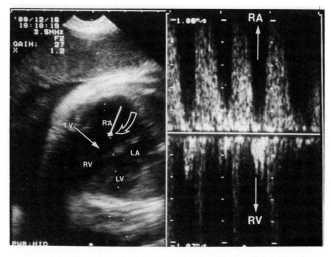

Figure 7–5. Pulsed Doppler demonstration of tricuspid insufficiency in a third-trimester fetus that was referred for fetal echocardiography because of obvious enlargement of the right atrium and ventricle (RA, RV). The sampling gate (curved arrow) is positioned within the right atrium just above the tricuspid valve. A high-velocity (more than 1 m/s) regurgitant jet in systole is clearly demonstrated. (*Reprinted with permission from Reece EA, Hobbins JC, Mahoney J, et al, eds. Medicine of the Fetus and Mother. Philadelphia: JB Lippincott, 1992.*)

and 3) M-mode sampling of the ventricular inlet or inferior vena cava.[24–26]

Premature Atrial and Ventricular Contractions

Premature atrial and ventricular contractions are the most common types of dysrhythmias.[25] Premature atrial contractions may result in an increased or decreased ventricular rate, depending on whether the impulse is conducted to the ventricles or is blocked. Premature atrial and ventricular contractions are considered to be benign conditions[25] and generally are not associated with pathologic conditions. Most disappear in utero or soon after birth. Serial monitoring of the fetal heart during pregnancy is suggested because of the possibility that an ectopic beat will trigger a re-entrant tachyarrhythmia.[25]

Prenatal diagnosis of fetal extrasystoles can be accomplished readily using M-mode ultrasonography (Fig. 7–6), whereas pulsed Doppler ultrasound can be evaluated and used in fetuses with premature beats to demonstrate the postextrasystolic potentiation (Fig. 7–7).[1,21]

Supraventricular Tachyarrhythmias

Included in the supraventricular tachyarrhythmias are supraventricular paroxysmal tachycardia (SVT) and atrial flutter and fibrillation. An atrial frequency of 200 to 300 bpm and a 1-to-1 rate of atrioventricular conduction are characteristic of SVT (Fig. 7–8),[1] which can be caused by irritable ectopic focus; or electrical activity at the level of the sinoatrial node inside the atrium,

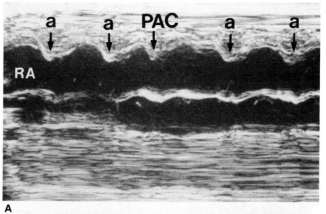

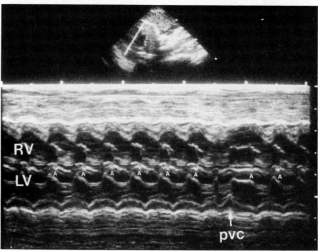

Figure 7–6. (A) TM-mode evaluation of the movement of the wall of the right atrium in a fetus with supraventricular extrasystoles. Regular atrial rhythm (a) is interrupted by a premature atrial contraction (PAC). **(B)** In this fetus, TM-mode reveals a premature ventricular contraction (pvc) that is not preceded by atrial systole (absence of the a wave on the mitral valve). This indicates ventricular extrasystoles. (*Reprinted with permission from Reece EA, Hobbins JC, Mahoney J, et al, eds. Medicine of the Fetus and Mother. Philadelphia: JB Lippincott, 1992.*)

at the atrioventricular node, or in the His–Purkinje system. An aberrant atrioventricular pathway, such as the Kent pathway in the Wolff–Parkinson–White syndrome, may lead to reentry rhythms and thus tachycardia.

Atrial flutter and atrial fibrillation, which often occur alternately in the same fetus are believed to arise from similar mechanisms, including circus movement of the electrical impulse, ectopic formation, multiple reentry, and formation of multifocal impulse.[1] As Pilu[1] points out, in atrial flutter, the rate ranges between 300 and 460 bpm, and because of varying degrees of atrioventricular (AV) block, the ventricular rate ranges between 60 and 200 bpm (Fig. 7–9). In fibrillation, the atrial rate is greater than 400 bpm, and the ventricular rate is 120 to 200 bpm.

Immediate auscultation is the easiest method of detecting fetal tachyarrhythmia. The heart rate and the

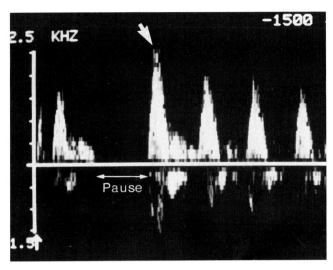

Figure 7–7. Blocked atrial extrasystoles in a second-trimester fetus. Doppler ultrasound evaluation of the ascending aorta reveals increased peak velocity (arrow) following a ventricular pause. This observation suggests the presence of the Frank-Starling mechanism. (*Reprinted with permission from Reece EA, Hobbins JC, Mahoney J, et al, eds.* Medicine of the Fetus and Mother. *Philadelphia: JB Lippincott, 1992.*)

sequence of atrioventricular contractions can be identified with M-mode or pulsed Doppler.[1]

Fetal tachyarrhythmia can lead to nonimmune hydrops[27,28] if the ventricular response is rapid and results in suboptimal filling of the ventricle. This process will lead to reduced cardiac output, overload of the right atrium, congestive heart failure, and, eventually, to nonimmune hydrops (Fig. 7–10).[28] In utero treatment of tachyarrhythmias is often successful by administering drugs, such as digoxin, verapamil, propranolol, quinidine, and procainamide, to the mother.

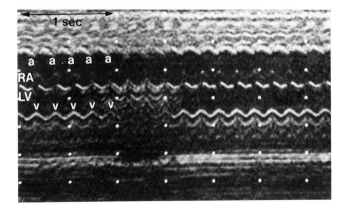

Figure 7–8. Supraventricular tachycardia in a third-trimester fetus. The TM-mode sonogram indicates an atrial rhythm of about 220 bpm and a 1:1 ventricular response (v). Return to a normal sinus rhythm was noted after maternal administration of a daily dose of 240 mg of verapamil. Digoxin and procainamide had been administered previously without any beneficial effect. (*Reprinted with permission from Reece EA, Hobbins JC, Mahoney J, et al, eds.* Medicine of the Fetus and Mother. *Philadelphia: JB Lippincott, 1992.*)

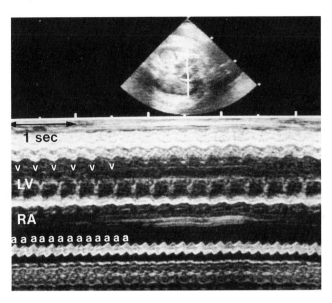

Figure 7–9. Atrial flutter. The TM-mode sonogram reveals an atrial rate (a) of about 440 bpm and a 2:1 ventricular response. This 36-week-old infant converted spontaneously to a normal sinus rhythm a few hours after this sonogram was obtained. Wolff-Parkinson-White syndrome was diagnosed after vaginal delivery at term. (*Reprinted with permission from Reece EA, Hobbins JC, Mahoney J, et al, eds.* Medicine of the Fetus and Mother. *Philadelphia: JB Lippincott, 1992.*)

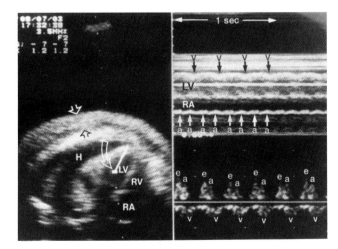

Figure 7–10. Simultaneous real-time, TM-mode, and duplex sonography in a third-trimester fetus with atrial flutter. The TM-mode sonogram reveals an atrial rate of 480 bpm and a ventricular rate of 240 bpm. Doppler ultrasound reveals an inversion between the size of the e and a peaks (compare with the normal sonograph displayed in Fig. 7–4) that is thought to represent failure of diastolic filling. Real-time sonography demonstrates polyhydramnios, pleural effusion (H), and subcutaneous edema (arrowheads). The curved arrow represents the dilated left ventricle. Although sinus rhythm could never be obtained, a significant reduction of the frequency with amelioration of hydropic manifestation was observed after maternal administration of amiodarone. Digoxin, procainamide, and verapamil were ineffective. The infant was delivered by cesarean section at 34 weeks and survived. (*Reprinted with permission from Reece EA, Hobbins JC, Mahoney J, et al, eds.* Medicine of the Fetus and Mother. *Philadelphia: JB Lippincott, 1992.*)

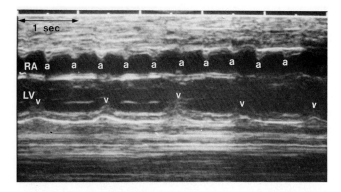

Figure 7–11. Complete atrioventricular block. The TM-mode sonogram reveals a regular atrial activity (a) with a frequency of about 120 bpm and a slow, independent ventricular activity (v) with a frequency of about 60 bpm. This infant was delivered at term by cesarean section. A pacemaker had to be installed on the third day of life. (*Reprinted with permission from Reece EA, Hobbins JC, Mahoney J, et al, eds.* Medicine of the Fetus and Mother. *Philadelphia: JB Lippincott, 1992.*)

Atrioventricular Block

Atrioventricular (AV) block can be partial or complete. First-degree AV block corresponds to a simple conduction delay and is associated with prolongation of the PR interval on the electrocardiogram.

Second-degree AV block is subdivided into Mobitz types I and II. Mobitz type I is a progressive prolongation of the PR interval that finally leads to the block of one atrial impulse (the Luciani–Wenckebach phenomenon). In Mobitz type II, the ventricular rate is a submultiple of the atrial rate (eg 2 to 1, 3 to 1).

In third-degree (complete) AV block, the atria and ventricles are disassociated, and ventricular activation typically is slow and independent (Fig. 7–11).[1] Third-degree AV block is associated with CHD in more than 50% of cases.[29] Furthermore, it may be associated with circulating autoantibodies, such as those seen in lupus. These antibodies presumably lead to inflammation and damage of the conduction system and result in fetal heart rate disorders. Although anti-SSA skin-sensitizing antibodies have been reported in more than 80% of mothers who delivered infants with AV block, only 30% of these mothers have clinical evidence of connective tissue disease, usually lupus erythematosus.[30–32] Carpenter et al[33] used a pacemaker in one case in an attempt to achieve intrauterine ventricular pacing for secondary hydrops. A regular ventricular frequency was obtained, but the fetus died a few hours later.

Ordinarily, no significant hemodynamic disturbance is associated with either first- or second-degree AV block. Third-degree block, however, can severely compromise the fetus by slowing the heart rate, which reduces cardiac output and leads to congestive heart failure.[25,27]

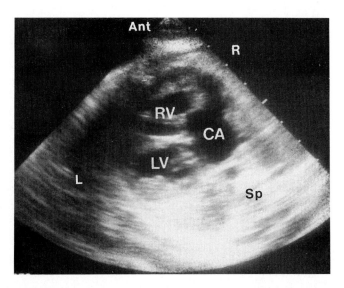

Figure 7–12. Partial atrioventricular septal defect in a third-trimester fetus with complex congenital heart disease. A common atrium (CA) is demonstrated. The two atrioventricular valves insert at the same level on the ventricular septum. (Other abbreviations are identified in earlier figures.) (*Reprinted with permission from Reece EA, Hobbins JC, Mahoney J, et al, eds.* Medicine of the Fetus and Mother. *Philadelphia: JB Lippincott, 1992.*)

STRUCTURAL ABNORMALITIES

Atrial and Ventricular Septal Defects

Atrioventricular septal defects can range from the minor to the extremely severe—complete atrioventricular defects (Figs. 7–12 and 7–13). They usually involve an atrial septal defect (ASD), a ventricular septal defect (VSD), and a common atrioventricular valve.

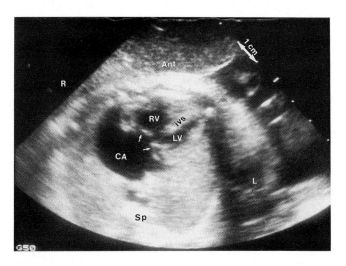

Figure 7–13. Complete atrioventricular septal defect. A common atrium (CA) is demonstrated in association with a common atrioventricular valve with central opening (arrows) and a large ventricular septal defect. (Other abbreviations are identified in earlier figures.) (*Reprinted with permission from Reece EA, Hobbins JC, Mahoney J, et al, eds.* Medicine of the Fetus and Mother. *Philadelphia: JB Lippincott, 1992.*)

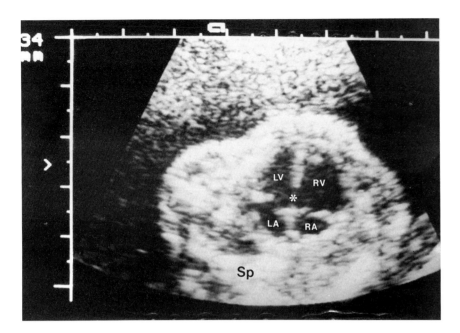

Figure 7–14. Four-chamber view in a second-trimester fetus with a large perimembranous ventricular septal defect (*). (Other abbreviations are identified in earlier figures.) The evidence indicates that ventricular septal defects are well tolerated during intrauterine life. However, in our experience, large defects are often associated with some degree of enlargement of the right ventricle. Color Doppler has revealed that, in these cases, a left-to-right shunt is a frequent finding even before birth. (*Reprinted with permission from Reece EA, Hobbins JC, Mahoney J, et al, eds.* Medicine of the Fetus and Mother. *Philadelphia: JB Lippincott, 1992.*)

More than 50% of infants with trisomy 21 have both atrioventricular septal and canal defects.[15,34]

The simplest form of atrioventricular septal defect, the primum type, is easy to detect in utero. The secundum type, the most common form of ASD, is difficult to detect because of patency of the foramen ovale. Atrial septal defects do not impair cardiac function in utero because normal fetuses have a large right-to-left shunt at the atrial level. In fact, most newborn infants with ASDs lack symptoms.

Ventricular septal defects apparently are the most common form of CHD and, like ASDs, do not cause hemodynamic compromise in the fetus. Because pressures in the right and left ventricles are assumed to be equal in utero,[35] even a large communication between the ventricles probably causes only small bidirectional shunts. Like infants with ASDs, most infants with VSDs are asymptomatic in the immediate neonatal period, unless the shunt is large.[1,36] Fetal echocardiography can diagnose these lesions, especially those larger than 2 mm, whereas smaller ones 1 to 2 mm (Fig. 7–14) fall below the resolution power of current ultrasound equipment and escape detection.

Because complete atrioventricular septal defects are usually large, the pressures between chambers tend to equalize, resulting in bidirectional shunting through the septal defects, which in turn may lead to congestive heart failure (Fig. 7–15).[37] Pulsed Doppler should be used to evaluate these defects because it can identify the regurgitant jet.[1,17]

Pulmonary and Aortic Stenoses

In pulmonary stenosis (Fig. 7–16), the obstruction can occur at various points along the outflow tract of the right ventricle. The increased resistance to right ven-

tricular outflow results in pressure overload and subsequently to myocardial hypertrophy. If extremely severe, the pressure overload may damage the tricuspid valve and result in congestive heart failure.

Aortic stenosis includes three lesions: valvular stenosis, supravalvular stenosis (rare), and subaortic stenosis (including the asymmetric form). The latter two lesions are generally not clinically evident in neonates.[1] One form of subaortic stenosis often found in infants of diabetic mothers is the result of hypertrophy of the ventricular septum and the free left ventricular walls.

When aortic stenosis is severe, pressure overload in the left ventricle and reduced coronary perfusion can result in early impairment of heart function in utero and, ultimately, to mitral valve insufficiency and to regurgitation in systole.[38] According to Reynolds,[39] an extremely high incidence of intrauterine growth retardation is the indirect result of the hemodynamic disturbance that occurs after aortic stenosis.

Diagnosis of pulmonic and aortic stenosis in utero is difficult: Only a few, extremely severe cases have been described, and those were characterized by enlargement of the ventricles or by poststenotic enlargement or hypoplasia of the great vessels.[38,40] Diagnosis of pulmonic and aortic stenosis after birth depends on real-time ultrasound to detect doming of the cusps and on Doppler to detect poststenotic turbulence.[41]

Tetralogy of Fallot

A large VSD in the perimembranous area, pulmonic stenosis (see Fig. 7–16), an aortic valve that overrides the ventricular septum, and a hypertrophic right ventricle are characteristic of the tetralogy of Fallot.[1,9,42] In most cases, the disorder does not lead to hemody-

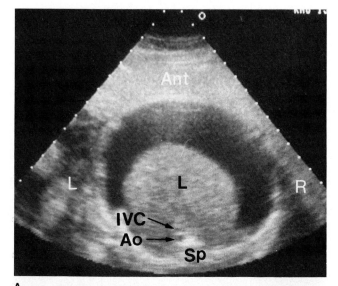

A

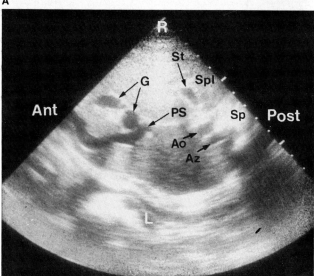

B

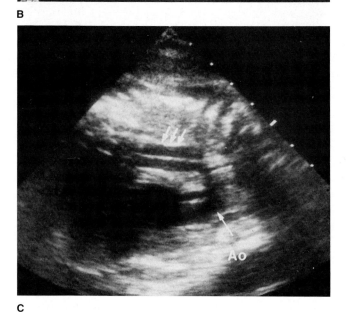

C

Figure 7–15. (A) Asplenia syndrome in a fetus with complex heart disease and nonimmune hydrops. A large layer of ascites delineates a symmetric liver (black L), and both the inferior vena cava (IVC) and descending aorta (Ao) are demonstrated on the same side of the spine (Sp). (Other abbreviations are identified in earlier figures.) **(B)** Polysplenia syndrome (same case as in Fig. 7–12). A transverse section of the upper abdomen reveals a considerable alteration in the topographic disposition of abdominal organs. The stomach (St) was seen on the right side as well as a splenic mass (Spl). The umbilical vein, left portal vein, and portal sinus (PS) are tortuous. The main abdominal vessels are seen on the same side of the spine (Sp). Careful sonographic examination along different planes revealed the most anterior vessel to be the descending aorta (Ao). The posterior vessel was eventually identified as an enlarged anomalous azygos vein (Az). Absence of the inferior vena cava with an azygos vein draining the lower portion of the body is pathognomonic of left isomerism, or polysplenia syndrome. **(C)** Longitudinal section of the fetal chest (same case as in panel B). A large vessel (arrow) in which pulsed Doppler sonography revealed venous blood flow is seen coursing within the thorax posterior to the descending aorta (Ao). This venous vessel can be positively identified with an anomalous azygos vein draining the lower portion of the body. Such a finding is pathognomonic of the absence of the inferior vena cava and left isomerism. (*Reprinted with permission from Reece EA, Hobbins JC, Mahoney J, et al, eds.* Medicine of the Fetus and Mother. *Philadelphia: JB Lippincott, 1992.*)

namic compromise in the fetus. Echocardiogram demonstrating normal growth in affected fetuses[41] supports the notion that even in the presence of a severe infundibular stenosis or pulmonary atresia, blood from both ventricles flows toward the aorta and the pulmonary vascular bed is supplied by reverse flow through the ductus arteriosus. Newborns rarely experience congestive heart failure; when they do, the pulmonary valve is probably absent.

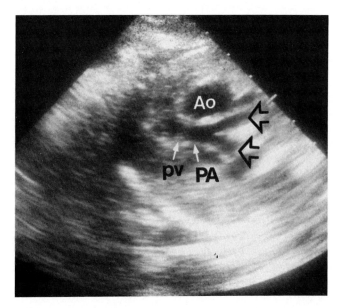

Figure 7–16. Pulmonic stenosis is a constant finding in tetralogy of Fallot. In this third-trimester fetus, a typically small pulmonary artery is seen (PA). The aortic root is relatively large. (pv = pulmonary valve; black outline arrows indicate the right and left pulmonary artery.) (Other abbreviations are identified in earlier figures.)

Tetralogy of Fallot can be diagnosed prenatally by visualizing the aorta overriding the ventricular septum (Fig. 7–17)[9,27] and by observing a greatly enlarged ascending aorta on real-time examination.

Transposition of the Great Arteries

In most cases of transposition of the great arteries (TGA), the aorta and pulmonary artery arise from the wrong ventricle, but atrioventricular blood flow is normal. Other types of transposition include transposition with an intact ventricular septum, with or without pulmonic stenosis; transposition with VSD; and transposition with VSD and pulmonic stenosis.[1]

Fetal echocardiography reveals that the two great vessels arise parallel from the base of the heart. As is shown in Figure 7–18, careful scanning allows identification of the aorta and pulmonary artery and their relationship to the ventricles. Transposition of the great arteries can be diagnosed by visualizing the moderator and papillary muscles, the insertion of the atrioventricular valves, and the structural characteristics of the ventricles. Pilu[1] states that the atrioventricular connection can be examined more closely by visualizing the systemic and pulmonary venous return. In addition, he points out that hemodynamic compromise in utero does not occur in the presence of uncomplicated complete TGA and that postnatal survival depends on the persistence of the fetal circulation.

Hypoplastic Left Heart Syndrome

In hypoplastic left heart syndrome (HLHS), any or all of the following may be hypoplastic, stenotic, or atretic: the left atrium, mitral valve, left ventricle, aortic valve, and the aorta. The right ventricle, right atrium,

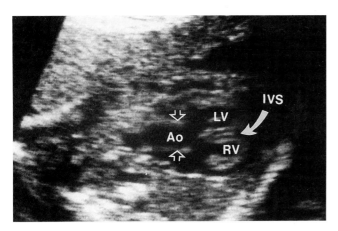

Figure 7–17. Tetralogy of Fallot. A large aortic root (Ao) is clearly seen overriding the ventricular septum (IVS) by almost 50%. (Other abbreviations are identified in earlier figures.) (*Reprinted with permission from Reece EA, Hobbins JC, Mahoney J, et al, eds. Medicine of the Fetus and Mother. Philadelphia: JB Lippincott, 1992.*)

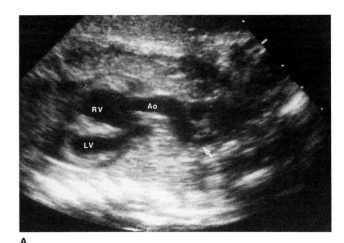

A

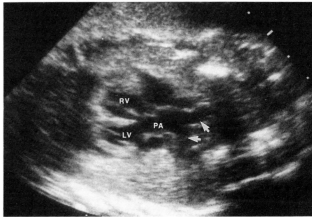

B

Figure 7–18. Evaluation of ventriculoarterial connections in a fetus with complete transposition of the great arteries. **(A)** The vessel that is connected to the right ventricle (RV) has a long upward course and gives rise to the brachiocephalic vessels (arrow). This finding allows one to identify this vessel with the aorta (Ao). **(B)** The vessel that arises from the left ventricle (LV) bifurcates (arrows), which indicates that this vessel is the pulmonary artery (PA). (*Reprinted with permission from Reece EA, Hobbins JC, Mahoney J, et al, eds. Medicine of the Fetus and Mother. Philadelphia: JB Lippincott, 1992.*)

and pulmonary artery are usually enlarged. This syndrome is frequently accompanied by an ASD, through which pulmonary venous return flows into the right atrium, and by a patent ductus arteriosus that feeds the descending aorta.[43]

The prognosis for HLHS is poor. Affected fetuses often succumb to heart failure, and most neonates, if untreated, die within a few days. Palliative procedures have been proposed, and long-term survivors have been reported.[44] In addition, heart transplants have been attempted in recent years.

Because ultrasound demonstrates the underdeveloped left ventricle and the incompletely developed or underdeveloped ascending aorta (see Fig.

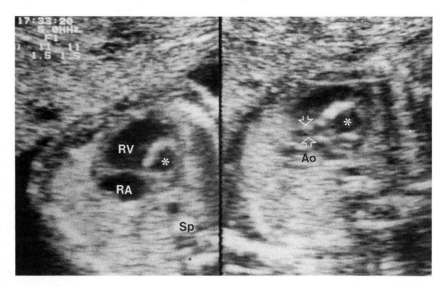

Figure 7–19. In this second-trimester fetus, the demonstration of a diminutive left ventricle (*) connected with an extremely small ascending aorta (Ao), within which Doppler ultrasound revealed no blood flow, prompted the diagnosis of hypoplastic left heart syndrome. (Other abbreviations are identified in earlier figures.) (*Reprinted with permission from Reece EA, Hobbins JC, Mahoney J, et al, eds.* Medicine of the Fetus and Mother. *Philadelphia: JB Lippincott, 1992.*)

7–19),[1,45,46] diagnosis is not difficult. If tricuspid insufficiency is present, Doppler may demonstrate retrograde blood flow in the ascending aorta and a systolic regurgitant jet within the right atrium.

Univentricular Heart

Two types of defects are grouped under the term univentricular heart: The first group is characterized by two atrial chambers that are connected to a main ventricular chamber by two atrioventricular valves or by a common atrioventricular valve (the "double-inlet" single ventricle). The second, relatively common, group is characterized by tricuspid or mitral atresia and thus an underdeveloped or absent ventricular chamber.[41] Prenatal diagnosis is relatively easy, and the hemodynamic alteration can vary from mild to severe (Fig. 7–20).

CARDIOMYOPATHIES

Cardiomyopathies generally are classified as either obstructive or nonobstructive. Both types tend eventually to produce congestive heart failure resulting from pump failure, valvular regurgitation, or both or from obstructed ventricular outflow. Although rare, heart failure in utero has been reported.[9,47] Most newborns are asymptomatic initially.

Inborn metabolic errors, muscular dystrophies, and infections are causes of the nonobstructive type. Diagnosis in utero requires echocardiographic documentation of cardiomegaly and poor contractility of the ventricle.[47]

Obstructive cardiomyopathies include hypertrophic cardiomyopathy in infants of diabetic mothers and asymmetric septal hypertrophy.[48] This type is as-

sociated with a thickening of the interventricular septum and free ventricular walls (see Fig. 7–21).[49,50]

OBSTETRICAL MANAGEMENT OF STRUCTURAL CONGENITAL HEART DISEASE

Because most cardiac defects such as VSDs, tetralogy of Fallot, and transpositions do not cause a significant degree of hemodynamic compromise until birth, vaginal delivery is not contraindicated, and corrective surgery usually produces positive results. If such defects are diagnosed before birth, the mother can be referred

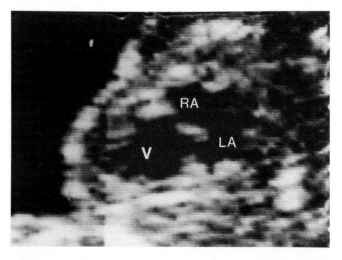

Figure 7–20. Double-inlet single ventricle in a second-trimester fetus. Two distinct atrioventricular valves are seen emptying into a single ventricular cavity (V). (Other abbreviations are identified in earlier figures.) (*Reprinted with permission from Reece EA, Hobbins JC, Mahoney J, et al, eds.* Medicine of the Fetus and Mother. *Philadelphia: JB Lippincott, 1992.*)

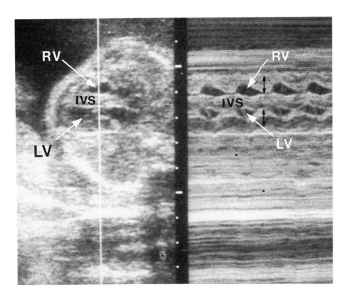

Figure 7–21. Hypertrophic cardiomyopathy in a second-trimester fetus. Thickened free walls of the ventricles and ventricular septum (IVS) are clearly demonstrated in both real-time and TM-mode sonograms. The size of the ventricular cavities (RV, LV) is significantly reduced. (*Reprinted with permission from Reece EA, Hobbins JC, Mahoney J, et al, eds.* Medicine of the Fetus and Mother. *Philadelphia: JB Lippincott, 1992.*)

to a tertiary institution for delivery and immediate neonatal care by a skilled perinatology/neonatology team. It remains unclear whether early diagnosis of severe defects that lead to heart failure in utero (eg complete AV block, complete atrioventricular septal defects, and cardiomyopathies) will improve the prognosis of these conditions.

In any case, in utero detection of cardiac lesions permits evaluation of the remainder of the fetal anatomy to exclude other structural malformations. Karyotypic analysis also is recommended. This additional information is extremely useful because it can dictate the types of obstetrical management required, including the mode of delivery.

CONCLUSION

Routine prenatal ultrasound examination should include, at the least, the four-chamber view of the heart. By so doing, the antenatal detection rate of dysrhythmias and structural cardiac lesions is expected to increase. This, in turn, is expected to improve the prognosis for many affected infants.

REFERENCES

1. Pilu G. Congenital heart disease and fetal echocardiography: In: Reece EA, Hobbins JC, Mahoney J, et al, eds. *Medicine of the Fetus and Mother.* Philadelphia, Pa: JB Lippincott; 1992:533–549.
2. Mitchell SC, Korones SB, Berendes HW. Congenital heart disease in 56,109 births: incidence and natural history. *Circulation.* 1971;43:323–332.
3. Hoffman JI, Christianson R. Congenital heart disease in a cohort of 19,502 births with long-term follow-up. *Am J Cardiol.* 1978;42:641–647.
4. Gerlis LM. Cardiac malformations in spontaneous abortions. *Int J Cardiol.* 1985;7:29–46.
5. Nora JJ, Nora AH. *Genetics and Counseling in Cardiovascular Disease.* Springfield, Ill: Charles C Thomas; 1978.
6. Nora JJ, Nora AH. Maternal transmission of congenital heart disease: new recurrence risk figures and the questions of cytoplasmic inheritance and vulnerability to teratogens. *Am J Cardiol.* 1987;59:459–463.
7. De Luca I, Ianniruberto A, Colonnan L. Aspetti ecografici del cuore fetale. *G Ital Cardiol.* 1978;8:776–784.
8. Kleinman CS, Hobbins JC, Jaffe CC, et al. Echocardiographic studies of the human fetus: prenatal diagnosis of congenital heart disease and cardiac dysrhythmias. *Pediatrics.* 1980;65:1059–1067.
9. Allan LD, Crawford DC, Anderson RH, et al. Echocardiographic and anatomical correlates in fetal congenital heart disease. *Br Heart J.* 1984;52:542–548.
10. Copel JA, Pilu G, Greene J, et al. Fetal echocardiographic screening for congenital heart disease: the importance of the four-chamber view. *Am J Obstet Gynecol.* 1987;157:648–656.
11. Allan LD, Joseph MC, Boyd EGCA, et al. M-mode echocardiography in the developing human fetus. *Br Heart J.* 1982;47:573–583.
12. DeVore GR, Donnerstein RL, Kleinman CS, et al. Fetal echocardiography, I. Normal anatomy as determined by real-time directed M-mode ultrasound. *Am J Obstet Gynecol.* 1982;144:249–260.
13. DeVore GR, Siassi B, Platt LD. Fetal echocardiography, IV. M-mode assessment of ventricular size and contractility during the second and third trimester of pregnancy in the normal fetus. *Am J Obstet Gynecol.* 1984;150:981–988.
14. St. John Sutton MG, Gewitz MH, Shah B, et al. Quantitative assessment of growth and function of the cardiac chambers in the normal human fetus: a prospective longitudinal echocardiographic study. *Circulation.* 1984;69:645–654.
15. Stewart PA, Tonge HM, Wladimiroff JW. Arrhythmias and structural abnormalities of the fetal heart. *Br Heart J.* 1983;50:550–554.
16. Huhta JC, Strasburger JF, Carpenter RJ, et al. Pulsed Doppler fetal echocardiography. *J Clin Ultrasound.* 1985;13:247–254.
17. Silverman NH, Kleinman CS, Rudolph AM, et al. Fetal atrioventricular valve insufficiency associated with nonimmune hydrops: a two-dimensional echocardiographic and pulsed Doppler ultrasound study. *Circulation.* 1985;72:825–832.
18. Reed KL, Sahn DJ, Scagnelli S, et al. Doppler echocardiographic studies of diastolic function in the human fetal heart: changes during gestation. *J Am Coll Cardiol.* 1986;8:391–395.

19. Kenny JF, Plappert T, Doubilet P, et al. Changes in intracardiac blood flow velocities and right and left ventricular stroke volumes with gestational age in the normal human fetus: a prospective Doppler echocardiographic study. *Circulation.* 1986;74:1208–1214.

20. Reed KL, Meijboom EJ, Sahn DJ, et al. Cardiac Doppler flow velocities in human fetus. *Circulation.* 1986;73:41–46.

21. Lingman G, Marsal K: Circulatory effects of fetal cardiac arrhythmias. *Pediatr Cardiol.* 1986;7:67–74.

22. Kenny JF, Plappert T, Doubilet P, et al. Effects of heart rate on ventricular size, stroke volume, and output in the normal human fetus: a prospective Doppler echocardiographic study. *Circulation.* 1987;76:52–59.

23. Machado MVL, Chita SC, Allan LD. Acceleration time in the aorta and pulmonary artery measured by Doppler echocardiography in the midtrimester normal human fetus. *Br Heart J.* 1987;58:15–18.

24. Allan LD, Anderson RH, Sullivan ID, et al. Evaluation of fetal arrhythmias by echocardiography. *Br Heart J.* 1983;50:240–245.

25. Kleinman CS, Donnerstein RL, Jaffe CC, et al. Fetal echocardiography: a tool for evaluation of in utero cardiac arrhythmias and monitoring of in utero therapy: analysis of 71 patients. *Am J Cardiol.* 1983;1:237–242.

26. De Vore GR, Siassi B, Platt LD. Fetal echocardiography, II. the diagnosis of cardiac arrhythmias using real-time directed M-mode ultrasound. *Am J Obstet Gynecol.* 1983;146:792–796.

27. Kleinman CS, Donnerstein RL, DeVore GR, et al. Fetal echocardiography evaluation of in utero congestive heart failure: a technique for study of non-immune fetal hydrops. *N Engl J Med.* 1982;306:568–575.

28. Kleinman CS, Copel JA, Weinstein EM, et al. In utero diagnosis and treatment of fetal supraventricular tachycardia. *Semin Perinatol.* 1985;9:113–129.

29. Griffiths SP. Congenital complete heart block. *Circulation.* 1971;43:615–619.

30. Chameides L, Truex RC, Vetter V, et al. Association of maternal systemic lupus erythematosus with congenital complete heart block. *N Engl J Med.* 1977;297:1204–1207.

31. McCue CM, Mantakas ME, Tingelstad JB, et al. Congenital heart block in newborns of mothers with connective tissue disease. *Circulation.* 1977;56:82–90.

32. Singsen BH, Akther JE, Weinstein MM, et al. Congenital complete heart block and SSA antibodies: obstetric implications. *Am J Obstet Gynecol,* 1985;152:655–658.

33. Carpenter RJ, Strasburger JF, Garson A, et al. Fetal ventricular pacing for hydrops secondary to complete atrioventricular block. *J Am Coll Cardiol.* 1986;8:1434–1439.

34. Rowe RD, Uchida IA. Cardiac malformation in mongolism: a prospective study of 184 mongoloid children. *Am J Med.* 1961;31:726–732.

35. Rudolph AM. *Congenital Disease of the Heart.* Chicago: Year Book Medical Publisher; 1974.

36. Hoffman JIE, Rudolph AM. The natural history of ventricular septal defects in infancy. *Am J Cardiol.* 1965;16:634–638.

37. Fink BW. *Congenital Heart Disease: A Deductive Approach to Its Diagnosis.* 2nd ed. Chicago: Year Book Medical Publisher; 1985.

38. Allan LD, Little D, Campbell S, et al. Fetal ascites associated with congenital heart disease: care report. *Br J Obstet Gynecol.* 1981;88:453–455.

39. Reynolds JL. Intrauterine growth retardation in children with congenital heart disease: its relation to aortic stenosis. *Birth Defects Original Articles Series.* 1972;8:143–148.

40. Huhta JC, Carpenter RJ, Moise KJ, et al. Prenatal diagnosis and postnatal management of critical aortic stenosis. *Circulation.* 1987;75:573–578.

41. Feigenbaum H. *Echocardiography.* 3rd ed. Philadelphia, Pa: Lea & Febiger; 1981.

42. Lev M, Rimoldi HJA, Rowlatt UF. The quantitative anatomy of cyanotic tetralogy of Fallot. *Circulation.* 1964;30:531–536.

43. Seward JB, Tajik AJ, Edwards WD, et al. *Two Dimensional Echocardiographic Atlas, I. Congenital Heart Disease.* New York, NY: Springer Verlag; 1987.

44. Norwood WI, Lang P, Hansen DD. Physiologic repair of aortic atresia—Hypoplastic left heart syndrome. *N Engl J Med.* 1983:308:23–27.

45. Sahn DJ, Shenker L, Reed KL, et al. Prenatal ultrasound diagnosis of hypoplastic left heart syndrome in utero associated with hydrops fetalis. *Am Heart J.* 1982; 104:1368–1372.

46. Silverman NH, Enderlein MA, Golbus MS. Ultrasonic recognition of aortic valve atresia in utero. *Am J Cardiol.* 1984;53:391–392.

47. Bovicelli L, Picchio FM, Pilu G, et al. Prenatal diagnosis of endocardial fibroelastosis. *Prenat Diagn.* 1984;4:67–72.

48. Walther FJ, Siassi B, King J, et al. Cardiac output in infants of insulin-dependent diabetic mothers. *J Pediatr.* 1985;107:109–114.

49. Stewart PA, Buise-Liem T, Verwey RA, et al. Prenatal ultrasonic diagnosis of familial asymmetric septal hypertrophy. *Prenat Diagn.* 1986;6:249–256.

50. Robero R, Pilu G, Jeanty P, et al. Cardiomyopathies. In: *Prenatal Diagnosis of Congenital Anomalies.* Norwalk, Conn: Appleton & Lange; 1987:178–180.

8

The Normal and Abnormal Fetal Spine

The Normal Fetal Spine

INTRODUCTION

Technical developments over the past decade have permitted better detection of fetal conditions prenatally.[1] Accurate prenatal diagnosis of defects involving the bony spine or the spinal cord, however, will require a thorough knowledge of the sonographic appearance of the normal fetal spine.

Three scanning planes are used in the evaluation of the fetal spine:[2] 1) sagittal plane (Fig. 8–1), 2) coronal plane, and 3) transverse plane (Fig. 8–2).

Sagittal plane. The spine appears as two parallel lines in the sagittal plane (Fig. 8–3, Fig. 8–4, and Fig. 8–5)

running from the base of the head to the sacrum, with the typical S-shape formation of the bony spine. The two parallel lines represent the articular facets of the vertebrae. The soft tissues behind the spine can be visualized in this plane.

Coronal plane. The fetal spine in the coronal plane appears as three parallel lines, with the additional third line representing the body of the vertebrae. The soft tissue can be seen on either side of the fetal spine in this plane.

Transverse plane. The neural canal appears as a closed circle in the transverse, or cross-sectional, plane of the

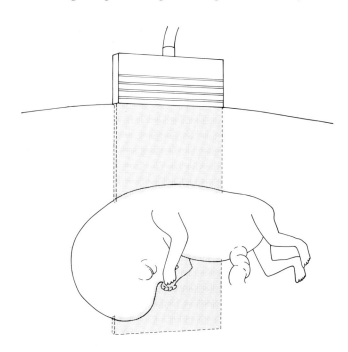

Figure 8–1. Diagrammatic representation of a fetus in the occipital–anterior position and sagittal scan of the fetal spine and back.

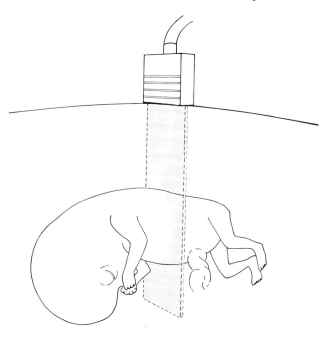

Figure 8–2. Schematic and sonographic representation of a transverse scan of the fetal abdomen. This view is best used to describe the abdominal circumference.

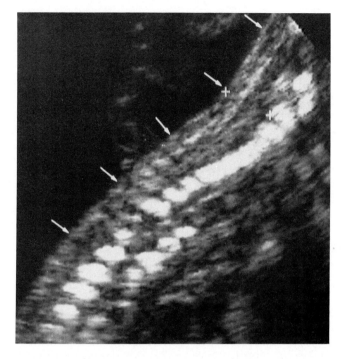

Figure 8–3. Second-trimester transabdominal ultrasound exam of the fetal spine demonstrating the echodense articular facets of the vertebral column in the cervical and thoracic areas. The calipers are placed at the levels of the neck(x's), and the small arrows outline the soft tissue and skin.

fetal spine. This canal is lined anteriorly by the ossified vertebral body and posteriorly by the ossified vertebral laminae. The three ossification centers of the vertebra (body and two lamina) give a triangular appearance covered by soft tissue (Fig. 8–6). The cross-sectional plane is the most informative (Fig. 8–7). Scanning of the spine should be done very carefully, from the level of the posterior fossa of the fetal head to the sacrum. The examiner should attempt to visualize

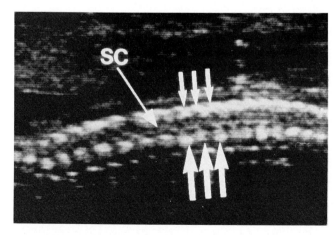

Figure 8–4. Sagittal ultrasound examination demonstrating a normal fetal spine. The groups of arrows indicate the articular facets that line up in a parallel pattern like a railroad track. The spinal cord (sc) can be seen within the spinal column.

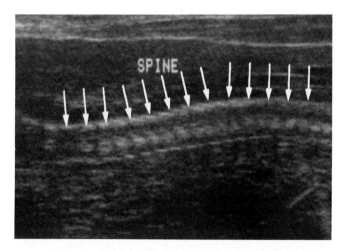

Figure 8–5. Normal scan of the fetal spine demonstrating the vertebral column of the fetus. The small arrows outline the soft tissue and skin of the fetal back, below which can be seen the vertebral bodies.

each vertebra of the spine, looking for continuity and general integrity.

Assessment of the fetal spine should also include a scan of the posterior fossa and observation of the general shape of the fetal head. The normal appearance of the cerebellum and head [3–6] and of the cisterna magna [7] provide additional information about spinal development. The status of the lateral ventricles can also be associated with spinal development.[8,9] Ventriculomegaly, for example, may be associated with spina bifida. Thus the morphologic and the biometric evaluation of the lateral ventricles should always be obtained.

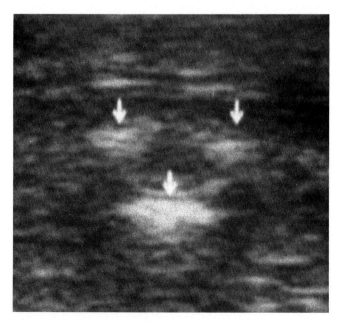

Figure 8–6. This cross-sectional view of the fetal spine demonstrates the central echolucent canal with the three surrounding ossification sites.

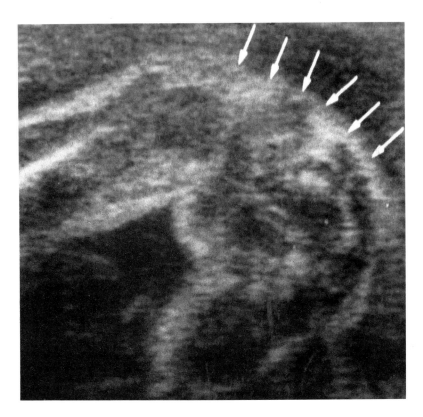

Figure 8–7. Transabdominal ultrasound scan of a fetus in the second trimester at the level of the buttocks and lower spine. This scan demonstrates the continuity of skin over these areas.

The Abnormal Fetal Spine

INTRODUCTION

One of the most common anomalies in spinal development is failure to close (spina bifida) with or without saccular protrusion of the spinal meninges or cord.[10] Spina bifida can be open (no skin covering) or closed (skin covering). The open variety is the most important and the most significant defect for the purposes of the prenatal diagnosis. The defect is usually located in the posterior or dorsal aspect of the vertebrae.

The dorsal defect of spina bifida can be open (aperta) or closed (occulta). Spina bifida occulta, characterized by small defects in the spine covered by skin, represents 15% of the cases. This condition is asymptomatic in most cases. Open spina bifida represents 85% of the cases. This defect is covered either by a thin membrane or is completely uncovered. The lesion frequently appears as a cystic sac containing the meninges (a meningocele) or containing the neural tissue (a myelomeningocele).[11]

Spina bifida is a fairly common malformation of the central nervous system. The incidence of this anomaly is variable, depending on factors, such as geographic location, ethnic origin, or seasonal variation.[10,12,13] It is common in the British Isles and uncommon in the Eastern world,[13] rare in blacks and orientals[14] and more frequent in whites; more frequent in December and January, and less common at other times of the year. Neural tube defects occur in 1.4 to 1.6 per 1,000 live births.[10] Approximately 6,000 infants with this lesion are born each year in the United States. Most defects of the neural axis are divided between spina bifida and anencephaly.[15,16]

Etiopathology

The central nervous system is derived from the neural plate, and the latter from dorsal ectoderm. At the 16th day after conception an invagination occurs, leading to the formation of the neural groove. At the 21st day the neural groove begins to close in the midportion of the embryo and advances caudally and rostrally. The rostral opening (rostral neuropore) of the spine closes at about day 24, while the caudal neuropore that corresponds to the lumbar area closes at about day 28. The two main causes of the formation of spina bifida are failure of closure of the caudal neuropore and an imbalance between the production rate and the reabsorption rate of the cerebrospinal fluid in the embryonic period. The absence of skin and muscles immediately above the defect results from failure of induction of the ectodermal and mesodermal tissue.[5,17–20]

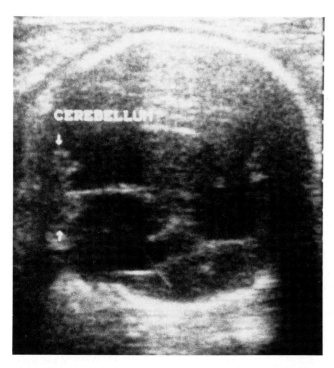

Figure 8–8. Scan of fetal head depicting subnormal transverse cerebral diameter (arrows).

The commonly accepted etiology for spina bifida appears multifactorial. This implies a genetic predisposition—probably due to several interacting genes—and other unknown environmental conditions or agents. There are geographic, ethnic, and racial variations in the frequency of these malformations. A neural tube defect may be one of a number of malformations present in fetuses and infants with chromosomal abnormalities. These abnormalities are observed in triploidy, trisomies 18 and 13, and in a number of cases involving partial duplication or deficiency of chromosomal segments.[10,21] Several malformation syndromes that include a neural tube defect follow a pattern of mendelian inheritance. Meckel's syndrome appears most commonly among these.

Almost all cases of open spina bifida are associated with abnormality of the posterior fossa, a condition called Arnold–Chiari type II malformation. This condition is characterized by herniation of the cerebellar vermis through the foramen magnum, causing the fourth ventricle to be displaced downward and posteriorly inside the neural canal.[22–24] This malformation often results in obstructive hydrocephaly secondary to lack of egress of the cerebrospinal fluid from the ventricular system.[8] The posterior fossa is usually shallow in these cases.[25–27] The pathogenesis of the Arnold–Chiari malformation is unclear. Several hypotheses about its etiology include tethering of the spinal cord with downward traction of the brain stem and cerebellum within the neural canal, overgrowth of the neural tissue, and a primary disturbance in the develop-

ment of the embryonic cerebellum.[25,28] Arnold–Chiari type II malformation results in hypoplasia of the cerebellum.[29] In an autopsy study of 100 infants with spina bifida, none had a cerebellar weight reaching the normal mean.[30]

Babcock and Han[9] reported that 23 of 29 infants had a small posterior fossa during the postnatal period. Goodwin and Quisling[7] documented a reduction in size of the cisterna magna and downward placement of the cerebellum within the cervical canal. Dislocation of the hip and foot are frequently seen in association with spina bifida, since the muscles corresponding to the involved peripheral nerves are affected.[31]

Prenatal Diagnosis
The first step in prenatal diagnosis is the sonographic assessment of the fetal head. Abnormalities of the posterior fossa in infants with spina bifida were described in the 19th century by Cleland, Chiari, Arnold, and Schwalbe and Greding.[25,32–34]

The transverse cerebellar diameter associated with spina bifida was found to be either below the normal size for the same gestational age or not visible (Fig. 8–8).[3] The cisterna magna is usually located posteriorly to the cerebellar vermis and is usually poorly visualized sonographically due to the low position of the cerebellum (Fig. 8–9 and Fig. 8–10). Nicolaides and Campbell[35] recently reported an abnormal configuration of the cerebellum, the "banana" sign and abnormal shape of the cranium, the "lemon" sign (Fig. 8–11).

Disappearance of one of the parallel lines in a

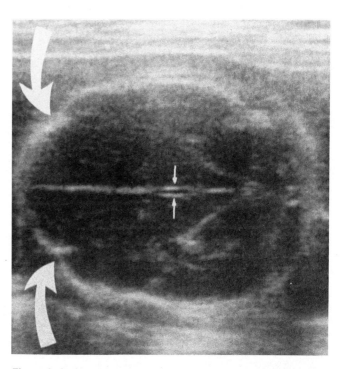

Figure 8–9. Abnormal configuration of fetal head depicting the "lemon" sign. Small arrows indicate third ventricle.

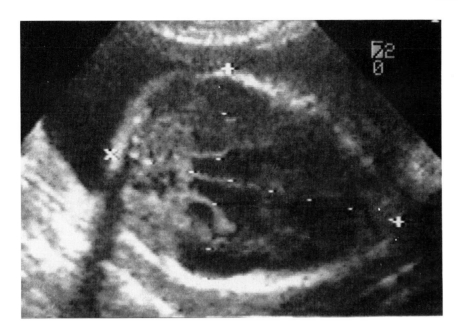

Figure 8–10. Scan depicting butterfly-like structure in posterior aspect of fetal head representing the cerebellum. The cisterna magna represents an echolucent space posterior and inferior to the cerebellum. With spina bifida the cisterna magna is often not seen.

sagittal scan plane of the fetal spine (Fig. 8–12 and Fig. 8–13) is highly indicative of a vertebral defect and should evoke a transverse evaluation at that site. If there is disappearance of the middle line or the "enlargement" of the spine, or widening of the two lateral or external lines during a coronal scan, the examiner should suspect an abnormality (Fig. 8–14 and Fig. 8–15).

The posterior ossification centers will be absent in a scan of the cross-sectional plane (Fig. 8–16 and Fig. 8–17). If spina bifida is present, it will form a typical v shape, u shape, or w shape. The skin and the muscles will also be absent. Scanning the fetus from the head to the sacrum repeatedly is desirable, since the examiner should be confident that enough sections of the fetal spine have been taken. If a defect is present, a scan will permit accurate determination of the level of the defect and the number of vertebrae affected. The more information the examiner obtains, the more information the parents will have. The cross-sectional plane is the most important for the detection of spina bifida. The spinal scan is sometimes difficult in breech presentation or oligohydramnios. A transvaginal scan, in addition to a transabdominal scan, can be informative. Instillation of physiologic water into the amniotic cavity can improve the image quality of the spine.

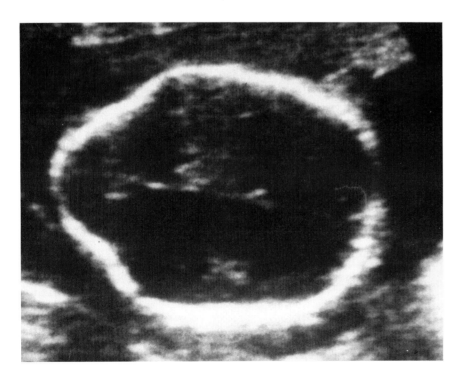

Figure 8–11. Scan of fetal head depicting a more pronounced "lemon" sign.

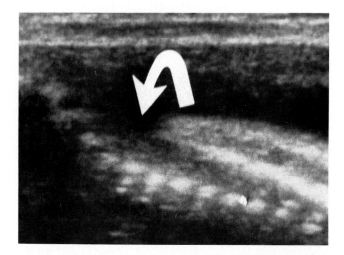

Figure 8–12. Sagittal scan of a second-trimester fetus by transabdominal ultrasound. This scan reveals the loss of one side of the vertebral column, as indicated by the curved arrow. These findings are indicative of a fetus with spina bifida.

In cases of spina bifida there may be paralysis of the corresponding pelvic organs.[31] For example, the lower extremities may be paralyzed and the bladder overdistended. Although these signs are not reliable, the recognition of clubfoot should increase the need to rule out fetal spine abnormality.

The detection of spina bifida in utero is one of the most difficult ultrasound diagnoses involving the central nervous system. These examinations are done, therefore, in special ultrasound laboratories by experienced sonographers and sonologists.

Maternal serum alpha-fetoprotein has become a routine test during pregnancy in many states, aiding in the identification of fetuses with ventral or dorsal wall defects or both.[36–39] This test, however, has a high false-positive rate. Investigators have reported different accuracies for the prenatal diagnosis of spina bifida. Allen et al[36] cites patients at high risk for neural tube defect, a diagnostic rate of 87% for ongoing affected cases. Robert et al.[6] in two studies, one performed between 1977 and 1980, found a sensitivity of 30%, and in the other study done in the following 3 years found a sensitivity of 80%. (Table 8–1)

Spina bifida is a severe congenital anomaly[40–42] (Fig. 3–1 and Fig. 8–18) with a stillbirth rate of 25%.[11]

TABLE 8–1. ACCURACY OF ULTRASOUND IN THE PRENATAL DIAGNOSIS OF SPINA BIFIDA

Reference	n	Prevalence	Sens	Specifi	PPV	NPV
Allen et al[36]	374	2.1	87	99	87	99
Roberts et al[6]	1,261	1.4	30	96	92	99
Roberts et al[6]	1,991	1.7	80	99	80	99
Persson et al[37]	10,147	0.1	40	100	100	99

Sens = sensitivity, Specifi = specificity, PPV = positive predictive value, NPV = negative predictive value.

Most affected and untreated infants die within the first few years of life.[28] At 7 years of age 40% of the treated infants were available for evaluation. Twenty-five percent of these infants were totally paralyzed; 25% almost totally paralyzed; 25% required intense rehabilitation; and only 25% had no significant lower limb dysfunction. Seventeen percent of the infants at late follow-up had normal continence.[11,28] Thus, an effort

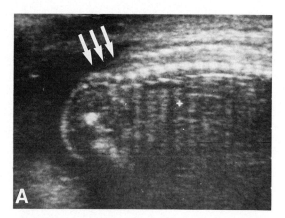

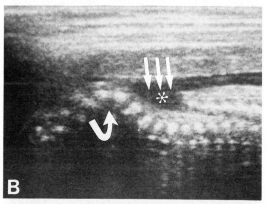

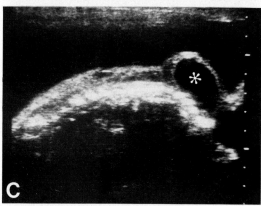

Figure 8–13. Transabdominal ultrasound examination of a fetus in the second trimester of pregnancy depicting neural tube defects at different levels of the spine. **(A)** A lumbosacral defect. Three small arrows point to the absence of the anterior aspect of the vertebral column. **(B)** A lumbar defect is indicated by three small arrows and an asterisk. The curved arrow refers to an abnormal curvature of the lumbosacral region. **(C)** A cervical mengingocele is indicated by an asterisk.

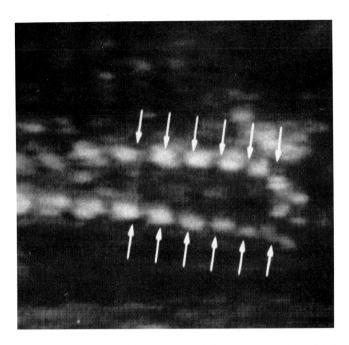

Figure 8–14. Second-trimester transabdominal scan of the fetal spine demonstrating a suspicious lumbar area, as outlined by the small arrows. Note the divergence of the articular facets to form a larger lumen in the lower area compared with the upper area. These findings suggest a neural tube defect.

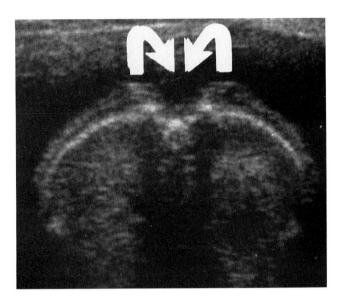

Figure 8–16. Cross-sectional view of a fetus suspected of having a neural tube defect on longitudinal scan. This scan reveals a V-shaped defect as indicated by double curved arrows. Not only is there lack of continuity of the spine in this view, but the skin is absent in this area.

should be made to define the defect in utero, not only qualitatively but also quantitatively. Prognostic signs include 1) the level of the defect, 2) the number of vertebrae involved, 3) deformity of the spine, 4) the severity of the hydrocephaly, and 5) the abnormality of the posterior fossa (Fig. 8–19, Fig. 8–20, and Fig. 8–21).[43]

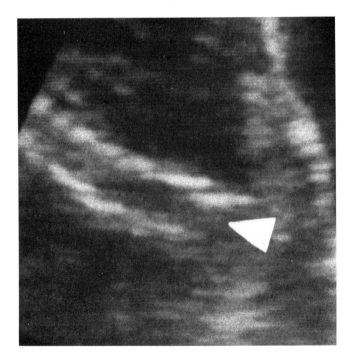

Figure 8–15. Second-trimester transabdominal examination of the fetal spine. It demonstrates a rather abrupt termination; the articular facets do not come to an apex as is normally seen in the sacral area. The arrowhead outlines the point of a neural tube defect at the level of the lumbosacral area.

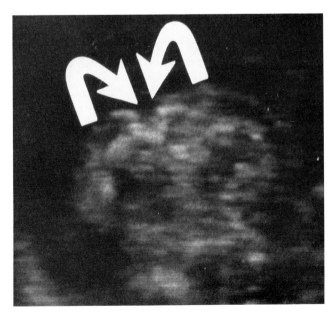

Figure 8–17. Cross-sectional scan of a second-trimester fetus using transabdominal ultrasound. The curved arrows indicate the open neural tube defect with loss of skin covering as well as bony and soft tissue covering in this area.

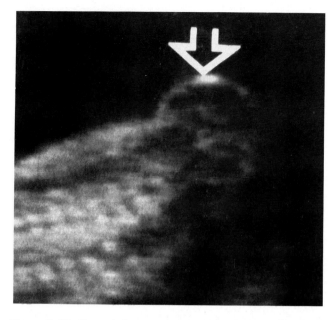

Figure 8–18. Second-trimester transabdominal ultrasound examination of a fetus with a mengingocele protruding from the lower spine (arrow).

Management and Outcome

Termination of pregnancy may be offered to parents if the diagnosis of spina bifida is made before viability. Otherwise, management should be cautious. In cases of isolated spina bifida diagnosed in the third trimester, the choice regarding mode of delivery and the follow-up sonographic examinations are important. In cases of spina bifida, a possible developmental hydrocephaly and macrocrania can result. Delivery thus should be accomplished when lung maturity is present. Delivery should be effected at term if spina bifida is isolated. Vaginal delivery may traumatize the neural cord with exposure of the neural elements to the infected delivery canal.[44–47] The ideal route of delivery has not been scientifically proven, however.

The most common risk factor is the family history. The recurrence risk is 1.7% to 1.8%.[21,48] When there are two affected siblings, risks for recurrence of neural tube defects rise from 5.7% to 12%.[2,49–52]

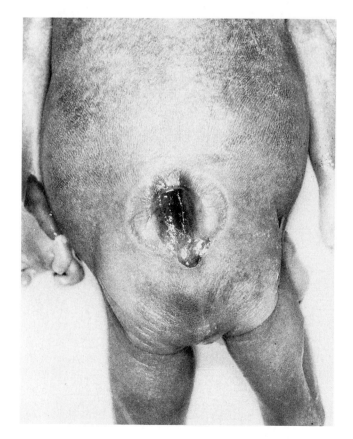

Figure 8–19. Gross examination of a malformed fetus with a lower lumbar neural tube defect involving about four vertebral segments.

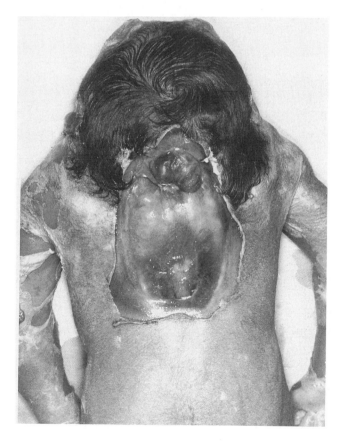

Figure 8–20. Gross examination of a malformed fetus with upper cervical–thoracic neural tube defect.

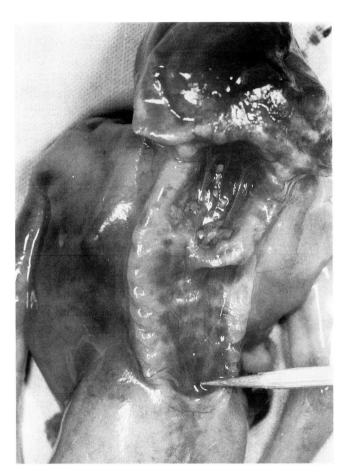

Figure 8–21. Gross examination of an abortus with a severe open neural tube defect extending from the lumbar region to the head. This type of severe deformity is referred to as a rachischisis. There is also abnormal curvature of the spine, causing severe lordosis and other skeletal deformities.

REFERENCES

1. Hobbins JC, Venus I, Tortora M, et al. Stage III ultrasound examination for the diagnosis of fetal abnormalities with an elevated amniotic fluid alpha-fetoprotein concentration. *Am J Obstet Gynecol.* 1982;142:1026–1029.
2. Milunsky A. Prenatal detection of neural tube defects: VI. Experience with 20,000 pregnancies. JAMA. 1980; 244: 2731–2735.
3. Goldstein I, Reece EA, Pilu F, et al. Sonographic evaluation of the normal developmental anatomy of fetal cerebral ventricles: I. The frontal horn. *Obstet Gynecol.* 1988;72:588–592.
4. McLeary RD, Kuhns LR, Barr M. Ultrasonography of the fetal cerebellum. *Radiology.* 1984;151:439–442.
5. Pearce JM, Little D, Campbell S. The diagnosis of abnormalities of the fetal central nervous system. In: Samders RC, James AE, eds. *The Principles and Practice of Ultrasound in Obstetrics and Gynecology.* Norwalk, Conn: Appleton-Century-Crofts; 1985:243–256.
6. Roberts, CJ, Hibbard BM, Roberts EE, et al. Diagnostic effectiveness of ultrasound in detection of neural tube defect. *Lancet.* 1983;2:1068–1069.
7. Goodwin L, Quisling RG. The neonatal cisterna magna: ultrasonic evaluation. *Radiology.* 1983;149:691–695.
8. Lorber J. Systematic ventriculographic studies in infants born with meningomyelocele and encephalocele: the incidence and development of hydrocephalus. *Arch Dis Child.* 1961;36:381.
9. Babcock DS, Han BK, Caffey award: cranial sonographic findings in meningomyelocele. *AJR.* 1981;136:563–569.
10. Main M, Mennuti MT. Neural tube defects: issues in prenatal diagnosis and counselling. *Obstet Gynecol.* 1986;67:1–16.
11. Blocklehurst G. Spina bifida. In: Vinken PJ, Bruyn GW, eds. *Handbook of Clinical Neurology.* vol 32. Amsterdam: Elsevier/North Holland; 1978:519–578.
12. Guthkelch AN. Studies in spina bifida cystica, III: seasonal variations in the frequency of spina bifida birth. *Br J Prev Soc Med.* 1962;16:159.
13. Laurence KM, Carter CO, David PA. Major central nervous system malformations in South Wales, I: Incidence, local variations and geographical factors. *Br J Prev Soc Med.* 1968;22:146.
14. Neel JV. A study of major congenital defects in Japanese infants. *Am J Hum Genet.* 1958;10:398.
15. Windham GC, Edmonds LD: Current trends in the incidence of neural tube defects. *Pediatrics.* 1982;70:333–337.
16. Alter M. Anencephalus, hydrocephalus, and spina bifida: epidemiology with special reference to a survey in Charleston. *Arch Neurol.* 1962;7:411.
17. Hamilton WJ, Boyd JD, Mossman HW. *Human Embryology.* 2nd ed. Baltimore, Md: Williams & Wilkins.
18. O'Rahilly R, Gardner E: The developmental anatomy and histology of the human central nervous system. In Vinken GW, Bruyn PJ, eds. *Handbook of Clinical Neurology.* vol 32. Amsterdam: Elsevier/North Holland, 1978:15–40.
19. Patten BM. Embryological stages in the establishment of myeloschisis with spina bifida. *Am J Anat.* 1953;93:365.
20. Gardner WJ. Myelomeningocele: the result of rupture of the embryonic neural tube. *Cleve Clin Q.* 1960;27:88.
21. Holmes LB, Driscoll SG, Atkins L. Etiologic heterogeneity of neural tube defects. *N Engl J Med.* 1976;294:365–369.
22. Naidich TP, Pudlowski RM, Naidich JB, et al. Computed tomographic signs of the Chiari II malformation, I: skull and dural partitions. *Radiology.* 1980;134:65–71.
23. Naidich TP, Pudlowski RM, Naidich JB. Computed tomographic signs of Chiari II malformation, II: midbrain and cerebellum. *Radiology.* 1980;134:391–398.
24. Naidich TP, Pudlowski RM, Naidich JB. Computed tomographic signs of the Chiari II malformation, III: ventricles and cisterns. *Radiology.* 1980;134:657–663.
25. Chiari H. Uber Veranderungen des Kleinhirns infolge von Hydrocephalie des Grosshirns. *Deutsch Med Wochenschr.* 1891;17:1172.
26. Penfield W, Coburn DF. Arnold-Chiari malformation and its operative treatment. *Arch Neurol Psychiatry.* 1938;40:328.
27. Carmel PW. Management of the Chiari malformations in childhood. *Clin Neurosurg.* 1983;30:385–406.
28. Lorber J. Results of treatment of myelomeningocele: an

analysis of 524 unselected cases, with special reference to possible selection for treatment. *Dev Med Child Neurol.* 1971;13:279–303.

29. Emery JL, MacKenzie N. Medullo-cervical dislocation deformity (Chiari II deformity) related to neurospinal dysraphism (meningomyelocele). *Brain.* 1973;96:155–162.

30. Variend S, Emery JL. The weight of the cerebellum in children with myelomeningocele. *Dev Med Child Neurol.* 1973;(Suppl 15)29:77–83.

31. Sharrad WJW. The mechanism of paralytic deformity in spina bifida. *Dev Med Child Neurol.* 1962;4:310.

32. Cleland J. Contribution to the study of spina bifida, encephalocele and anencephalus. *J Anat Physiol.* 1983;17:257.

33. Arnold J. Myelocyste, Transposition von Gewebskeimen und Sympodie. *Beitrage Pathol Anat.* 1894;16:1.

34. Schwalbe E, Gredig M. Uber Entwicklungsstorungen des Kleinhirns, Hirnstamms und Halsmarks bei Spina Bifida. *Beitrage Pathol Anat.* 1907;40:132.

35. Nicolaides KH, Campbell S, Gabbe SG, et al. Ultrasound screening for spina bifida: cranial and cerebellar signs. *Lancet.* 1986;2:72–74.

36. Allen LC, Doran TA, Miskin M, et al. Ultrasound and amniotic fluid alphafetoprotein in the prenatal diagnosis of spina bifida. *Obstet Gynecol.* 1982;60:169–173.

37. Persson PH, Kullande S, Gennser G, et al. Screening for fetal malformations using ultrasound and measurements of alpha-fetoprotein in maternal serum. *Br Med J.* 1983;286:747–749.

38. Polanska N, Burgess DE, Hill P. Screening for neural tube defect: false positive findings on ultrasound and in amniotic fluid. *Br Med J.* 1983;287:24.

39. Slotnick N, Filly R, Callen PW, et al. Sonography as a procedure complementary to alpha-fetoprotein testing for neural tube defects. *J Ultrasound Med.* 1982;1:319–322.

40. Mapstone TB, Rekate HL, Nielsen FE, et al. Relationship of CSF shunting and IQ in children with myelomeningocele: a retrospective analysis. *Child's Brain.* 1984; 11:112–118.

41. McCullough DC, Balzer-Martin LA. Current prognosis in overt neonatal hydrocephalus. *J Neurosurg.* 1982; 57:378–383.

42. McKeown T, Record RG. Malformations in a population observed 5 years after birth. In: Wolstenholme WGW, O'Connor CM, eds. *Ciba Found Symp Congenital Malformations.* London: Churchill; 1960:2–14.

43. Romero R, Pilu G, Jeanty P, et al. The central nervous system. In: *Prenatal Congenital Abnormalities.* Norwalk, Conn: Appleton & Lange 1988:1–11.

44. Chervenak FA, Duncan C, Ment L, et al. Perinatal management of meningomyelocele. *Obstet Gynecol.* 1984;63:376–380.

45. Ralis ZA. Traumatizing effect of breech delivery on infants with spina bifida. *J Pediatr.* 1975;87:613–616.

46. Ralis Z, Ralis HM. Morphology of peripheral nerves in children with spina bifida. *Dev Med Child Neurol.* 1972;14:109–112.

47. Stark G, Drummond M. Spina bifida as an obstetric problem. *Dev Child Neurol.* 1970;22(suppl 22):157

48. Janerich DT, Piper J. Shifting genetic patterns in anencephaly and spina bifida. *J Med Genet.* 1978;15:101–105.

49. Carter CO. Recurrence risks for common malformations *Practitioner.* 1974;213:667–674.

50. Cowchock S, Ainbender E, Prescott G, et al. The recurrence risk of neural tube defects in the United States: a collaborative study. *Am J Med Genet.* 1980;5:309–314.

51. Williamson EM. Incidence and family aggregation of major congenital malformations of the central nervous system. *J Med Genet.* 1965;2:161.

52. Smith C. Computer programs to estimate recurrence risks for multi-factorial familial disease. *Br Med J.* 1972;1:495–497.

9

The Fetal Abdomen

Normal Gastrointestinal Tract

INTRODUCTION

The ultrasound appearance of the normal fetal bowel is highly variable; however, there is considerable overlap between normal and abnormal patterns. Appreciation of the wide range of variation in the appearance of the gastrointestinal tract is important to ensure accurate interpretation of the ultrasound images. It is important to be familiar not only with the various pathologic entities detectable but also with the wide range of sonographic patterns attributable to the normal fetal bowel, to optimize interpretation of images of the fetal gastrointestinal system. Normal growth and development of the fetal stomach, small intestine, and colon are described here.

EMBRYOLOGY

The primitive gut forms during the fourth week of gestation and is divided into three parts: the foregut, the midgut, and the hindgut. The derivatives of the foregut are the esophagus, stomach, duodenum, pharynx, liver, pancreas, and lower respiratory tract.[1]

Esophagus. Initially the esophagus is very short, but it elongates rapidly, reaching its final relative length by about 7 weeks' gestation. Elongation of the esophagus results mainly from cranial body growth, that is, from ascent of the pharynx rather than from descent of the stomach.[2]

Stomach. The stomach first appears at about 4 weeks' gestation as a fusiform dilatation of the caudal part of the foregut. The latter enlarges and broadens ventrodorsally. At about 6 weeks' gestation it descends into the abdomen, and by about 11 weeks' gestation the muscles of the stomach are capable of contracting. The dorsal border grows faster than the ventral border of the greater curvature during the following weeks. The stomach slowly rotates 90 degrees in a clockwise di-

rection around its longitudinal axis as it acquires its adult shape.[1,3]

Duodenum. Early in the fourth week of gestation the duodenum develops from the caudal part of the foregut and the cranial part of the midgut. The junction and the two parts grows rapidly and form a C-shaped loop. The lumen of the duodenum becomes reduced and may be temporarily obliterated by epithelial cells during the fifth and sixth weeks of gestation, but it normally recanalizes by the end of the embryonic period.[3]

Small Intestine and Colon. The intestine elongates more rapidly than the embryo as a whole and begins to form a loop that protrudes into the umbilical cord during the 5- to 8-mm stage. The small intestine rotates around the axis of the superior mesenteric artery between the 8- and 16-mm stage. Subsequently, rapid elongation and coiling, beyond the capacity of the slower-growing abdominal cavity, force the bulk of the developing intestine into the umbilical cord, forming a physiologic umbilical herniation. At about 10 weeks of gestation the intestine reenters the abdominal cavity, which has gained in capacity not only in growth but also by regression of the mesonephros and reduced hepatic growth. The bowel elongates approximately 1,000-fold from the 5th to 40th weeks of gestation; the small intestine measures six times the length of the colon. The small intestine, at birth, is approximately three times the crown–heel length of the infant.[3]

The colon enters last into the abdominal cavity, with fixation of the cecum. Later development of the colon leads to elongation and establishment of the hepatic flexure and loose transverse colon.[3] The embryologic development of the colon occurs along with that of the small intestine. The cecum is identified in the seventh week of gestation and is followed closely by a period of rapid growth, elongation, and eventual fixation of the cecum in the right lower quadrant. The ascending colon and the hepatic flexure become distinct from the transverse colon as the liver decreases in size. The rectum is derived separately as a subdivision of the cloaca and joins the digestive tube by the eighth week of gestation. Failure to complete this union, as in the case of an imperforate anus, is associated with rectovaginal or rectovesicular fistula.[1,3]

SONOANATOMY

The Fetal Stomach

The fetal stomach is identified sonographically at the upper portion of the fetal abdomen. Goldstein et al[4] studied the fetal stomach with the earliest sonographic visualization possible at 9 weeks' gestation; measurements were consistently obtainable after 10 weeks of gestation. The fetal stomach could be seen as an echolucent organ that appeared elliptical on a longitudinal plane and spherical on a transverse plane. The characteristic anatomy of the stomach, including the greater curvature, the lesser curvature, the fundus, the body, and the pylorus, were identified at about 14 weeks' gestation. A prominent echodense structure was seen later at the lesser curvature of the stomach, representing the incisura angularis ventriculi.[4]

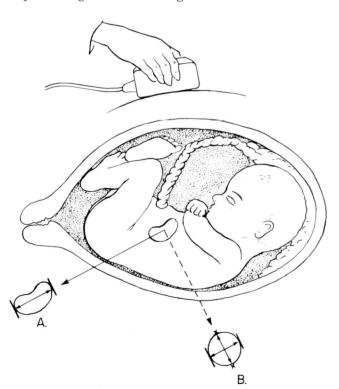

Figure 9–1. A schematic representation of a fetus undergoing ultrasound examination. **(A)** The longitudinal scan of the fetal stomach; **(B)** a cross-sectional view of this organ. (*Reproduced with permission from Goldstein I, Reece EA, Yarkoni S, et al. Growth of the Fetal Stomach in Normal Pregnancies. Obstet Gynecol. 1987;70:641–44.*)

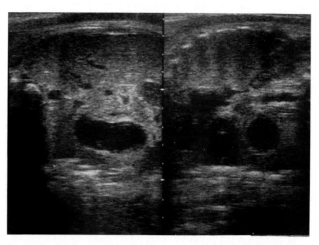

Figure 9–2. An ultrasound picture of a second-trimester fetus showing the stomach. Right: longitudinal view; left: cross-sectional view.

The fetal spine is identified after determination of the fetal position. The transducer is rotated into a cross-sectional plane until the fetal heart rate is visualized; then the transducer passes caudally, and the fetal stomach is identified in the upper portion of the abdomen.

Measurements are obtained in longitudinal, anteroposterior, and transverse planes, from outer-to-outer margins of the fetal stomach (Fig. 9–1, Fig. 9–2, Fig. 9–3, and Table 9–1).

Clinical Application

The fetal stomach must be seen in every sonographic examination. Inability to detect the fetal stomach by the very early second trimester should alert the examiner to the possibility of a noncommunicating type of esophageal atresia. A small fetal stomach may be vi-

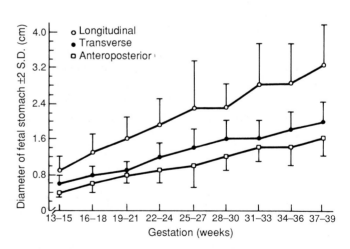

Figure 9–3. Figure depicting growth of the fetal stomach throughout pregnancy assessed by measurements in the longitudinal, transverse, and anteroposterior dimensions. (*Reproduced with permission from Goldstein I, Reece EA, Yarkoni S, et al. Growth of the Fetal Stomach in Normal Pregnancies. Obstet Gynecol. 1987;70:642.*)

TABLE 9–1. THE MEASUREMENTS OF THE DIAMETERS OF THE FETAL STOMACH ± 2 SD

Gestational Age (wk)	Anteroposterior (cm)		Transverse (cm)		Longitudinal (cm)			Volume	
	Mean	± 2 SD	Mean	± 2 SD	Mean	± 2 SD	n	Mean	± 2 SD
13–15	0.4	0.1	0.6	0.2	0.9	0.3	12	0.1	0.1
16–18	0.6	0.2	0.8	0.2	1.3	0.4	29	0.4	0.3
19–21	0.8	0.2	0.9	0.2	1.6	0.5	17	0.6	0.5
22–24	0.9	0.3	1.8	0.3	1.9	0.6	11	1.2	0.9
25–27	1.0	0.5	1.9	0.5	2.3	1.0	8	2.0	2.7
28–30	1.2	0.3	1.6	0.4	2.3	0.5	15	2.4	1.2
31–33	1.4	0.3	1.6	0.4	2.8	0.9	15	3.7	2.5
33–36	1.4	0.4	1.6	0.4	2.8	0.9	15	3.6	2.3
36–39	1.6	0.4	2.0	0.4	3.2	0.9	13	6.1	3.6

From Goldstein I, Reece EA, Yarkoni S, et al. Growth of the fetal stomach in normal pregnancies. Obstet Gynecol. 1987; 70:641–644, with permission.

sualized sonographically in communicating types of esophageal atresia and, possibly, in the noncommunicating types in which gastric secretions may distend this organ. A longitudinal study of the fetal stomach was attempted to assess the variability of the fetal stomach as a function of time. Serial evaluations of the fetal stomach size during a 3-hour period revealed that there were no significant changes in the fetal stomach dimension during this short period of time.[4]

The Fetal Small Intestine

The small intestine can be identified sonographically at 12 weeks' gestation as an echodense mass in the lower abdomen[5–7] (Fig. 9–4). Semi-quantitative evaluation of the nature of small-intestinal peristalsis was studied by Goldstein et al,[8] It was graded as follows:

Grade 0: Small-intestinal peristalsis is absent.
Grade I: There is sporadic small-intestinal peristalsis in one to three discrete areas, present for a short duration—less than 3 seconds.

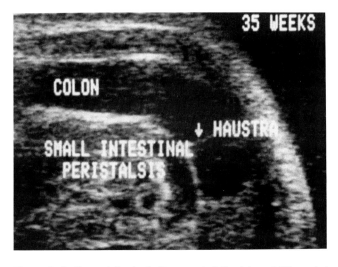

Figure 9–4. Transabdominal ultrasound of the fetus at 35 weeks' gestation; it demonstrates the colon, with its echodense pattern, outside of the small intestine.

Grade II: There are moderate waves of small-intestinal peristalsis in more than three discrete areas, present for a longer duration of greater than 3 seconds.
Grade III: Active waves of small-intestinal peristalsis are seen throughout the observational interval (Fig. 9–4).

In this study,[8] the authors visualized intestinal peristalsis sonographically as early as 18 weeks' gestation. Early peristalsis was characterized by sporadic and fleeting movements, with a duration of less than 3 seconds. Later peristaltic waves were more vigorous, ubiquitous, and of longer duration. The diameter of the loops of the small intestine is variable in dimension and in its changes during observation. There was a relationship between the activity of the small-intestinal peristalsis and gestational age. After 37 weeks' gestation the small-intestinal peristalsis was grade III in 80% of the cases. Grade II small-intestinal peristalsis, however, characterized 81% of fetuses of gestational age 33 to 34 weeks.[8]

The Fetal Colon

Semi-quantitative evaluation of the nature of the fetal colon was also studied by Goldstein et al.[8] The echogenicity of the colon was assessed and graded in comparison with the bladder and liver echogenicity:

Grade 0: The abdomen is uniform in appearance; the colon cannot be identified (Fig. 9–5).
Grade I: The colonic contents are echo-free in appearance. The echogenicity is essentially identical to that of the bladder and the stomach, and colonic haustra may be identified (Fig. 9–6).
Grade II: The echogenicity is intermediate, more dense than the bladder, but less than the liver (Fig. 9–7).
Grade III: The colonic contents are echodense, essentially equal to the echogenicity of the liver (Fig. 9–8 and Fig. 9–9).

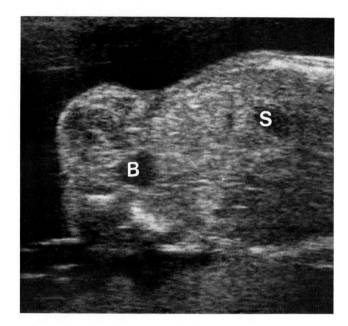

Figure 9–5. The colon is not clearly visualized. The bladder (B) and the stomach (S) can be seen. (Grade 0)

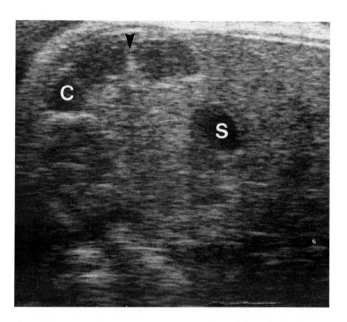

Figure 9–7. The stomach (S) is represented by an echolucent structure, and dilated loops of colon (C) with a heterogenous pattern (arrowhead) can be seen. The echogenicity of the bowel is intermediate; it is not as clear as that shown in grade I but is somewhat hazy in its appearance. This represents grade II.

Meconium first accumulates in the small bowel at 13 to 14 weeks of gestation, after which the distal segment of the small intestine begins to fill with meconium. The anal sphincter is closed at 22 weeks' gestation; therefore the colon is filled with meconium. By birth the entire colon is filled with 69 to 200 mL of meconium, presumably reflecting the variation in

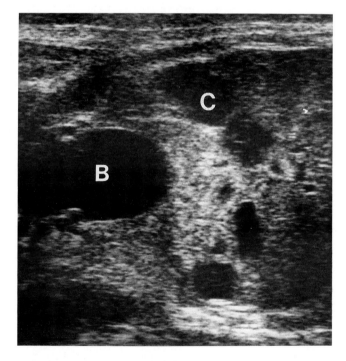

Figure 9–6. Ultrasound demonstrates the colonic grading system. The fetus is shown in a sagittal plane, with the bladder clearly seen as an echolucent structure in the lower pelvis. The echogenicity of the colon (C) and the bladder (B) are similar. This represents grade I.

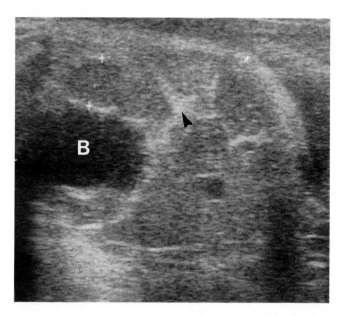

Figure 9–8. The echolucent cystic area represents the fetal bladder (B). The fairly echodense pattern of the fetal bowel (arrowhead) demonstrates the maturing pattern of the bowel from the rather echolucent appearance of grade I to the echodense state of grade III.

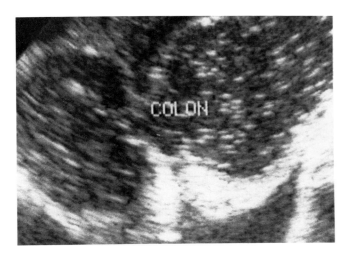

Figure 9–9. Transabdominal ultrasound of a third-trimester fetus depicting dilated colon with echodense material throughout the colon. These findings are indicative of meconium.

TABLE 9–2. TRANSVERSE COLONIC DIAMETER ACROSS GESTATIONAL AGE

Gestational Age (wk)	Percentile (cm)		
	10th	*50th*	*90th*
26	0.1	0.5	0.9
27	0.2	0.5	0.9
28	0.3	0.6	1.0
29	0.4	0.7	1.1
30	0.4	0.8	1.1
31	0.5	0.8	1.2
32	0.6	0.9	1.3
33	0.6	1.0	1.3
34	0.7	1.1	1.4
35	0.8	1.1	1.5
36	0.9	1.2	1.6
37	1.0	1.3	1.7
38	1.1	1.4	1.8
39	1.2	1.5	1.9
40	1.3	1.6	2.0
41	1.4	1.7	2.1
42	1.5	1.9	2.2

From Goldstein I, Lockwood C, Hobbins JC: Ultrasound assessment of fetal intestinal development in the evaluation of gestational age. Obstet Gynecol. 1987; 70:682, with permission.

echogenicity during gestation.[3] Despite the elasticity of the colon, the presence of active peristalsis, and the variable quantities of meconium, there appears to be a high degree of correlation between the maximal transverse diameter of the colon and the gestational age (Table 9–2). This presumably reflects the continual accumulation of colonic meconium that is not discharged into the amniotic fluid under physiologic circumstances. Abrupt sonographic appearance of haustra can be identified at 30 weeks' gestation, providing an independent marker for gestational age.[9]

The colon can be identified in the lower abdomen, usually close to the fetal bladder, and measurement can be obtained after 26 weeks' gestation. Measurements are obtained from the midpoints of colonic echogenicity (Fig. 9–8 and Fig. 9–10).

Clinical Application

A semi-quantitative characterization and evaluation of growth and the function of the small bowel and colon becomes an adjunct to standard biometric assessments of fetal gestational age. The normal pattern of growth and development can be applied in intestinal pathologic conditions, including Hirschsprung's disease, intestinal atresia, volvulus, intussusception, cystic fibrosis, and meconium ileus.

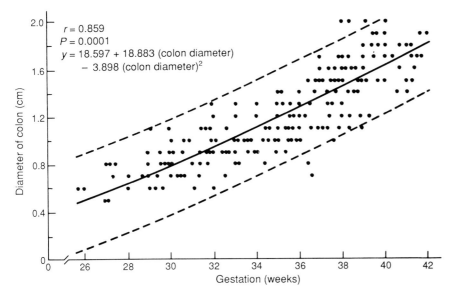

$r = 0.859$
$P = 0.0001$
$y = 18.597 + 18.883 \text{ (colon diameter)} - 3.898 \text{ (colon diameter)}^2$

Figure 9–10. The growth of the colon measured in width throughout pregnancy. This figure demonstrates a curvilinear relationship with time. (*Reproduced with permission from Goldstein I, Lockwood C, Hobbins JC. Ultrasound Assessment of Fetal Intestinal Development in the Evaluation of Gestational Age. Obstet Gynecol. 1987;70:682–686*)

REFERENCES

1. Moore KL. *The digestive system.* In: *The Developing Human: Clinically Oriented Embryology. 3rd ed.* Philadelphia, Pa: WB Saunders Co; 1982:227–230.
2. Arey LB. *Developmental Anatomy: The Digestive Tube and Associated Glands.* Philadelphia, Pa: WB Saunders Co; 1965: 249–262.
3. Grand RJ, Watkins JB, Tori FA. Development of human gastrointestinal tract. *Gastroenterology.* 1976;70:790–810.
4. Goldstein I, Reece EA, Yarkoni S, et al. Growth of the fetal stomach in normal pregnancies. *Obstet Gynecol.* 1987; 70:641–644.
5. Nyberg DA, Mack LA, Patten RM, et al. Fetal bowel: normal sonographic findings. *J Ultrasound Med.* 1987;6:3–6.
6. Zilianti M, Fernandez S. Correlation of ultrasonic images of fetal intestine with gestational age and fetal maturity. *Obstet Gynecol.* 1983;62:569–573.
7. Lee TG, Warren BH. Antenatal ultrasonic demonstration of fetal bowel. *Radiology.* 1977;124:471–474.
8. Goldstein I, Lockwood C, Hobbins JC. Ultrasound assessment of fetal intestinal development in the evaluation of gestational age. *Obstet Gynecol.* 1987;70:682–686.
9. Pace JL. The age of appearance of the haustra of the human colon. *J Anat.* 1981;109:75–80.

Fetal Liver

Fetal growth and development has been measured, and normal values have been established throughout gestation for various fetal body measurements. These parameters are used currently to evaluate pregnancies associated with aberrant fetal growth patterns, for ex-

ample, intrauterine growth retardation, macrosomia, and Rh sensitization. The first organ to be affected by such conditions is the fetal liver.[1] Fetal liver ultrasound measurements and some clinical applications are presented.

Embryology
The liver arises as a ventral bud from the foregut early in the fourth week of gestation. This hepatic diverticulum extends into the septum transversum as a rapidly proliferating cell. It soon enlarges and divides into two parts as it grows between the layers of the ventral mesentery. The liver grows rapidly and soon fills most of the abdominal cavity. The right and the left lobes are initially about the same size, but the right lobe eventually becomes much larger.

Sonoanatomy
The fetal liver can be imaged using the following technique: the fetal aorta is identified in the longitudinal plane; then the transducer is moved parallel to the plane until both the right hemidiaphragm and the tip of the right lobe of the liver is visualized. The fetal liver size is represented by the length of the liver from the tip of the right lobe to its base, where the right hemidiaphragm is used to reflect the same boundary (Fig. 9–11).

Clinical Application
In the assessment of fetal nutrition the most important measurement is the abdominal circumference, which reflects liver mass and the quantity of the subcutaneous tissue within the abdominal wall. A relationship between the abdominal circumference and fetal age and weight has been reported, and the abdominal circumference is shown to be the first measurement to be affected by asymmetric fetal growth retardation, causing a decrease in fetal mass.

The fetal liver undergoes rapid growth in the third trimester, while growth of most other fetal parameters slows considerably (Fig. 9–12). The fetal liver size can potentially be used as a marker to predict the growth-retarded fetus syndrome, and its measurement can differentiate the symmetric and asymmetric growth retardation patterns as well as evaluation of the early fetal effects of various abnormal maternal conditions. It is possible that ultrasonography-determined abnormalities of fetal liver size might precede the abdominal circumference changes that accompany fetal growth abnormalities. Investigators[1] reported a study of 16 fetuses with abnormal growth. Ten were growth-retarded (birth weight below the 10th percentile). The ultrasound fetal liver measurements were abnormally decreased in all growth-retarded fetuses, and abnormally increased in all the macrosomic fetuses. Direct liver measurements, however, are less routinely useful

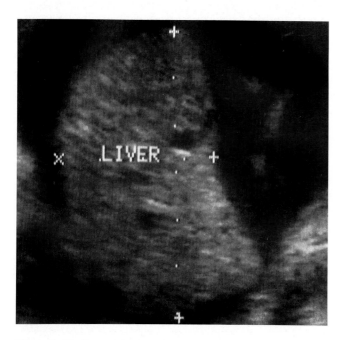

Figure 9–11. Scan of the fetal liver showing the precise outline. The calipers(+'s) indicate the limits of the organ measured in both length and width.

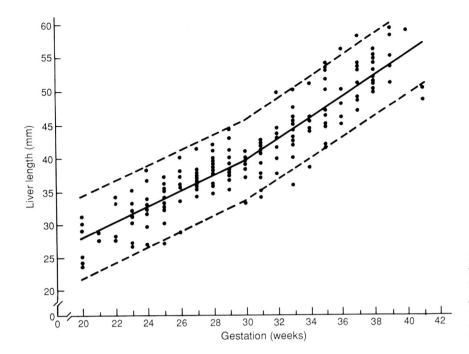

Figure 9–12. Figure depicting growth of the fetal liver throughout pregnancy as assessed by ultrasound measurements. (*Reproduced with permission from Vintzileos AM, Neckles S, Campbell WA, et al. Fetal liver ultrasound measurements during normal pregnancy. Obstet Gynecol. 1985;66:447.*)

than the traditional abdominal circumference measurements (Table 9–3).

In addition, both severe Rh sensitization and congestive heart failure of the fetus are conditions associated with hepatomegaly. In erythroblastosis fetalis the most sensitive and reproducible sonographic findings seem to be serial measurements of the fetal liver size.[2] One group[1] reported that the diagnosis of hepatomegaly occurred in fetuses with Rh sensitization without ascites or edema, while the abdominal circumference measurements were still within normal limits for gestational age.[3]

There are several common causes of intraabdominal calcification in the fetus. The most common condition is associated with meconium ileus,[4] a condition nearly always associated with cystic fibrosis.[5] Calcifications within the fetal liver can be caused in other conditions, such as transplacental infections, primary and metastatic tumors, and vascular accidents.[6–8] Most available information about causes of fetal liver calcification comes from a newborn series. Prenatal infections with cytomegalovirus,[6] herpes,[7] and toxoplasmosis[7] have been reported as causes of neonatal liver calcification. Benign and malignant childhood liver tumors are calcified.[8] Vascular accidents can also cause neonatal liver calcifications.[9] Note that some cases of liver calcifications have been associated with multiple anomalies, including aneuploidy.[9]

TABLE 9–3. ULTRASOUND MEASUREMENT* OF THE FETAL LIVER FROM 20 WEEKS' GESTATION TO TERM

Gestational Age (wk)	No. of measurements	Arithmetic mean (mm)	± 2 SD (mm)
20	8	27.3	6.4
21	2	28.0	1.5
22	4	30.6	6.7
23	13	30.9	4.5
24	10	32.9	6.7
25	14	33.6	5.3
26	10	35.7	6.3
27	20	36.6	3.3
28	14	38.4	4.0
29	13	39.1	5.0
30	10	38.7	5.0
31	13	39.6	5.7
32	11	42.7	7.5
33	14	43.8	6.6
34	11	44.8	7.1
35	14	47.8	9.1
36	10	49.0	8.4
37	10	52.0	6.8
38	12	52.9	4.2
39	5	55.4	6.7
40	1	59.0	
41	2	49.3	2.4

SD = standard deviation.
*Mean length ± 2 SD.
From Vintzileos AM, Neckles S, Campbell WA, et al. Fetal liver ultrasound measurements during normal pregnancy. Obstet Gynecol. 1985; 66:477, with permission.

REFERENCES

1. Vintzileos AM, Campbell WA, Storlazzi E, et al. Fetal liver ultrasound measurements in isoimmunized pregnancies. *Obstet Gynecol.* 1986;68:162–167.
2. Weiner S. *The Isoimmunized Pregnancy: Perinatal Medicine*

Management in the High Risk Fetus and Neonate. 2nd ed. Belognese RJ, Scwartz RH, Schneider J, eds. Baltimore, Md: Williams & Wilkins; 1978:267–289.

3. Hadlock FP, Deter RL, Harris RB, et al. Fetal abdominal circumference as a predictor of menstrual age. *AJR.* 1982;139:367–370.

4. Lince DM, Pretorius DH, Manco-Johnson ML, et al. The clinical significance of increased echogenicity in the fetal abdomen. *AJR.* 1985;145:683–686.

5. Muller F, Aubry MC, Gasser B, et al. Prenatal diagnosis of cystic fibrosis, II: meconium ileus in affected fetuses. *Prenatal Diagn.* 1985;5:109–117.

6. Alix D, Castel Y, Gouedard H. Hepatic calcification in congenital cytomegalic inclusion disease. *J Pediatr.* 1978; 92:856.

7. Shackelford GD, Kirks DR. Neonatal hepatic calcification secondary to transplacental infection. *Radiology.* 1977; 122:753–757.

8. Smith WL, Franken EA, Mitros FA. Liver tumors in children. *Semin Roentgenol.* 1983;18:136–148.

9. Friedman AP, Haller JO, Boyer B, et al. Calcified portal vein thromboemboli in infants: radiography and ultrasonography. *Radiology.* 1981;140:381–382.

THE FETAL SPLEEN

Embryology

The fetal spleen is a complex organ located in the left upper quadrant of the abdomen. This organ arises as an aggregation of reticular mesenchymal cells in the dorsal mesentery of the stomach between the sixth and seventh weeks' gestation. The left surface of the mesogastrium fuses with the peritoneum over the left kidney as the stomach rotates. The spleen acquires its characteristic shape early in the fetal period. Hematopoietic activity of the spleen begins by 12 weeks' gestation. After 24 weeks' gestation the bone marrow normally begins to produce hematopoietic cells; the liver and spleen concomitantly decrease their production. The splenic reticulum is infiltrated in later pregnancy by lymphocytes that multiply to form the lymph follicles.[1,2]

Sonoanatomy

The normal fetal spleen can be seen sonographically as a well-circumscribed echogenic mass. On a transverse or slightly oblique scan, the spleen is seen in the fetal abdomen below the diaphragm, lateral to the spine, and, depending on the fetal position, either anteriorly or posteriorly to the fluid-filled stomach. Anteriorly, the spleen reaches up to the midaxillary line. The spleen is homogeneous and echodense in appearance with an echogenicity similar to that of the liver. The diaphragm, spine, and stomach are useful landmarks for identification of the fetal spleen.

Schmidt et al studied the sonographic measure-

TABLE 9–4. FETAL SPLEEN DIAMETERS AND THE CALCULATED VOLUME AND PERIMETER

Gestational Age (weeks)	No. of Patients	Diameters (mm)									Volume (cm³)			Perimeter (mm)		
		Length			Sagittal			Transverse								
		15th	Mean	95th	15th	Mean	95th	5th	Mean	95th	5th	Mean	95th	5th	Mean	95th
18	2	0.7	1.4	2.1	0.3	0.8	1.1	0.4	0.9	1.3	—	0.7	0.73	2.3	3.5	4.7
19	3	1.2	1.6	2.3	0.4	0.8	1.2	0.4	0.9	1.4	0.4	0.9	1.4	2.7	3.9	5.1
20	3	1.1	1.8	2.6	0.5	0.8	1.2	0.5	1.0	1.5	0.5	1.0	1.5	3.3	4.5	5.7
21	2	1.2	2.0	2.7	0.5	0.9	1.3	0.6	1.1	1.6	0.8	1.3	1.8	3.5	4.7	5.9
22	3	1.5	2.2	2.9	0.6	1.0	1.3	0.7	1.2	1.6	1.2	1.7	2.2	4.1	5.3	6.5
23	4	1.6	2.3	3.1	0.7	1.0	1.4	0.8	1.2	1.7	1.4	2.0	2.5	4.5	5.7	6.9
24	3	1.9	2.5	3.2	0.7	1.1	1.5	0.8	1.3	1.8	1.6	2.2	2.8	4.9	6.1	7.2
25	3	1.9	2.6	3.3	0.7	1.1	1.5	0.9	1.4	1.9	1.9	2.5	3.1	5.3	6.4	7.7
26	3	2.0	2.7	3.4	0.8	1.2	1.5	1.0	1.5	1.9	2.1	2.8	3.5	5.5	6.7	7.9
27	5	2.2	2.9	3.7	0.9	1.3	1.7	1.0	1.5	2.0	2.0	3.0	4.1	5.9	7.1	8.3
28	3	2.4	3.1	3.8	1.0	1.3	1.7	1.1	1.6	2.1	2.2	3.4	4.6	6.2	7.4	8.6
29	3	2.5	3.3	4.0	1.0	1.4	1.8	1.2	1.7	2.1	2.4	3.8	5.3	6.5	7.7	8.9
30	4	2.7	3.4	4.1	1.1	1.5	1.9	1.3	1.7	2.2	2.6	4.3	6.1	6.9	8.1	9.3
31	4	3.0	3.6	4.3	1.2	1.5	1.9	1.3	1.8	2.3	2.9	5.0	7.0	7.3	8.5	9.7
32	3	3.1	3.8	4.5	1.2	1.6	2.0	1.4	1.9	2.4	3.3	5.7	8.1	7.7	8.9	10.1
33	3	3.3	4.0	4.7	1.3	1.6	2.0	1.5	2.0	2.4	3.8	6.6	9.2	8.1	9.3	10.5
34	4	3.5	4.3	5.0	1.3	1.7	2.1	1.6	2.0	2.5	4.5	7.6	10.7	8.6	9.8	11.0
35	4	3.8	4.5	5.2	1.4	1.8	2.2	1.6	2.1	2.6	5.2	8.8	12.3	9.1	10.3	11.5
36	5	4.1	4.8	5.5	1.5	1.9	2.2	1.7	2.2	2.7	6.1	10.1	14.1	9.7	10.9	12.1
37	6	4.4	5.1	5.8	1.5	1.9	2.3	1.8	2.3	2.7	7.3	11.8	16.2	10.4	11.6	12.8
38	3	4.7	5.4	6.2	1.6	2.0	2.3	1.8	2.3	2.8	8.6	13.6	18.6	11.1	12.3	13.4
39	3	5.1	5.8	6.5	1.7	2.0	2.4	1.9	2.4	2.9	10.1	15.6	21.1	11.8	13.0	14.2
40	3	5.5	6.2	7.0	1.7	2.1	2.5	2.0	2.5	2.9	11.8	17.9	24.1	12.7	13.8	15.1

From Schmidt W, Yarkoni S, Jeanty P, et al. Sonographic measurements of the fetal spleen; clinical implications. J Ultrasound Med. *1985; 4:667–672, with permission.*

ments of the fetal spleen.[3] They measured the longitudinal diameter of the spleen from the apex of the highest part lateral to the spine to the highest part close to anterior abdominal wall. The coronal diameter was measured at the level of the fetal stomach (Table 9–4).

REFERENCES

1. Kyriazis AA, Esterly JR. Development of lymphoid tissues in the human embryo and early fetus. *Arch Pathol.* 1970;90:348–353.
2. Moore KL. *The Developing Human: Clinically Oriented Embryology.* 3rd ed. Philadelphia, Pa: WB Saunders Co; 1982:203–206.
3. Schmidt W, Yarkoni S, Jeanty P, et al. Sonographic measurements of the fetal spleen: Clinical implications. *J Ultrasound Med.* 1985;4:667–672.

THE ADRENAL GLANDS

Embryology

The cortex and the medulla of the adrenal glands have different origins. The cortex develops from mesoderm, and the medulla forms from neuroectoderm. The cortex is first indicated by aggregation of mesenchymal cells on each side between the root of the dorsal mesentery and the developing gonad. The fetal cortex is derived from cells of the coelomic epithelium lining the posterior abdominal wall, whereas the cells that form the medulla are derived from an adjacent sympathetic ganglion, which, in turn, arises from the neural crest. These cells form a cellular mass on the medial side of the fetal cortex and are encapsulated by the fetal cortex, while the neural crest cells differentiate into the chromaffin cells of the adrenal medulla.[1]

Sonoanatomy

The adrenal gland of the human fetus is 10 to 20 times larger than the adult gland relative to body weight and is large compared with the kidneys. After birth, the adrenal glands decrease in size during the first 3 to 4 extrauterine months.

The fetal adrenals can be imaged because of their relatively large intrauterine size, and perhaps because of the relative paucity of the surrounding retroperitoneal fat. The in utero adrenal glands are triangular and can be imaged as early as 21 weeks of gestation (Fig. 9–13).[2]

The fetal adrenals can be identified by localizing the fetal kidneys in the axial plane as the transducer passes slightly more cephalad. They can be imaged as an ovoid mass, closer to the spine and placed slightly more anteriorly than the kidney. The transducer is turned 90 degrees in order to scan the long axis of the

fetal body through the flank. Once the scan plane is adjusted to allow identification of the long axis of the kidney, slight medial angulation of the transducer toward the spine allows adrenal gland identification. The normal structures identified adjacent to the fetal kidney and adrenals were the spine, abdominal aorta, and less frequently, the inferior vena cava.

Biometry

The length of the long axes of the fetal adrenal glands between 30 and 39 weeks' gestation measure 14 to 22 mm. Lewis[3] et al measured the fetal adrenal to kidney length ratio and found the range between 0.46 and 0.66.

Adrenal Pathology

Hyperplasia of the fetal adrenal cortex during the fetal period usually results in female pseudohermaphroditism. Congenital adrenal hyperplasia is caused by a genetically determined deficiency of adrenal cortical enzymes that are necessary for the synthesis of various steroid hormones. The reduced hormone output results in an increased release of adrenocorticotropic hormone (ACTH), which causes adrenal hyperplasia and overproduction of androgens by the hyperplasic adrenal glands. This causes masculinization in females. The excess androgens may cause precocious sexual development in males.

Sonographic studies of adrenogenital syndrome were reported on newborn infants.[4] The adrenals were found to be enlarged in three infants, at the upper

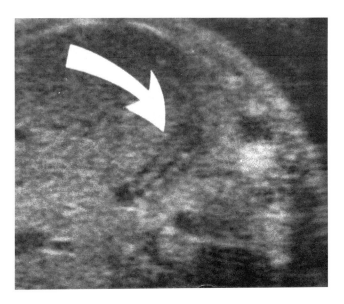

Figure 9–13. Cross-sectional view of the lower fetal abdomen at the level of the stomach. Curved arrow shows a narrow echodense structure bordered entirely by a thin echolucent line. This structure represents the fetal adrenal glands. Slight angulation upward, or cephalad, of the transducer brings the fetal kidney into focus.

limit of normal in three infants, and in two infants the adrenals were within the normal limits in size.[4]

REFERENCES

1. Moore KL. *The Developing Human: Clinically Oriented Embryology.* 3rd ed. Philadelphia, Pa: WB Saunders Co; 1982:269–271.
2. Rosenberg ER, Bowie JD, Andreotti RF, et al. Sonographic evaluation of the fetal adrenal glands. *AJR.* 1982; 139:1145–1147.
3. Lewis E, Kurtz AB, Dubbins PA, et al. Real-time ultrasonographic evaluation of normal fetal adrenal glands. *J Ultrasound Med.* 1982;1:265–270.
4. Bryan PJ, Caldamone AA, Morrison SC, et al. Ultrasound findings in adreno-genital syndrome. *J Ultrasound Med.* 1988;7:675–679.

Abnormal Gastrointestinal Tract

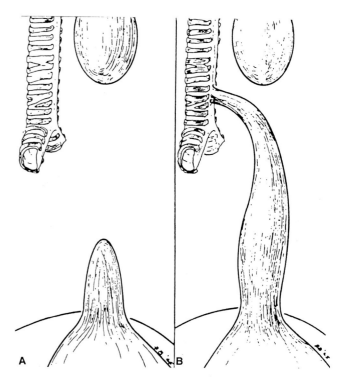

Figure 9–14. (A) A schematic representation of esophageal atresia. **(B)** With distal tracheoesophageal fistula. (*Reproduced with permission from Holder TM, Ashcraft KW. Esophageal Atresia. In: Bergsma D, ed.* Birth Defects Compendium, *2nd ed. New York: AR LISS; 1979:414.*)

INTRODUCTION

A wide variety of abnormalities of the fetal gastrointestinal tract can be detectable sonographically. The fetus swallows amniotic fluid and passes it into the gastrointestinal tract. Any obstruction along this tract, however, may result in impairment in the passage of amniotic fluid with dilatation proximal to the stenosis or the occlusion. The following are the main obstructive processes affecting the gastrointestinal tract:

1. Esophageal atresia and tracheoesophageal fistula
2. Duodenal atresia
3. Small-bowel obstruction
4. Meconium ileus and peritonitis
5. Large-bowel obstruction

Esophageal Atresia

Etiopathology
Esophageal atresia can result from failure of the esophagus to recanalize during the embryologic period, and it can also occur from deviation of the tracheoesophageal septum in the posterior direction. Esophageal atresia is associated with tracheoesophageal fistula[1] (Fig. 9–14) in 90% of cases.

Prenatal Diagnosis
The sonographic diagnosis of esophageal atresia is based on 1) the presence of polyhydramnios, associated with 2) inability to detect the fetal stomach (Fig. 9–15).[2]

The fetal stomach can be seen sonographically at 10 weeks' gestation,[3] and consistently from 12 weeks' gestation and beyond. Failure to see fluid in the stom-

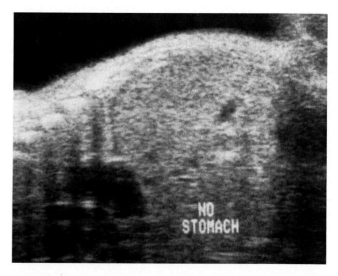

Figure 9–15. Fetus in the second trimester examined on a sagittal scan demonstrating the fetal chest with the ribs and the fetal heart, below which no stomach bubble can be identified. The findings suggest a diagnosis of esophageal atresia.

ach in normal fetuses is rare beyond this stage. Poly-hydramnios occurs in approximately 60% to 90% of gestations associated with esophageal atresia, but such a disorder accounts for only a small proportion of cases of polyhydramnios.[4] Although visualization of the stomach might be expected in cases of esophageal atresia associated with a tracheoesophageal fistula, the stomach, in fact, is not seen in up to one third of these fetuses. Thus, it seems that amniotic fluid flows into the stomach through some, but not all, fistulas.[5,6,7] The presence of polyhydramnios and the absence of the fetal stomach are the classic features of esophageal atresia; direct visualization of a dilated proximal esophageal pouch, which may be seen alternatively to fill and empty, and observation of fetal vomiting has been reported.[5,7]

Associated anomalies are present in 60% of cases of esophageal atresia. They include cardiac, chromosomal, gastrointestinal, genitourinary, and central nervous system lesions.[6,8,9] The VACTERL complex of vertebral, anal, cardiovascular, tracheal, esophageal, renal, and limb malformations is a well-known group of fetal malformations.[2,6]

Management and Outcome

A careful search for associated congenital anomalies is indicated. Fetal karyotyping and fetal echocardiography should be included. Termination of pregnancy may be offered to the parents before viability. After viability, no intervention is necessary, except amniotic fluid drainage in severe polyhydramnios.[6]

The prognosis of esophageal atresia with or without tracheoesophageal fistula depends on three factors: 1) associated anomalies, 2) respiratory complication, 3) gestational age and weight at delivery. In cases of isolated esophageal atresia and term delivery, the outcome is good. In cases of birth weights of more than 1,800 g and less than 2,500 g, however, or moderate respiratory complications, the mortality rate is approximately 40%. The survival rate is approximately 6% in cases of very low birth weight fetuses from severe respiratory complications.[6]

REFERENCES

1. Moore KL. The digestive system. In: The Developing Human: Clinically Oriented Embryology. 3rd ed. Philadelphia, Pa: WB Saunders Co; 1982:227–230.
2. Hertzberg B, Bowie JD. Fetal gastrointestinal abnormalities. Radio Clin North Am. 1990;28:103–105.
3. Goldstein I, Reece EA, Yarkoni S, et al. Growth of the fetal stomach in normal pregnancies. Obstet Gynecol. 1987; 70:641–644.
4. Eyheremendy E, Pfister M. Antenatal real-time diagnosis of esophageal atresias. J Clin Ultrasound. 1983;11:395–397.
5. Pretonius DH, Drose JA, Dennis MA. Tracheoesophageal fistula in utero: twenty-two cases. J Ultrasound Med. 1987; 6:509–513.
6. Romero R, Pilu G, Jeanty P, et al. Esophageal atresia with or without tracheoesophageal fistula. In: Prenatal Diagnosis of Congenital Anomalies, Romero R, Pilu G, Jeanty P, et al, eds. Norwalk, Conn: Appleton & Lange; 1982:235–236.
7. Bowie JD, Clair MR. Fetal swallowing and regurgitation: observation of normal and abnormal activity. Radiology. 1982;144:877–878.
8. Landing BH. Syndromes of congenital heart disease with tracheoesophageal anomalies. AJR. 1975;123:679–686.
9. Greenwood RD, Rosenthal A. Cardiovascular malformation associated with tracheoesophageal fistula and esophageal atresia. Pediatrics. 1976;57:87–91.

DUODENAL ATRESIA

Introduction

Duodenal atresia is the most common form of congenital small-bowel obstruction, with an incidence of 1 in 2,710 to 1 in 10,000 live births.[1] This lesion results either from incomplete recanalization of the duodenum or from external pressure from the pancreas or peritoneal bands.[2]

Etiopathology

The vast majority of the cases of duodenal atresia affect the second portion of the duodenum. The condition results from failure of luminal recanalization by the 11th week. At the fifth week of gestation the epithelial lining of the primitive duodenum rapidly proliferates, resulting in complete obliteration of the lumen by epithelial cells. Vacuoles appear subsequently and coalesce. Luminal patency is normally restored by the 11th week. Aberrant vacuolization presumably results in segmental obstruction or stenosis.[2]

Duodenal obstruction may be a consequence of processes extrinsic or intrinsic to the bowel. Extrinsic obstruction is rare in the duodenum. Duodenal obstruction, when present, results from compression by or rotation about aberrant blood vessels (anterior portal vein), or from peritoneal bands, produced by abnormal retroperitonealization.[3] Intrinsic obstructions are categorized into four major anatomic subgroups: 1) web 41%, 2) cordlike 38%, 3) mesenteric 5%, and 3) multiple 21%[3] (Fig. 9–16). The defects virtually always occur in the proximal duodenum and may be preampullary (24%), producing bilious meconium, or postampullary (76%), resulting in bilious gastric contents.[4] Incomplete formation can result in duodenal stenosis with partial patency and variable degrees of obstruction in web or cordlike defects. Stenosis accounts for 12% of congenital duodenal lesions. Annular pancreas in 20% of cases is found in association with type II cordlike duodenal atresia. It does not appear to have a

Type I (web or diaphragm)
Results from a mucosa-lined diaphragm in continuity with muscularis of proximal and distal segments of involved bowel

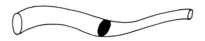

Type II (cordlike)
Proximal and distal lumens separated by fibrous cord

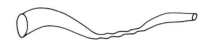

Type III (mesenteric)
Associated with mesenteric defects (IIIa)—Complete separation of proximal and distal lumens, with corresponding V-shaped mesenteric defect

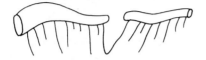

(IIIb)—Extensive small-bowel atresia from distal duodenum to proximal ileum, as consequence of superior mesenteric artery occlusion, giving appearance of long, spiraling "apple peel"

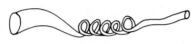

Type IV (multiple)
Multiple atretic secretions, generally diaphragmatic lesions

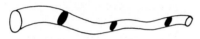

Figure 9–16. A schematic representation of the four types of congenital duodenal atresia. (*Reproduced with permission from Lockwood C. How to spot duodenal atresia. Cont.* Obstet Gynecol. *1986: 28:28*)

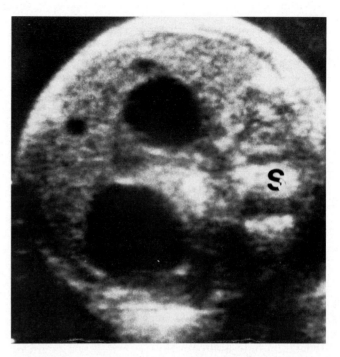

Figure 9–17. Transverse scan of the fetal abdomen demonstrating two echolucent structures representing the dilated fetal stomach and proximal duodenum. These findings are diagnostic of duodenal atresia. Note the spine (S) and the surrounding fluid in the periphery suggestive of polyhydramnios.

role in the formation of the duodenal lesion; instead it is a consequence of a common developmental field defect.[5]

The high incidence of associated malformations and chromosomal aneuploidy in fetuses with duodenal atresia supports the hypothesis that an early gestational insult is causal. Duodenal atresia was noted in a high proportion of fetuses exposed to thalidomide between 30th and 40th day of gestation, a critical period in duodenal differentiation.[6]

Prenatal Diagnosis
Antenatal diagnosis is simple and relies on the sonographic image of the "double-bubble" sign in the transverse section of the fetal abdomen (Fig. 9–17). This image results from dilatation of the stomach and duodenum proximal to the atretic area. A connection between the two bubbles must be demonstrated. Otherwise, one cystic mass such as a choledochal cyst or omental cyst might be seen in association with a large stomach and confused with duodenal atresia. The double-bubble sign indicates the presence of an obstructive process in the duodenum. A coronal scan of a normal stomach can produce, on occasion, an image similar to that of duodenal atresia because of the presence of a prominent incisura angularis. Transverse scans will demonstrate the depth of the incisura and solve this diagnostic problem.[7]

The double-bubble picture is not always present before 24 weeks' gestation, leading to false-negative diagnoses in the second trimester. A number of case reports have described fetuses that had normal sonographic findings before 24 weeks' gestation and hydramnios and bowel dilatation early in the third trimester. Jouppila and Kirkinen[8] reported the sonographic diagnosis of duodenal atresia in eight fetuses, all at or after 24 weeks' gestation. Miro and Bard[5] reported 26 cases of congenital duodenal atresia. The mean gestational age at prenatal diagnosis was 33.7 weeks of gestation (range 27 to 37 weeks). One of the cases was suspected at 20 weeks but was not confirmed until 35 weeks. Romero et al[9] reported 11 cases of duodenal atresia; the gestational age at diagnosis was between 22 and 36 weeks of gestation. Balcar et al[7] also reported a case where the diagnosis was made at 22 weeks' gestation. These reports conflict with others that suggest that even serial scans may fail to reveal the diagnosis until the third trimester.[4] These reports illustrate the possibility of making the diagnosis before the third trimester; exclusion, however, may not be entirely feasible.

Associated Anomalies
Duodenal atresia is associated with other anomalies in 23% to 48% of cases,[5,6] especially with Down syndrome and polyhydramnios. Moreover, in karyotyp-

ing otherwise normal fetuses with duodenal atresia there is increased incidence of other malformations. Vertebral anomalies are present in 37% of all cases; esophageal atresia with tracheoesophageal fistulas is associated in 7%; and congenital heart disease was reported in 36% of fetuses with duodenal atresia, particularly endocardial cushion or ventricular septal wall defects.[6] Polyhydramnios is associated with 44% of fetuses affected with duodenal atresia.

Management and Outcome

Once a positive diagnosis of duodenal atresia is made, a careful search for other anomalies is necessary. Early diagnoses of duodenal atresia decrease the delay before operating and morbidity from metabolic complications, such as dehydration, electrolyte imbalance, or aspiration pneumonia.[9] Karyotyping and fetal echocardiography are indicated in cases of duodenal atresia. Recognition of trisomy 21 before viability offers the parents the option of pregnancy termination. After viability, a diagnosis of trisomy 21 may not alter obstetric management, but the parents may benefit from knowing in advance that they have a chromosomally abnormal infant, and the pediatric team can be prepared to handle a sick child by making any necessary arrangements for surgery should that be needed.[9,10]

REFERENCES

1. Duenhoelter JH, Santos-Ramos, R. Rosenfeld CR, et al. Prenatal Diagnosis of Gastro-intestinal tract obstruction. Obstet Gynecol. 1976;47:618–620.
2. Moore KL. The Developing Human: Clinically Oriented Embryology. 3rd ed. Philadelphia, Pa: WB Saunders Co; 1982:232–233.
3. Fonkalsrud EW, deLorimier AA, Hays DM. Congenital atresia and stenosis of duodenum: a review compiled from members of surgical section of American Academy of Pediatrics. Pediatrics. 1969;43:79–83.
4. Aubrespy P, Derlon S, Seriant-Gautier B. Congenital duodenal obstruction: a review of 82 cases. Prog Pediatr Surg. 1978;11:109–124.
5. Miro J, Bard H. Congenital atresia and stenosis of duodenum: the impact of a prenatal diagnosis. Am J Obstet Gynecol. 1988;158:555–559.
6. Young DG, Wilkinson AW. Abnormalities associated with neonatal duodenal obstruction. Surgery. 1968; 63:832–836.
7. Balcar I, Grant DC, Bieber FA. Antenatal detection of Down's syndrome by sonography. AJR. 1984;143:29–30.
8. Jouppila P, Kirkinen P. Ultrasonic and clinical aspects in the diagnosis and prognosis of congenital gastrointestinal anomalies. Ultrasound Med Biol. 1984;10:465–472.
9. Romero R, Ghidini A, Costigan K, et al. Prenatal diagnosis of duodenal atresia: does it make any difference? Obstet Gynecol. 1988;71:739–741.
10. Nelson LH, Clark CE, Fishburne JI, et al. Value of serial sonography in the in utero detection of duodenal atresia. Obstet Gynecol. 1982;59:657–660.

ATRESIA AND STENOSIS OF THE SMALL INTESTINE

Introduction

The incidence of jejunal and ileal atresia has been reported as 1 in 330 to 1 in 1,500 live births,[1, 2] occurring more frequently than duodenal or colonic atresia.[3] It can be diagnosed sonographically because of the characteristic features of small-intestinal peristalsis and dilatation of the intestinal tract proximal to the atresia.

There are four types of obstructions: 1) type 1: a septum; 2) type 2: a fibrous strand; 3) type 3A: a mesenteric defect with or without a fibrous strand—the length of the bowel is subnormal; type 3B: the "apple peel" or "Christmas tree" atresia; 4) type 4: multiple obstructions.[1–3]

Most small-bowel atresias develop after organogenesis, such as duodenal atresia, which develops between the fifth and eighth week of gestation. The latter thus often occurs in combination with other congenital malformations.[4] Gastrointestinal anomalies are associated with other defects in approximately 45% of cases and include bowel malrotation (23%), intestinal duplication (3%), microcolon and esophageal atresia (3%). Extragastrointestinal anomalies are less frequent.[4–6]

Etiopathology

Narrowing, stenosis, obstruction, and atresia of the small intestine is probably caused by interruption of blood supply to the loop of the fetal intestine, which occurs during the 10th week of life when the intestines return to the abdomen.[7] This was confirmed by an experimental animal study, interfering with the blood supply of the fetal animal bowel, partly by ligation of the arterial branches supplying it and partly by creating strangulation. After 2 days, disintegration of the fetal bowel was observed. There was correlation between the diameter of the obstructed vessel and the extent of the atresia. A mobile loop of the intestine may become twisted, thereby interrupting its blood supply and leading to necrosis of the bowel involved. This segment later becomes a fibrous cord connecting the proximal and the distal ends of normal intestine.[2] Another possibility is failure of an adequate number of vacuoles to form during recanalization.[7]

Jejunal and ileal atresias are less frequently associated with nongastrointestinal malformations than is duodenal atresia, supporting the theory of a late onset fetal insult causing this obstruction. Occlusion of the fetal superior mesenteric artery or its major branches

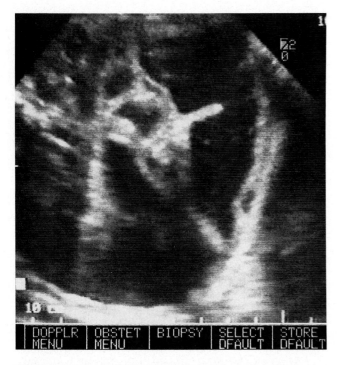

Figure 9–18. Excessively dilated loops of bowel are shown in a cross-sectional view. This finding is indicative of an obstructive lesion in the lower small intestine.

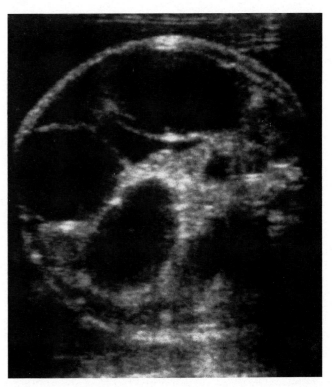

Figure 9–20. Dilated fetal bowel indicative of lower small-bowel obstruction or atresia.

can result in a severe apple peel (type IIIb) atresia extending from the distal duodenum to the proximal ileum[8,9] (Fig. 9–18 and Fig. 9–19). Vascular interruption, however, is generally not a cause of proximal duodenal lesions.

Prenatal Diagnosis

The diagnosis of fetal intestinal obstruction is characterized by consistently dilated sonolucent masses that occupy the fetal abdominal cavity asymmetrically (Fig. 9–20). Polyhydramnios is associated with intestinal

obstruction but is rare in distal obstructions[5] and upper gastrointestinal obstructive lesions.[5] Dilated loops filling the abdominal cavity suggest obstruction of the small bowel.[10–14] Extension of the loops into the pelvis is indicative of large-bowel obstruction. The differential diagnosis includes conditions capable of producing intra-abdominal echo-free images, such as ovarian or mesenteric cysts. The loops are seen on the sonogram to be extremely dilated, with active peristalsis and meconium floating inside the lumen of the intestinal loops. The abdominal circumference is above the

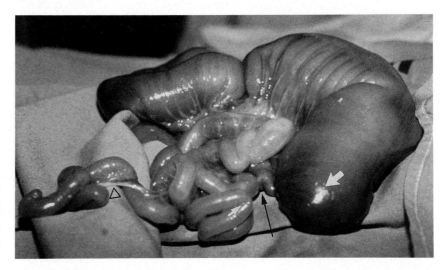

Figure 9–19. The atretic small bowel is shown by a small white arrow; the black outlined arrow indicates the small intestine distal to the obstruction, which appears to be otherwise normal, and the triangular arrowhead indicates atretic area of the small intestine. This finding is diagnostic of an apple peel atresia type IIIb.

95th percentile, and the head to abdominal circumference ratio is below the fifth percentile for the same gestational age. A careful examination of the stomach, bladder, and kidneys is necessary. In the second trimester, however, the colonic loops (grade 1) show increased echo-free pattern in the lower fetal abdomen, which is a normal characteristic image. The differential diagnosis between small- and large-intestinal obstruction is difficult. The examiner should suspect small-intestinal obstruction in virtually all such cases of bowel dilation, since small-intestinal atresia is more frequent than colonic obstruction.

Another possibility is determination of disaccharidase activity in the amniotic fluid.[13] This enzyme originates from the fetal bowel. The disaccharidase activity decreases if the lower part of the bowel is obstructed. This determination must be performed before the 22nd week of gestation because after this period the fetus stops defecating. Disaccharidase activity then drops abruptly.[4,13]

Management and Outcome

Although the intestinal loops are remarkably dilated and the abdominal circumference is above the 95th percentile, obstetrical management should be without early intervention. Term newborn infants with normal weights have a better prognosis. Vaginal delivery is preferable.

The most common cause of death of infants with jejunal atresia is infection related to pneumonia, peritonitis, sepsis, or leakage of the suture line, and disturbances of wound healing.[1,15] The prognosis depends on the site of the obstruction, the length of the remaining bowel, birth weight, meconium peritonitis, delayed diagnosis, and associated anomalies. The survival rate of proximal, distal, and midbowel atresia was reported by some authors to be between 62% and 100%.[2] The more distal the obstruction, the greater the prognostic improvement. An increase in mortality is observed with multiple atresia, apple peel variety of small-bowel atresia, and the atresia associated with meconium ileus or meconium peritonitis.

REFERENCES

1. Phelhan JT. Jejunal atresia and stenosis. *Pediatr Surg.* 1959;46:470–475.
2. De Lorimier A, Fonkalsrud EW, Hays DM. Congenital atresia of the jejunum and ileum. *Surgery.* 1969;65:819–827.
3. Evans CH. Atresia of gastrointestinal tract. *Surg Gynecol Obstet.* 1951;92:1–6.
4. Bergmans MGM, Merkus JMW, Baars AM. Obstetrical and neonatalogical aspects of a child with atresia of the small bowel. *J Perinatol Med.* 1984;12:325–329.
5. Flowers WK. Hydramnios and gastrointestinal atresia: a review. *Obstet Gynecol Survey.* 1983;38:685–688.
6. Delmer DL, Poynter CWM. Congenital occlusion of the intestines. *Surg Gynecol Obstet.* 1922;34:35–41.
7. Moore KL. *The Developing Human: Clinically Oriented Embryology.* 3rd ed. Philadelphia, Pa: WB Saunders Co; 1982:232.
8. Zivkovic S, Milosevlc VR. Duodenal and jejunal atresia with agenesis of dorsal mesentery: "apple peel" small bowel. *Am J Surg.* 1979;137:676–678.
9. Fletman D, McQuown D, Kanchanapoom V, et al. "Apple peel" atresia of the small bowel: prenatal diagnosis of the obstruction by ultrasound. *Pediatr Radiol.* 1980; 9:118–119.
10. Lyrenas S, Lindberg CB. Fetal jejunal atresia and intrauterine volvulus: a case report. *J Perinatal Med.* 1982; 10:247–248.
11. Bahgat O, Lev-Gur M, Divon MY. Prenatal ultrasound diagnosis of intestinal obstruction: a case report. *Am J Perinatol.* 1989;6:324–325.
12. Duenhoelter J, Santos-Ramos R, Rosenfeld C, et al. Prenatal diagnosis of gastrointestinal tract obstruction. *Obstet Gynecol.* 1976;47:618–620.
13. Morin PR, Potier M, Dallaire L, et al. Prenatal detection of intestinal obstruction: deficient fluid disaccharidases in affected fetuses. *Clin Genet.* 1980;18:217–222.
14. Jouppila P, Kirkinen P. Ultrasonic and clinical aspects in the diagnosis and prognosis of congenital gastrointestinal anomalies. *Ultrasound Med.* 1984;10:465–472.
15. Nixon HH, Tawes R. Etiology and treatment of small intestinal atresia. *Surgery.* 1971;69:41–51.

COLONIC ATRESIA

Introduction

Atresia or stenosis of the colon is a rare cause of intestinal obstruction, accounting for less than 10% of all atresias or stenoses of the bowel.[1,2] Meconium ileus appears to be the most common.

Etiopathology

Colonic atresia is believed to result from a local intrauterine vascular accident and not from a general disturbance in the development of the embryo. Associated anomalies are rare.[2]

Prenatal Diagnosis

The diagnosis of colonic stenosis or atresia is based on the detection of enlarged echo-free colonic loops in the lower abdomen, with active peristalsis of the small-intestinal bowel. The biometric measurement of the colon is above the 95th percentile. Polyhydramnios is more frequently present when the lesion is proximal. The abdominal circumference is above the 95th percentile, and the head to abdominal circumference ratio is below the fifth percentile. The fetal stomach and urogenital tract should be observed carefully.

Management and Outcome
The outcome is good.[2] The prenatal diagnosis is highly important for immediate treatment to the newborn.

REFERENCES

1. Coran AG, Eraklis AJ. Atresia of the colon. *Surgery.* 1969; 65:828–831.
2. Freeman NV. Congenital atresia and stenosis of the colon. *Br J Surg.* 1966;53:595–599.

MECONIUM ILEUS AND PERITONITIS

Introduction

The incidence of meconium peritonitis is approximately 1 in 35,000 live births,[1] and results from perforation of the gut in the prenatal or neonatal period. Extravasation of sterile meconium into the peritoneal cavity causes an intense peritoneal reaction, resulting in characteristic calcification.[1,2]

Etiopathology
Meconium is composed primarily of mucopolysaccharide and water, largely representing the residual of gastrointestinal secretion.[1] Swallowing of amniotic fluid begins in the 3-month-old fetus, leading to the eventual formation of meconium in the small intestine at 4 months of age.

The abnormal meconium causing the syndrome is formed as a result of two factors: 1) pancreatic insufficiency, causing deficient digestion of protein in normal meconium and; 2) excessive amounts of abnormal, tenacious mucus produced by the intestinal goblet cells. Meconium ileus appears in approximately 70% of patients with Hirschsprung's disease. Meconium peritonitis[3–5] is a complication of meconium ileus.

A wide spectrum of sonographic findings is associated with meconium peritonitis. Sterile meconium leads to formation of dense fibrotic tissue. The latter often calcifies, resulting in the characteristic intraperitoneal calcification identified by ultrasound, which depicts the calcification as a highly echogenic area in the abdomen or pelvis.[2]

Prenatal bowel perforation usually occurs proximal to the obstruction. Intestinal stenosis, or atresia and meconium ileus account for 65% of the cases. Other causes include volvulus, internal hernia, and Meckel's diverticulum.[3] Meconium escapes into the peritoneal cavity and forms a calcified mass at the site of the perforation, or spreads to cause a calcified fibroadhesive peritonitis, which may obliterate the peritoneal space.[5] If the bowel perforation remains patent, a cystic form of meconium peritonitis termed meconium pseudocyst may result.[2] Meconium pseudocyst forms secondary to continued spillage of intestinal contents into the cavity of the bowel loops and fibrous tissue matted around the perforation.

Prenatal Diagnosis
Meconium peritonitis results from perforation of the bowel in utero, with spillage of gastrointestinal contents into the peritoneal space. The sonographic image of meconium peritonitis reveals a calcified intra-abdominal mass, balloon-shaped structure with echogenic walls, or fetal ascites and peritoneal echoes.[2,5–7] Associated features of meconium peritonitis include polyhydramnios and fetal bowel obstruction.[4] Meconium peritonitis may give rise to intra-abdominal calcification and may take a variety of forms, depending on the time sequence of the perforation.

The differential diagnosis of a cystic mass in the fetal abdomen or pelvis is wide, including a possible ovarian cyst, pelvic teratoma, and omental cyst. Cystic fibrosis is associated with meconium peritonitis in approximately 40% of cases.[3]

Management and Outcome
Early clinical awareness allows preparation for complications of labor such as dystocia due to fetal abdominal distension, respiratory distress, and disseminated intravascular coagulation. These conditions commonly accompany massive fetal ascites; surgical repair of the bowel perforation (bacterial contamination of the sterile peritonitis may occur rapidly following birth); and testing to exclude cystic fibrosis.[3,8] The mortality rate of treated infants is 62%.[8]

REFERENCES

1. Hertzberg BS, Bowie JD. Fetal gastrointestinal abnormalities. *Radiol Clin North Am.* 1990;28:101–104.
2. McGraham JP, Hanson F. Meconium peritonitis with accompanying pseudocyst: prenatal sonograhpic diagnosis. *Radiology.* 1983;148:125–126.
3. Finkel LI, Solvis TL. Meconium peritonitis, intraperitoneal calcification and cystic fibrosis. *Pediatr Radiol.* 1982; 12:92–93.
4. Samuel N, Dicker D, Landman J, et al. Early diagnosis and intrauterine therapy of meconium plug syndrome in the fetus. *J Ultrasound Med.* 1986;5:425–428.
5. Dunne M, Haney P, Sun J. Sonographic features of bowel perforation and calcific meconium peritonitis in utero. *Pediatr Radiol.* 1983;13:231–233.
6. Nancarrow PA, Mattrey R, Edwards DK, et al. Fibroadhesive peritonitis: in utero sonographic diagnosis. *J Ultrasound Med.* 1985;4:213–215.
7. Brugman SM, Bjelland JJ, Thomasson JE, et al. Sonographic findings with radiologic correlation in meconium peritonitis. *J Clin Ultrasound.* 1979;7:305–306.
8. Blumenthal DH, Rushovich AM, Williams RK, et al. Prenatal sonographic findings of meconium peritonitis with pathologic correlation. *J Clin Ultrasound.* 1982;10:350–352.

ABDOMINAL WALL DEFECTS

Introduction

Defects of the abdominal wall are fairly easily identifiable by ultrasound. Each disorder is characterized by a distinct embryologic origin, gross appearance, and clinical presentation. A thorough understanding of these differences will aid in the interpretation of ultrasound findings and development of a perinatal management plan.

Omphalocele. Omphalocele, estimated to occur in approximately 1 in 5,800 live births, is defined as a membrane-covered herniation of intra-abdominal contents through a defect in the anterior abdominal wall, occurring at the site of umbilical cord insertion. The membrane is composed of amnion and peritoneum.[1-4]

Gastroschisis. Gastroschisis, a less frequent defect than omphalocele with an incidence ranging from 1 in 9,900 to 1 in 15,400, is a paramedian, full-thickness anterior abdominal wall defect. These defects are usually located to the right of a normally inserted umbilical cord. The absence of a covering membrane exposes abdominal viscera to the potentially irritating amniotic fluid.[3-5]

Etiopathology

Omphalocele. The critical process of transforming the flat trilaminar embryologic disk into the cylindrical fetus involves body folding, which occurs at 22 to 28 days postconception. The embryonic ectoderm is initially continuous with the amniotic ectoderm and forms the floor of the amniotic cavity, while the embryonic endoderm is contiguous with the yolk sac endoderm and forms the roof of the primitive yolk sac. The interposed mesoderm delaminates, or divides, to form the intraembryonic coelomic space. The lateral ventral mesoderm and underlying endoderm is designated as the splanchnopleure,[6] while the lateral dorsal mesoderm and overlying ectoderm form the somatopleure.

This period of embryogenesis is also marked by the excessive longitudinal growth of the embryo along the neural tube axis, creating cephalic and caudal bulges. Folding takes place along the three planes: cephalic, caudal, and lateral. The net effect is: 1) to close off the inner embryonic coelom, or peritoneal cavity, from the extraembryonic coelom, or chorionic cavity; 2) to allow the amniotic cavity to surround the growing embryo, obliterating the extraembryonic coelom; and 3) to develop the body stalk or umbilical cord.

Each fold gives rise to discrete anatomic structures. The splanchnic layer of the cephalic fold forms the primitive heart and superior foregut. The cephalic somatic layer produces the epigastric portion of the anterior abdominal wall, the anterior chest wall, and the primitive diaphragm. The caudal fold forms the primitive hindgut (splanchnic), hypogastrium, and urinary bladder (somatic). Lateral somatic folds give rise to the midabdominal wall. Failure of any of the folds to form appropriately results in distinct anatomic defects. Aberrant cephalic folding may result in any or all of the features of the pentalogy of Cantrell, including: 1) epigastric omphalocele, 2) defective lower sternum, 3) deficiency of the diaphragmatic pericardium, 4) defect in the ventral diaphragm, and 5) congenital intracardiac abnormalities. Caudal defects may produce any or all the features noted with so-called cloacal extrophy. The latter includes hindgut agenesis, bladder extrophy with intestinal fistulae, and hypogastric omphalocele.[6]

Gastroschisis. Multiple embryonic dysfunctions may account for the unique features of gastroschisis. The two principal theories suggest vascular compromise, abnormal umbilical vein involution, and intrauterine interruption of the omphalomesenteric artery.[6]

The human embryo initially bears both left and right umbilical veins. These vessels drain the abdominal wall and chorionic villi. There is involution of the right umbilical vein between 28 and 32 days postconception. Premature or delayed involution may lead to ischemia, with the resultant mesodermal and ectodermal defects.[6]

The omphalomesenteric arteries branch from the primitive dorsal aorta and extend to the right along the omphalomesenteric duct toward the yolk sac. The left omphalomesenteric artery involutes, while the right omphalomesenteric artery is transformed into the superior mesenteric artery superiorly. The terminal portion extends out into the extraembryonic coelom, now localized in the body stalk. Disruption of the distal segment could result in right-sided periumbilical ischemia and the paramedian defect observed in gastroschisis. Proximal disruption of the superior mesenteric artery may account for the high incidence of the jejunal atresia found in association with the gastroschisis.[6,7-9]

Prenatal Diagnosis

Omphalocele. The ultrasound diagnosis of the fetal omphalocele is based on the identification of the following features: 1) shallow abdominal cavity; 2) abdominal wall defect associated with a membranous sac, although in utero rupture may occur; 3) compact mass of normal intestinal loops within the sac and small-intestinal peristalsis can be seen; 4) high incidence of hepatic herniation; and 5) insertion of the umbilical cord into the apex of the membranous sac (Fig. 9–21 and Fig. 9–22).[5]

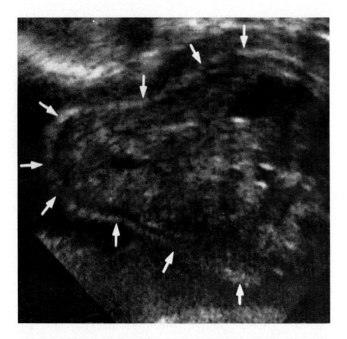

Figure 9–21. Transabdominal ultrasound exam of a fetus in a transverse, slightly oblique plane that reveals the stomach in the right lower area of the picture followed by herniation of the abdominal contents in the umbilical stalk. These findings are diagnostic of omphalocele. Note the membrane that surrounds the intra-abdominal contents without free-floating loops of bowel as seen in gastroschisis.

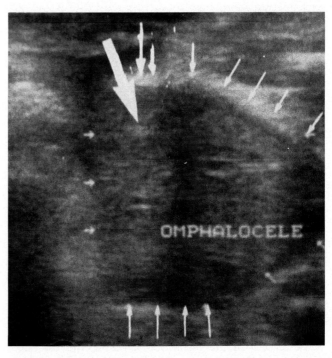

Figure 9–22. Transabdominal ultrasound examination of a fetus presenting with omphalocele.

Gastroschisis. Gastroschisis is characterized sonographically by the absence of a covering membrane and an umbilical cord insertion adjacent to the defect. The liver is rarely herniated, and the intestines have a characteristic "cauliflowerlike" appearance (Fig. 9–23). The bowel walls are highly echogenic, reflecting edema and inflammation (Fig. 9–24). The bowel may often be found floating freely in the amniotic cavity some distance from the fetal abdomen. Viewing the fetus with its right side toward the maternal spine allows observation of the umbilical cord insertion independent of the ventral wall defect, which is to the right of the cord insertion (Fig. 9–25, Fig. 9–26, and Fig. 9–27).

Associated Anomalies

Omphalocele. Associated anomalies include aneuploidy, congenital heart disease neural tube defect (6.5%), and pulmonary hypoplasia. Trisomy 13 and trisomy 18 may be associated with as high as a 40% incidence of omphalocele.[10] Cardiac defects are often severe; tetralogy of Fallot is the most frequent lesion identified.[11] Cephalic fold defects, including the complete pentalogy of Cantrell, are associated with a 78% mortality rate.[13] Associated anomalies must be

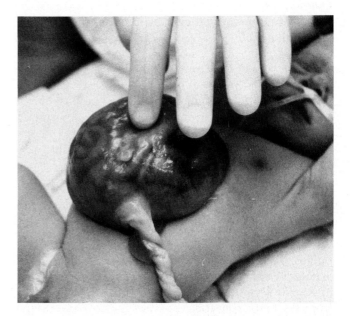

Figure 9–23. Infant lying supine with large cystic mass protruding from the abdomen and with the umbilical cord attached to the side of the fetal mass. These findings are diagnostic of an omphalocele, which represents the herniation of the intra-abdominal contents within the umbilical stalk. Failure of this physiologic bowel herniation to return to the abdomen results in this lesion. This condition is often associated with aneuploidy.

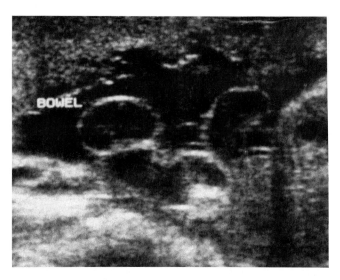

Figure 9–24. Ultrasound exam demonstrating the anterior placenta with free loops of bowel floating into the amniotic cavity. Findings are indicative of gastroschisis.

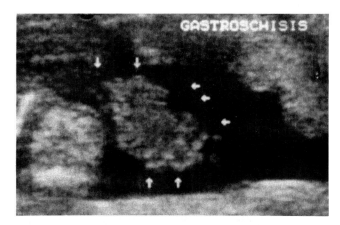

Figure 9–26. Transvaginal ultrasound exam of a fetus at 14 weeks' gestation demonstrating a cross-sectional view of the fetal abdomen; arrows demarcate a mass of free bowel loops. These findings are consistent with a diagnosis of gastroschisis. On a real-time ultrasound, bowel peristalsis may be seen.

searched for, including congenital heart defects, diaphragmatic hernia (cephalic fold defect), cleft lip and palate, polydactylism, and ectopic bladder and neural tube effect. Amniotic fluid acetylcholinesterase enzyme is usually present with neural tube defects and abdominal wall defects. The ratio of the acetylcholinesterase band to the pseudocholinesterase band in the electrophoretic gel is much lower for ventral wall defects than that observed with neural tube defects.[12] Enlargement of the tongue may be detected as can hepatosplenomegaly, making the diagnosis of Beckwith's syndrome more likely.[5]

Gastroschisis. Gastroschisis does not share the high association with major life-threatening congenital anomalies that is observed with omphalocele. There is,

however, a high frequency of intrauterine growth retardation. Meconium is commonly found in the amniotic fluid of these fetuses, but does not appear to be associated with fetal distress,[4] and probably reflects intestinal irritation.[4,14] At birth these infants have low serum albumin and total protein levels, possibly reflecting chronic sclerosing peritonitis[15] (Table 9–5 and Table 9–6).

Recurrence Risk

Omphalocele. The recurrence risk for isolated omphalocele is probably less than 1%. When omphaloceles are identified in association with trisomies, careful

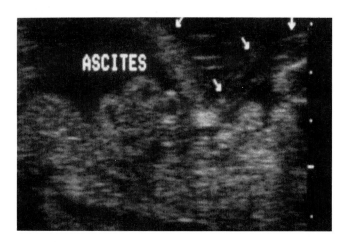

Figure 9–25. Transverse scan of the fetal abdomen demonstrating ascites within the abdominal cavity and herniation of the intraabdominal contents to the exterior.

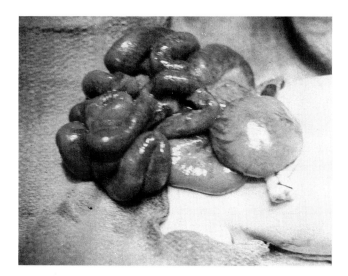

Figure 9–27. Fetus lying supine with a ventral wall defect and loops of bowel resting on the fetal legs. These finding are diagnostic of an omphalocele. The site of umbilical cord insertion is intact. In utero, the ventral wall defect is usually lateral to the cord insertion site, with egress of free loops of bowel into the amniotic fluid.

interpretation of the karyotype should exclude the possibility of balanced translocation, which could increase the recurrence risks to 10%.[16] The omphalocele of Beckwith–Wiedemann syndrome is accompanied by hypoglycemia, macroglossia, and enlargement of the abdominal viscera, including liver, pancreas, adrenal cortex, gonads, interstitial cells, and spleen.[17,18] While most cases are sporadic, an autosomal recessive inheritance pattern has been proposed. Familial clusters have been reported with omphalocele; inheritance patterns vary from autosomal to X-linked.[16]

Gastroschisis. Familial recurrence of gastroschisis has also been reported, and an autosomal dominant inheritance pattern, with variable expression from abdominal hernia to gastroschisis, is postulated.

Management and Outcome

If the diagnosis of omphalocele is suspected antenatally, amniocentesis for karyotyping as well as fetal echocardiography are recommended. Fetal heart rate testing should be initiated after 30 weeks' gestation in cases of gastroschisis because of the strong association with intrauterine growth retardation and in cases of omphalocele because of the high incidence of stillbirth and fetal distress in labor.

While there is no clear evidence to recommend either abdominal or vaginal delivery in pregnancies complicated by abdominal wall defects, possible advantages for abdominal delivery include the availability of maximal pediatric support and reduced risk of hepatic injury in cases of liver herniation with gastroschisis. Although there are theoretical advantages to abdominal delivery, many pediatric surgeons do not believe the delivery mode affects the outcome.

Omphalocele. The physical appearance of the neonate with omphalocele is remarkable. The umbilical cord dilates as it inserts into the shiny membrane-covered sac. The sac varies in size and may contain a single loop of bowel or the entire contents of the intraperitoneal cavity (Fig. 9–23).[14,19,20] Mortality is directly proportional to the size of the defect and to the presence and severity of associated anomalies.[11] Virtually all of the excess perinatal mortality in cases of omphalocele is a consequence of the high incidence of associated major congenital anomalies. The membranous sac protects the abdominal contents from the sclerosing effects of the amniotic fluid, simplifying the operative management of isolated omphalocele.

Gastroschisis. The gross appearance of gastroschisis (Fig. 9–27) differs markedly from that omphalocele due to lack of the covering membrane.[14,19] Contact with amniotic fluid results in intestinal edema, shortening, rigidity, and dilatation. The bowel is often matted together with the greenish "gelatinous matrix." The defect in gastroschisis is generally smaller (2 to 5 cm) than that observed with omphalocele (2 to 12 cm), and there is less risk for hepatic herniation (16% vs 47%). Mortality is independent size of the defect in gastroschisis.[11,21]

The etiology of jejunal atresia in association with fetal gastroschisis is uncertain. Proposed mechanisms include strangulation of the bowel secondary to small defect size, volvulus, and vascular interruption. Neonatal mortality in gastroschisis is primarily a consequence of gastrointestinal complications.[21]

The sonographic diagnosis of ventral wall defects is based on a careful visualization of the anterior abdominal wall. After the fetal position is determined the transducer is placed in a longitudinal plane, parallel to the fetal spine; then it is rotated at right angles, revealing a cross-sectional view. The motion of the fetal heart rate is seen; then the transducer passes caudally. The anterior abdominal wall is identified from the level of the four-chamber view of the heart, until the level of the fetal bladder is seen. Multiple cross-sectional planes are preferable to a longitudinal plane only. The most important view is the identification of the umbilical cord inserting into the anterior abdominal wall. If the fetus faces the maternal spine, the sonographer must wait until the fetus moves and the cord insertion is visible before considering the examination complete.

Patients are often brought to the clinician's attention because of elevated maternal serum alphafetoprotein, suspected fetal growth retardation, or an incidental finding on routine ultrasonography. Polyhydramnios is associated with intestinal obstruction if such is present; otherwise there are no other maternal complications associated with this condition.

Modern surgical techniques utilizing Silastic facial bridges have greatly improved the surgical management of infants with both omphalocele and gastroschisis. Meticulous neonatal management to avoid fluid loss, hypothermia of the bowel, or liver trauma, and the onset of sepsis have further improved survival. Optimal outcome, however, requires delivery at centers equipped to provide pediatric surgical intervention and intensive neonatal support.

Omphalocele. The prognosis in omphalocele is limited by the association of life-threatening congenital anomalies. Mortality is chiefly determined by the presence or absence of other anomalies. Proper antenatal surveillance and the identification of associated defects can expedite pediatric care and direct attention to the critical problem. Perinatal identification of trisomy 13 or 18, as well as anencephaly, allows termination or conservative management, since these disorders are incompatible with long-term survival.

Gastroschisis. Gastroschisis is seldom associated with non-gastrointestinal anomalies. Survival depends on neonatal management, appropriate surgical intervention, and the quality and quantity of the remaining bowel. Antenatal detection allows for delivery at appropriate tertiary facilities.

TABLE 9–5. ULTRASOUND DIAGNOSIS OF ABDOMINAL WALL DEFECTS

Omphalocele
1. Membranous sac enclosing abdominal contents
2. Umbilical insertion into omphalocele
3. Normal appearance of the bowel
4. High incidence of hepatic herniation
5. High incidence of associated anomalies

Gastroschisis
1. Absence of covering membrane
2. Insertion of the umbilical cord into normal portion of the abdominal wall
3. Echogenic bowel walls with distinct lumens assembled in a "cauliflower-like" arrangement
4. Bowel loops floating freely at a distance from the fetal abdomen

TABLE 9–6. CLINICAL PRESENTATION OF OMPHALOCELE AND GASTROSCHISIS

Characteristic	Omphalocele	Gastroschisis
Mean maternal age	25	20
Sex ratio M/F	1.6	1.1
Neonatal and infant mortality since 1970	34%	13%
Associated anomalies	60%	14%
Trisomies (13, 18, 21)	20%	0%
CHD	30%	5%
Intestinal abnormalities	11%	14%
Stillbirth rate	16%	5%
IUGR	20%	77%
Apgar score < 5	32%	8%

CHD = congenital heart disease, IUGR = intrauterine growth retardation.

Body Stalk Anomaly

Body stalk anomaly results in a severe abdominal wall defect, maldevelopment of the hindgut, and presence of a very rudimentary umbilical cord.

Etiopathology
During early intrauterine life the embryo is connected to the developing placenta by a body stalk composed of extraembryonic somatic mesoderm, two umbilical arteries, and one umbilical vein. The body stalk is intimately involved in the process of lateral body folding during the fourth to eighth weeks of embryonic life.

The umbilical cord is formed from both the body stalk and remnant yolk sac and covered by the amnion. Abdominal development of the body stalk might thus result in a severe abdominal wall defect, abnormal development of the hindgut, and the presence of a very rudimentary umbilical cord. The last two components differentiate this entity from the other two common body wall defects, gastroschisis and omphalocele. Agenesis or maldevelopment of a variety of abdominal organs derived from the hindgut are commonly seen with body stalk anomaly.

Body stalk anomaly is also associated with other anomalies. Mann[22] et al reported the occurrence of the skeletal and genitourinary abnormalities, intestinal atresia, neural tube defects, and cardiac anomalies in decreasing frequency.

Sonoanatomy
The diagnosis of body stalk anomaly should be strongly considered when there is a body wall defect or skeletal anomalies, such as severe lordosis and scoliosis of the spine, and when the umbilical cord is either absent or very rudimentary. The abdomen is extremely small, without a well-defined anterior abdominal wall. The liver and the intestine are in the membranous sac, which is attached to the placenta and the uterine wall. Intestinal peristalsis may be observed, and the umbilical cord is not visualized.

Management and Outcome
Since the body stalk anomaly is a lethal condition, even in the presence of normal chromosomes, termination of the pregnancy should be considered.

REFERENCES

1. Baird PA, MacDonald EC. An epidemiologic study of congenital malformations of the anterior abdominal wall in more than half a million consecutive live births. *Am J Hum Genet.* 1981;33:470–478.
2. deVries PA. The pathogenesis of gastroschisis and omphalocele. *J Pediatr Surg.* 1980;15:245–251.
3. Lindham S. Omphalocele and gastroschisis in Sweden 1965–76. *Acta Paediatr Scand.* 1981;70:55–60.
4. Carpenter MW, Curci MR, Dibbins AW, et al. Perinatal management of ventral wall defects. *Obstet Gynecol.* 1984;64:646–651.
5. Klein MD, Kosloske AM, Hertzler JH. Congenital defects of the abdominal wall. *JAMA.* 1981;245:1643–1646.
6. Moore KL. *The Developing Human: Clinically Oriented Embryopathy.* Philadelphia, Pa: WB Saunders Co; 1982:69–70.
7. Smith H. On the development of the superficial veins in the pig. *Am J Anat.* 1909;9:441–446.
8. Hoyme HE, Higginbottom MC, Jones KL. The vascular

pathogenesis of gastroschisis: intrauterine interruption of the omphalomesenteric artery. *J Pediatr.* 1981;98:228–231.

9. Hoyme HE, Jones MC, Jones KL. Gastroschisis: abdominal wall disruption secondary to early gestational interruption of the omphalomesenteric artery. *Semin Perinatol.* 1983;7:294–298.

10. Greenwood RD, Rosenthal A, Nadas AS. Cardiovascular malformations associated with omphalocele. *J Pediatr.* 1974;85:818–821.

11. Wald NJ, Barlow RD, Cuckle HS. Ratio of amniotic fluid acetylcholinesterase to pseudocholinesterase as an antenatal diagnostic test for exomphalos and gastroschisis. *Br J Obstet Gynaecol.* 1984;91:882–884.

12. Mayer T, Black R, Matlak ME, et al. Gastroschisis and omphalocele: an eight-year review. *Ann Surg.* 1980; 192:783–787.

13. Cantrell J, Haller J, Ravitch M. A syndrome of congenital defects involving the abdominal wall, sternum, diaphragm, pericardium, and heart. *Surg Gynecol Obstet.* 1958;107:602–609.

14. Seashore JH. Congenital abdominal wall defects. *Clin Perinatal.* 1978;5:61–77.

15. Meller JL, Reyes HM, Loeff DS. Gastroschisis and omphalocele. *Clin Perinatol.* 1989;16:113–122.

16. Czeizel A. Recurrence risk of omphalocele. *Lancet.* 1979; 2:470–473.

17. Beckwith J. Macroglossia, omphalocele, adrenal cytomegaly, gigantism and hyperplastic visceromegaly. *Birth Defects.* 1969;5:188–192.

18. Cohen M, Strom UL. Beckwith-Weidemann syndrome. In *Birth Defects: Compendium.* 2nd ed. Bergsma D, ed. New York, NY: Alan R. Liss; 1979:140–152.

19. Moore TC. Gastroschisis and omphalocele: clinical differences. *Surgery.* 1977;82:561–568.

20. Mahour GH, Weitzman JJ, Rosenkrantz JG. Omphalocele and gastroschisis. *Ann Surg.* 1972;177:478–482.

21. Kirk EP, Wah RM. Obstetric management of the fetus with omphalocele or gastroschisis: a review and report of one hundred twelve cases. *Am J Obstet Gynecol.* 1983; 146:512–518.

22. Mann L, Ferguson-Smith MA, Desai M., et al. Prenatal assessment of anterior abdominal wall defects and their prognosis. *Prenat Diagn.* 1984;4:427–435.

NONIMMUNE HYDROPS FETALIS

Introduction

Hydrops fetalis denotes generalized edema in a fetus; this condition may be accompanied by ascites, pleural effusion, pericardial effusion skin edema, abnormal thickness of the placenta, and polyhydramnios. It refers to a state of fetal hydrops in the absence of blood group incompatibility.

Incidence

The incidence of nonimmune hydrops fetalis is about 20%, compared with 85.7%[1] of all cases of fetal hy-

drops. It appears, however, that with the successful prophylaxis of Rh isoimmunization, the relative proportion of nonimmunologic hydrops fetalis has increased. The incidence of nonimmunologic hydrops fetalis varies from 1 in 3,478 to 1 in 7,000 live births.[2,3]

Etiopathology

Major fetal malformations are often present; they are frequently responsible for this condition. Investigators[2] found 44% of the cases were idiopathic, and 41% were associated with major malformations. The most common maternal complications in cases of nonimmune hydrops fetalis include polyhydramnios (75%), anemia (45%), preeclampsia (29%), and postpartum hemorrhage or difficulty in delivering the placenta (64%).[2]

Fetal edema and serous effusions have been associated with decreased osmotic pressure, anemia, and congestive heart failure in utero. Increased venous and capillary hydrostatic pressures resulting from chronic heart failure secondary to structural heart disease, arrhythmias, or anemia contribute to the development of the edema. Infants with anemia or infection may have increased capillary permeability due to chronic tissue hypoxia. There may also be decreased plasma colloid osmotic pressure secondary to hypoproteinemia. It is often difficult to confirm the cause-and-effect relationship in most cases, since none of these factors has been singularly or uniformly related to the formation of the edema (Table 9–7).[4]

Cardiovascular Disorders. The largest group of disorders of nonimmune hydrops fetalis that result in generalized edema in utero is cardiac failure: by obstruction, increased work secondary to shunting, arrhythmia, or abnormal contractility. A variety of congenital heart defects have been associated with nonimmune hydrops. Anomalies include those of the tricuspid and pulmonic valves, premature closure of the foramen ovale, atrioseptal and ventriculoseptal defects, tetralogy of Fallot, and hypoplastic heart. Other factors associated with nonimmune hydrops include intrauterine cardiac arrhythmias, disorders of myocardial contractility, congenital myocarditis, neoplasms, and congenital vascular tumors.[2,4–15]

Hematologic Disorders. Fetal anemia from a variety of causes, including hemolytic disease, chronic anemia associated with hypoproteinemia, alpha-thalassemia, and glucose-6-phosphate dehydrogenase deficiency, may cause nonimmune hydrops fetalis. Anemia severe enough to result in heart failure and hydrops may also result from acute intrauterine hemorrhage in the fetus.[4,7,9,16]

Pulmonary Disorders. Intrathoracic lesions, presumed to obstruct the return of blood to the heart,

TABLE 9–7. NONIMMUNE HYDROPS FETALIS: CAUSES AND ASSOCIATIONS

Hematologic
  Homozygous alpha-thalassemia
  Chronic fetomaternal transfusion
  Twin-to-twin transfusion (recipient or donor)
  Multiple gestation, with "parasitic" fetus
Cardiovascular
  Severe congenital heart disease (atrial septal defect, ventricular septal defect, hypoplastic left heart, pulmonary valve insufficiency, Ebstein's subaortic stenosis)
  Premature closure of foramen ovale
  Myocarditis
  Large arteriovenous malformation
  Tachyarrhythmias: paroxysmal SVT, atrial flutter
  Bradyarrhythmias: heart block
  Fibroelastosis
Pulmonary
  Cystic adenomatoid malformation of lung
  Pulmonary lymphangiectasia
  Pulmonary hypoplasia (diaphragmatic hernia)
Renal
  Congenital nephrosis
  Renal vein thrombosis
Intrauterine infections
  Syphilis
  Toxoplasmosis
  Cytomegalovirus
  Leptospirosis
  Chagas' disease
  Congenital hepatitis
Congenital anomalies
  Achondroplasia
  E trisomy
  Multiple anomalies
  Turner syndrome
Miscellaneous
  Meconium peritonitis
  Fetal neuroblastomatosis
  Dysmaturity
  Tuberous sclerosis
  Storage disease
  Small-bowel volvulus
Placental
  Umbilical vein thrombosis
  Chronic vein thrombosis
  Chorioangioma
Maternal
  Diabetes mellitus
  Toxemia
  Idiopathic

SVT = supraventricular tachycardia.
From Etches PC, Lemons JA. Non-immune hydrops fetalis: report from 22 cases including three siblings. Pediatrics. 1979; 64:326, with permission.

appear to be associated with nonimmune hydrops fetalis.[4,9]

Renal Disorders. Hydrops fetalis is occasionally reported with urinary obstruction (such as urethral or ureteral stenosis), congenital nephrosis (such as nephrotic syndrome of Finnish type), and congenital renal malformations (such as polycystic kidneys).[17]

Gastrointestinal and Hepatic Disorders. Intrauterine volvulus or obstruction of the small intestine has been associated with nonimmune hydrops fetalis. Liver abnormalities, including hepatic vascular tumors, and congenital infection such as rubella and syphilis, may compromise hepatic function sufficiently to result in hypoproteinemia, with resulting hydrops.[4,9]

Congenital Neoplasms. Hemangiomas, arteriovascular communication, and shunting of blood, with associated high-output cardiac failure, may result in hydrops. Tumors, such as Wilms' tumor, congenital neuroblastoma, and sacrococcygeal teratomas, may also result in hydrops (Fig. 9–28).[4,18]

Chromosomal Disorders. Turner syndrome, Down syndrome, trisomy 18, and triploidy may be associated with nonimmune hydrops fetalis, even without structural abnormalities.[19]

Heritable Disorders. A large variety of heritable disorders, such as Gaucher's disease, Hurler syndrome, and cystic fibrosis occur with nonimmune hydrops fetalis.[20]

Congenital Infections. Congenital syphilis, toxoplasmosis, cylomegalovirus, and rubella, all of which continue to be frequent transplacental infections, may be complicated by hydrops fetalis.[4,21]

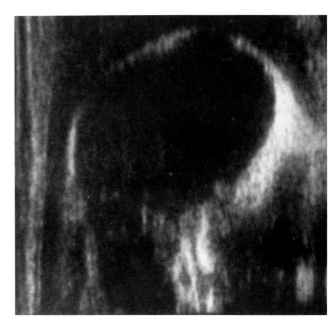

Figure 9–28. Ultrasound exam of the sacral area of the fetal spine demonstrating a large echolucent mass that protrudes from the lower spine. The vertebral column itself appears intact. These findings are indicative of a sacrococcygeal teratoma.

Disorders of Placenta and Cord. Chorioangioma of
the placenta is a common placental disorder associated with hydrops fetalis. Hydrops may result from
high-output heart failure. Aneurysm of the umbilical
artery has also been reported in association with hydrops fetalis.[9]

Gestational Disorders. Twin-to-twin transfusion may
produce volume overload in the recipient twin, causing high-output cardiac failure and hydrops, and simultaneously initiating hydrops in the donor twin
from acute blood loss.[2,3,22]

Prenatal Diagnosis

The antenatal diagnosis of hydrops fetalis is usually
suspected when the uterine growth increases dispro-
portionally to the gestational age. The diagnosis can be
made by an ultrasound examination that demonstrates
fetal skin edema (Fig. 9–29) greater than 5 mm.[1] The
associated findings often include fetal ascites (Fig.
9–30) and pleural effusions (Fig. 9–31), maternal hydramnios, and an abnormally thick placenta greater
than 6 mm.[1] An evaluation should be undertaken to
determine etiology once the diagnosis of fetal hydrops
is made. The antepartum diagnostic tests include:
blood type and antibody screen, serology, TORCH
(toxoplasmosis, rubella, cytomegalovirus, and herpes

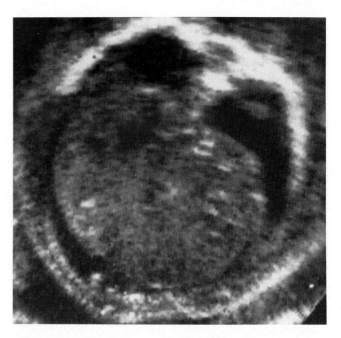

Figure 9–30. Transverse scan of the fetal abdomen demonstrating
ascites within the abdomen, and the liver, which appears to be free-
floating.

simplex), Kleihauer-Bethe test, glucose tolerance test,
ultrasonography to detect fetal malformations, and fetal echocardiography.[23]

It is important therapeutically to distinguish
isoimmune from nonimmune hydrops fetalis by blood
typing and complete antibody screening. Ultrasonography plays an important role in identifying anatomic

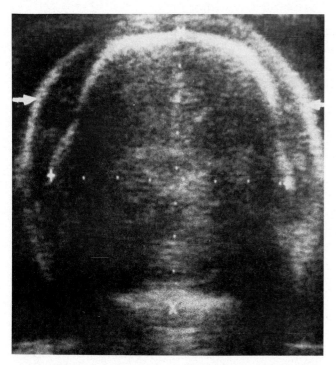

Figure 9–29. Coronal view of the fetal head demonstrating the skull
table, with scalp edema surrounding the head, as indicated by two
arrows bilaterally. The calipers(+'s) outline the limits of the normal
fetal head; the area beyond this represents scalp edema.

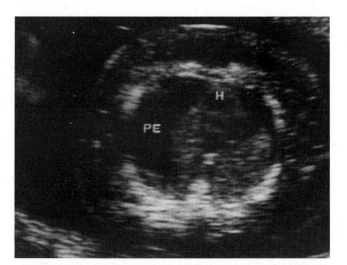

Figure 9–31. Transverse scan at the level of the fetal chest demonstrating the heart centally (H); anteriorly and to the left is pericardial effusion (PE); to the right is a large pleural effusion. In addition,
there is marked edema that covers the anterior and lateral walls of
the chest cavity.

anomalies that may be associated with nonimmune hydrops fetalis.[1] Fetal echocardiography provides diagnostic information about structural heart defects and cardiac arrhythmias resulting in fetal congestive heart failure.[10,11]

A complete ultrasound examination must be carried out in all patients at risk for hydrops. Sonographic assessment of gestational age by the usual biometric measurements includes biparietal diameter (BPD), head circumference, transverse cerebellar diameter, outer and inner orbital diameters, and long bone measurements. These measurements are useful in confirming the fetal age. The abdominal circumference in cases of fetal ascites is not useful in predicting the gestational age because of the ascites. The abdominal circumference measurement, however, may be important to monitor the collection of the fetal ascites.

Evaluation of the placenta by measuring the greatest placental width to determine placentomegaly in fetuses with hydrops fetalis may be useful. Evaluation of the amount of amniotic fluid can be undertaken by using either the amniotic fluid index or measurement of the greatest amniotic fluid pocket without umbilical cord or fetal limbs.

Assessment of the thickness of the fetal skin edema can be made by measuring the thickness of the skin tissue in addition to the assessment of either pericardial effusion, pleural effusion, or both. The next approach is to evaluate the fetal organs systematically, including the heart. Careful attention should be paid to the cardiovascular system, chest cavity, liver, kidneys, and lower abdomen. Attention should also be given to calcifications in the fetal head or tumors in the placenta or in the umbilical cord.

Management and Outcome

The timing and the mode of delivery may be influenced by fetal maturity, fetal well-being, and the history and outcome of a previous infant with nonimmune hydrops fetalis. It is recommended that from 30 weeks' gestation on, nonimmune hydrops fetalis should be managed by monitoring the lectin/sphingomyelin (L/S) ratio and by maternal treatment with a course of dexamethasone if fetal lungs are immature.[2] Termination of pregnancy may be required if fetal distress is detected. Aggressive evaluation should be undertaken, including fetal blood sampling, to exclude viral etiology. Delivery may sometimes prove difficult; and adding perinatal asphyxia and trauma to the already precarious perinatal situation may adversely affect the neonatal outcome. Some investigators have thus suggested delivery by cesarean section. Gough and et al[24] reported 31 pregnancies with nonimmune hydrops fetalis during an 8-year period. Thirty percent of the fetuses were delivered by cesarean sections; none survived. There are no conclusive

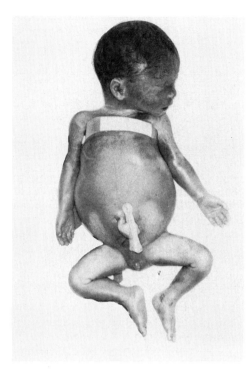

Figure 9–32. Fetus with evidence of massive ascites and pleural effusion demonstrating the dilated abdomen and chest. Prune belly syndrome is not uncommon in fetuses like these, who have a distended abdomen over a prolonged period of time.

data, however, that would support one route of delivery over the other.

Perinatal mortality for nonimmune hydrops has ranged from 50% to nearly 100%.[2,3] Hutchinson et al[2] have reported 61 cases of nonimmune hydrops with only one survivor. Etches and Lemons[3] reported a 50% survival in 22 cases of hydrops, suggesting that aggressive neonatal care might be rewarded with increased salvage. Survival in their series was much more frequent among idiopathic cases, encouraging an aggressive therapeutic approach in infants in whom no malformations or causes could be defined antenatally (Fig. 9–32).[25]

REFERENCES

1. Fleischer AC, Killam AP, Boehm FH, et al. Hydrops fetalis: sonographic evaluation and clinical implications. *Radiology.* 1981;141:163–168.
2. Hutchinson AA, Drew JH, Yu VYH, et al. Non-immunologic hydrops fetalis: a review of 61 cases. *Obstet Gynecol.* 1982;59:347–352.
3. Etches PC, Lemons JA. Non-immune hydrops fetalis: report of 22 cases including three siblings. *Pediatrics.* 64:326–332.
4. Turkel SB. Conditions associated with non-immune hydrops fetalis. *Clin Perinatol.* 1982;9:613–625.

5. Macafee CAJ, Fortune DW, Beischer NA. Non-immunological hydrops fetalis. *J Obstet Gynecol.* 1970; 77:226–237.

6. Altenburger KM, Jedziniak M, Roper WL, et al. Congenital complete heart block with hydrops fetalis. *J Pediatr.* 1977;91:618–620.

7. Becker MJ. Proceedings: Hydrops fetalis. *Arch Dis Child.* 1975;50:655.

8. Cooke RW, Mettau JW, Cappelle AW, et al. Familial congenital heart block and hydrops fetalis. *Arch Dis Child.* 1980;55:479–480.

9. Harkavy KL. Aetiology of hydrops fetalis. *Arch Dis Child.* 1977;52:338.

10. Kleinman CS, Donnerstein RL, DeVore GR, et al. Fetal echocardiography for evaluation of in utero congestive heart failure: a technique for study of non-immune fetal hydrops. *N Engl J Med.* 1982;306:568–575.

11. Klienman CS, Hobbins JC, Jaffe CC, et al. Echocardiographic studies of the human fetus: prenatal diagnosis of congenital heart disease and cardiac dysrhythmias. *Pediatrics.* 1980;65:1059–1067.

12. Leake RD, Strimling B, Emmanouilides GC. Intrauterine cardiac failure with hydrops fetalis: case report in twin with the hypoplastic left heart syndrome and a review of the literature. *Clin Pediatr.* 1973;12:649–651.

13. McCue CM. Congenital heart block in newborns of mothers with connective tissue disease. *Circulation.* 1977; 56:82–90.

14. Moller JH, Lynch RP, Edwards JE. Fetal cardiac failure resulting from congenital anomalies of the heart. *J Pediatr.* 1966;68:699–703.

15. Naeye RL, Blanc WA. Prenatal narrowing of closure of the foramen ovale. *Circulation.* 1964;30:736–739.

16. Bryan EM, Chaimongkol B, Harris DA. Alphathalassaemic hydrops fetalis. *Arch Dis Child.* 1981;56:476–478.

17. Linde NC. Neonatal ascites and urinary-tract obstruction. *Acta Pediatr Scand.* 1966;55:345–349.

18. Spahr RC, Botti JJ, MacDoland HM, et al. Non-immunologic hydrops fetalis: a review of 19 cases. *Int J Obstet Gynaecol.* 1980;18:303–307.

19. Bowman JM, Lewis M, deSa DJ. Hydrops fetalis caused by massive maternofetal transplacental hemorrhage. *J Pediatrics* 1984;104:769–72.

20. Gillan JE, Lowden JA, Gaskin K, et al. Congenital ascites as a presenting sign of lysosomal storage disease. *J Pediatrics.* 1984;104:225–231.

21. Bulova SI, Schwartz E, Harrer WV. Hydrops fetalis and congenital syphilis. *Pediatrics.* 1972;49:285–287.

22. Im SS, Rizos N, Joutsi P, et al. Non-immune hydrops fetalis *Am J Obstet Gynecol.* 1984;148:566–569.

23. Davis CL. Diagnosis and management of non-immune hydrops fetalis. *J Res Med.* 1982;27:594–600.

24. Gough JD, Keeling JW, Castle B, et al. The obstetric management of non-immunological hydrops. *Br J Obstet Gynaecol.* 1986;93:226–234.

25. Seeds JW, Herbert WNP, Bowes WA, et al. Recurrent idiopathic fetal hydrops: results of prenatal therapy. *Obstet Gynecol.* 1984;64:30S–32S.

10

The Urogenital Tract

Normal Fetal Urinary Tract

EMBRYOPHYSIOLOGY

The fetal urinary system begins development during the fifth week of gestation and starts to function about 6 weeks later. This system begins to function via urine production as early as 12 weeks' gestation. The latter was confirmed by Hewer.[1] Amniotic fluid is considered to be primarily a dialysate of fetal blood at the time when the fetal skin is permeable. After the 12th week of gestation, however, the skin begins the process of keratinization, which makes it more impermeable. Between the 12th and the 20th week of gestation the primary source of amniotic fluid gradually changes from permeable fetal skin, to the kidney. By the 16th to the 18th weeks of gestation, absent or nonfunctioning kidneys would invariably be associated with oligohydramnios. Wladimiroff[2] has shown that the hourly fetal urine production increases from 12 mL per hour at the 32nd week of gestation to 26 mL hour at term.

SONOANATOMY

The ultrasound examination of a fetus should incorporate the following: 1) identification of the kidneys and bladder with the assessment of textural and architectural appearance of the kidneys, 2) estimation of the size of the kidneys, and 3) estimation of the amniotic fluid volume.[3]

The fetal kidneys can first be recognized at the ninth week of gestation.[4] In cross-sectional views of the fetal abdomen the kidneys appear as sonolucent areas, homogeneous in texture on either side of the fetal spine. The renal sinus appears as an echogenic area in the central portion of the kidney at approximately 21 weeks of gestation.[5] At 30 to 32 weeks of gestation, the renal architecture becomes more distinct, and identification of 1) the echogenic rim of the cortex, 2) the renal sinus, and 3) the outline of the pyramids is more easily accomplished (Fig. 10–1). To-

ward the end of the third trimester of pregnancy these changes become even more evident.

The renal pelvis can be seen as early as 16 to 18 weeks' gestation and appears as a sonolucent rectangular area toward the medial aspect of the kidney. The fetal bladder can be seen in the lower aspect of the pelvis as a sonolucent area. It can be recognized as early as 9 weeks' gestation.[4] In the first half of the second trimester the bladder appears as a rectangular area with two dense echogenic borders. In the second half of the second trimester and in the third trimester the full bladder may assume an almost pearlike shape,

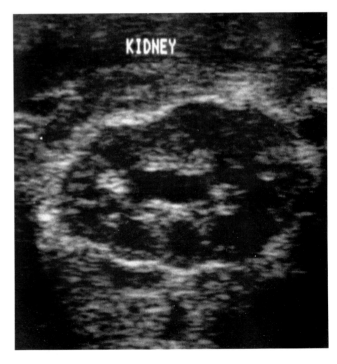

Figure 10–1. Transabdominal ultrasound examination of a fetus at the level of the kidney demonstrating the contours of the outer borders of the kidney with the calices shown as semicircular structures. The smaller echodense ring represents the outer margin of the renal pelvis. Except for a slight dilation of the renal pelvis, this is an otherwise normal kidney.

131

with the dome of the bladder more rounded. The bladder can be identified in either cross-sectional or longitudinal plane.

The dimensions of the normal fetal kidneys—anteroposterior, and transverse diameters—reflecting growth throughout gestation were first published by Grannum et al[3] (Table 10–1). The ratio of kidney circumference to abdominal circumference was found to be relatively constant throughout, for example, 0.27 to 0.30 in the normal fetus. This measurement is useful in identifying increased kidney size; for example, a ratio of 0.4 or greater is associated with markedly enlarged kidneys, as seen in patients with infantile polycystic kidney disease or in some types of dysplastic kidneys.

Abnormal Fetal Urinary Tract

Abnormal fetal kidneys are found in the following conditions:

1. Infantile polycystic kidney disease (IPKD)
2. Bilateral renal agenesis
3. Obstructive uropathy
4. Multicystic kidney disease (MKD)

INFANTILE POLYCYSTIC KIDNEY DISEASE (IPKD)

IPKD is an autosomal recessive disease with an incidence in the general population of 2 in 100,000 births and a recurrence risk of 25%. The fetal kidneys are bilaterally enlarged and are associated with oligohydramnios and the absence of a bladder. This disease can occur as an isolated anomaly, or it may be associated with other structural malformations. This association can also be seen in Meckel's syndrome.

Etiopathology
The kidneys of fetuses with IPKD appear uniformly enlarged and contain cylindrical cysts from the papillae to the cortex. These cysts represent proliferation and dilatation of the proximal collecting tubules.

Prenatal Diagnosis
The criteria used for a positive diagnosis of IPKD include: 1) oligohydramnios, 2) kidney circumference to abdominal circumference ratio greater than 2 standard

TABLE 10–1. FETAL KIDNEY AND ABDOMINAL PARAMETERS BY GESTATIONAL AGE GROUP IN NORMAL FETUSES

Variable	Gestational Age (wk)					
	<16 (n = 9)	17–20 (n = 18)	21–25 (n = 7)	26–30 (n = 11)	31–35 (n = 19)	>36 (n = 25)
Fetal kidney						
Anteroposterior (cm)						
Mean	0.84	1.16	1.49	1.93	2.20	2.32
SD	0.24	0.24	0.37	0.19	0.32	0.32
Transverse (cm)						
Mean	0.86	1.13	1.64	2.00	2.34	2.63
SD	0.14	0.25	0.40	0.28	0.42	0.50
Circumference (cm)						
Mean	2.79	3.80	5.40	6.58	7.86	8.42
SD	0.64	0.72	0.68	0.67	0.86	1.39
Fetal abdomen						
Anteroposterior (cm)						
Mean	2.92	3.73	5.12	6.74	8.50	8.88
SD	0.62	0.72	0.80	0.58	0.82	0.94
Transverse (cm)						
Mean	2.93	3.68	5.12	7.09	8.76	9.68
SD	0.59	0.56	0.49	0.61	0.89	1.44
Circumference (cm)						
Mean	9.66	12.37	17.36	22.03	28.11	30.45
SD	1.88	2.28	1.77	1.77	2.31	3.45
KC/AC ratio*						
Mean	0.28	0.30	0.30	0.29	0.28	0.27
SD	0.02	0.03	0.02	0.02	0.03	0.04

* Calculation of ratio used variables measured to eight decimal places.
From Grannum P, Bracken M, Silverman R, et al. Assessment of fetal kidney size in normal gestation by comparison of ratio of kidney circumference to abdominal circumference. Am J Obstet Gynecol. 1980; 136:249, with permission.

deviations (SD) above the mean (enlarged kidneys), and 3) a typical echogenic appearance of an infantile polycystic kidney (Fig. 10–2).

Blyth and Ockenden[6] have suggested that there are four subgroups based on age, onset, and the degree of renal involvement.

Fetal Disease. The onset of renal failure takes place in utero, or at birth, with 90% renal involvement and massively dilated kidneys.

Neonatal Disease. There is 60% renal involvement and smaller kidney size. There may be mild hepatic fibrosis; death follows within 1 year of birth.

Infantile Disease. This form presents 3 to 6 months after birth. There is 20% renal involvement with moderate hepatic fibrosis, hepatosplenomegaly, progressive chronic renal failure, hypertension, and portal hypertension.

Juvenile Disease. The disease presents 6 months to 1 year after birth. There is less renal involvement, and the course of the disease is similar to the infantile form.

Enlarged echodense kidneys are the principal findings in this disease. The kidney circumference to abdominal circumference ratio is usually equal to or greater than 0.4. The anteroposterior and the transverse kidneys measurements can also be useful in determining infantile polycycstic kidneys (Fig. 10–3).

Management and Outcome

Termination of pregnancy may be considered if diagnosis of this disease is made prior to 24 weeks; otherwise, management should be cautious. The prognosis for an affected fetus is poor; often, in the more severe form, death can occur in utero. Most of the neonates die of pulmonary hypoplasia shortly after delivery.

BILATERAL RENAL AGENESIS (BRA)

Bilateral renal agenesis (BRA) or Potter's syndrome, occurs in 3 in 10,000 births, and is accompanied by pulmonary hypoplasia, typical facies, and aberrant hand and foot positioning.[7,8]

Prenatal Diagnosis

Both kidneys can be visualized in 90% of the cases by the end of the first trimester of pregnancy. Both kidneys should almost always be seen during the early second trimester (beyond 13 weeks). If the kidneys and bladder are not seen in the presence of oligohydramnios, the diagnosis of bilateral renal agenesis should be strongly considered.

The fetal adrenal glands are often enlarged during the second trimester and can be misdiagnosed as

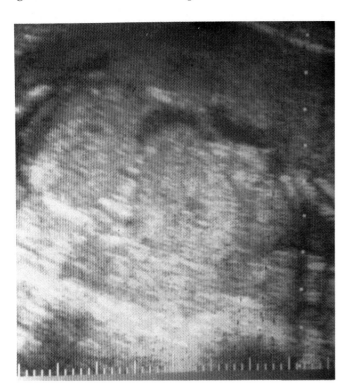

Figure 10–2. Transverse scan of a fetus in the second trimester demonstrating bilaterally enlarged echodense structures in the kidney area. These findings are consistent with a diagnosis of polycystic kidney disease.

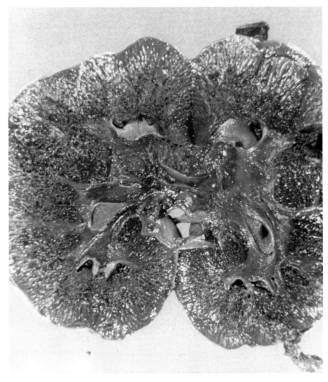

Figure 10–3. Macroscopic view of polycystic kidney disease.

being the fetal kidneys. The absence of a well-defined renal capsule and the inability to image the renal pelvis should alert the sonologist to the possibility that this structure is the adrenal gland masquerading as a kidney. When the diagnosis is difficult and a clinical decision needs to be made, instillation of sterile water via the intra-amniotic cavity is suggested to improve sonographic visualization.

Management and Outcome

BRA is a lethal congenital anomaly. Termination should thus be considered when the diagnosis is made. Aggressive care should be discouraged, in view of the dismal prognosis.

OBSTRUCTIVE UROPATHY

There are three different levels of obstructions:

1. High level: dilatation of the renal pelvis
2. Midlevel: ureteral dilatation with a nondistended bladder, with or without renal pelvis enlargement
3. Low level: dilatation of the bladder and urethra

HIGH LEVEL OF OBSTRUCTIVE UROPATHY

Etiopathology

Beck et al[9] reported that if ureteral obstruction occurred prior to day 70 of gestation in the sheep fetus (term is 147 to 150 days), renal dysplasia with large amounts of undifferentiated mesenchymal stroma, reduced glomeruli, and cystic dilatation of Bowman's capsule will result. If the obstruction took place after day 80 of gestation, the renal architecture remains well preserved despite the resulting hydronephrosis. These findings are compatible with experience in the human fetus, where, in the presence of complete bladder obstruction prior to the 20th week of gestation, there is likely to be failure of ampullary division. This, in turn, will lead to irreversible damage to the renal collecting system resulting in oligohydramnios and the development of pulmonary hypoplasia.

Prenatal Diagnosis

High level ureteral obstructions are usually located at the ureteropelvic junction (UPJ), resulting in sonographic findings such as hydronephrosis and type IV cystic dysplasia.

The sonographic findings in hydronephrosis may vary from a small dilated renal pelvis to a markedly distended retroperitoneal cystic structure on the medial aspect of the kidney (Fig. 10–4 and Fig. 10–5). Although the kidney may be enlarged to impressive

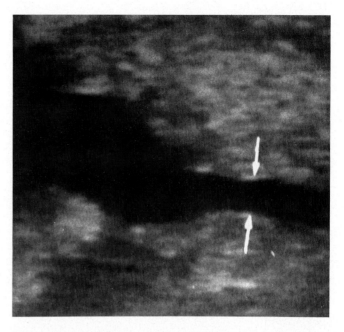

Figure 10–4. Sagittal scan of a fetus in the second trimester using transabdominal ultrasound reveals a dilated ureter (two small arrows) and dilated renal pelvis. These findings are consistent with a ureteropelvic junction obstruction.

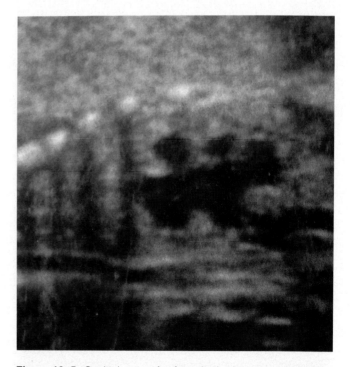

Figure 10–5. Sagittal scan of a fetus in the late second trimester demonstrating a kidney with a dilated renal pelvis as well as calyces. Note the semicircular structures that represent the calyces and open directly into the renal pelvis. These should be distinguished from kidneys in multicystic kidney disease, where these are neither semicircles nor empty into the renal pelvis but are complete circles or cysts. The ureter can be seen exiting the renal pelvis and draining toward the bladder at the inferior border of the kidney and coursing toward the right.

proportions, the renal architecture remains sonographically unremarkable. Caliectasis is often a normal feature, but in the early stages of hydronephrosis the individual calyces become more pronounced.

In type IV cystic dysplasia there is an increase in echogenicity and loss of renal architecture. The degree of dysplasia noted is a function of the severity and duration of the obstruction. The more severe the dysplasia, the poorer the renal function. There is an increased echogenicity in the renal cortices in early cystic dysplasia. Later, after the kidneys have been subjected to prolonged and increased pressures, echospared areas appear inside the enlarged renal capsule, representing sonographic evidence of significant renal compromise.

Management and Outcome

In fetuses with bilateral UPJ obstruction, the course of management can be based on the following: 1) the presence of cystic dysplasia in both kidneys, 2) the assessment of amniotic fluid volume, 3) the gestational age, and 4) fetal lung maturity.

When the diagnosis of bilateral cystic dysplasia and oligohydramnios is made, efforts should be made to deliver the fetus as soon as possible, hoping that there may be enough residual renal function to support life.

The prognosis is poor if UPJ is found early in the second trimester; thus termination of the pregnancy should be considered. It is very unusual, however, to have severe cystic dysplasia from a UPJ obstruction diagnosed early in pregnancy. Cautious management may be used for other variations in this fetal condition.

MIDLEVEL OBSTRUCTIVE UROPATHY

Prenatal Diagnosis

Obstruction in midlevel leads to dilatation of the ureter and development of hydronephrosis. The ureters can dilate to enormous proportions, losing their tubular shape and appearing sonographically as huge cystic structures in the fetal abdomen. This finding should be diagnostic of ureterovesical junction (UVJ) obstruction, although it may be confused with an intestinal obstruction.

Management and Outcome

Management should be conservative if there are no textural changes observed in the kidneys. Early delivery should be strongly considered in bilateral UVJ obstruction with signs of bilateral cystic dysplasia. If both kidneys appear normal, however, conservative management with frequent ultrasound examination is appropriate.

LOW-LEVEL OBSTRUCTIVE UROPATHY

Prenatal Diagnosis

Prenatal diagnosis of urethral obstruction (Fig. 10–6) is suggested by sonographic findings of oligohydramnios, a dilated fetal bladder, and sometimes, bilateral hydronephrosis. Bladder enlargement is usually present, but a normal-sized bladder does not exclude the diagnosis of partial urethral obstruction. Decreased urine production, secondary to renal dysplasia or spontaneous decompression of the urinary tract, can reduce the bladder volume.[10] Bladder size does not change during sonographic examination.[11] The precise cause may be posterior urethral valve obstruction in the male fetus or urethral obstruction in the female fetus.

Management and Outcome

Possible fetal treatment with shunting of the fetal bladder is suggested in those cases when the prenatal diagnosis is made prior to 20 weeks of gestation. If the diagnosis is made later, a determination should be made of fetal lung maturation status and delivery effected if mature. On the other hand, if delivery will be several weeks hence, assessment of fetal urine osmolality and electrolyte status may be useful before attempting fetal bladder shunting.

Urethral obstruction that occurs before the 20th week of gestation is likely to be associated with fetal pulmonary hypoplasia if severe oligohydramnios is present. The prognosis for fetuses with posterior urethral obstruction is poor.[11] In a review of obstructive uropathy by Hobbins et al[7] seven cases of fetal urethral obstruction were managed without in utero intervention or pregnancy termination. Of the seven live births, there were no neonatal survivors. An overall survival rate of 37% was reported by Mahony et al.[10] Specific information concerning obstetric management was not detailed.

MULTICYSTIC KIDNEY DISEASE (MKD)

MKD is an abnormal congenital development of the kidney tubules from the time of organogenesis. This disease is characterized by multiple cysts of varying size in the kidney, loss of renal architecture, nonvisualization of fetal bladder, and absence of amniotic fluid.[12]

Prenatal Diagnosis

The multicystic kidneys appear sonographically as echo-free areas of cysts of varying size and number scattered throughout the renal parenchyma (Fig. 10–7). The kidneys may be mildly or severely enlarged, or reduced in size in multicystic kidney disease. The

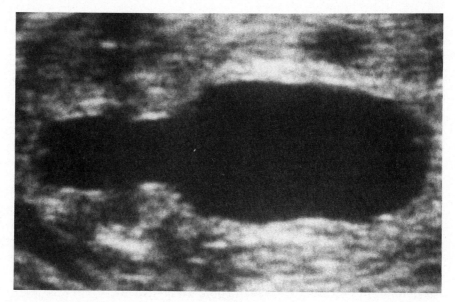

Figure 10–6. Sagittal scan of a fetus in the second trimester using transabdominal ultrasound. The figure reveals a bottle-shaped object: The neck of the bottle represents the dilated urethra; the remainder of the bottle represents the dilated bladder. These findings are consistent with a diagnosis of posterior urethral valve obstruction.

sonographic criteria useful for prenatal diagnosis include 1) several cystic masses separated by interfaces; 2) largest cysts are noncentral in location; 3) decreased renal parenchyma; 4) absence of fetal bladder; and 5) oligohydramnios.

Management and Outcome

In cases of bilateral multicystic kidney, as in cases of IPKD, the diagnosis can be aided by improved visualization resulting from the instillation of physiologic water into the amniotic cavity. Termination of pregnancy may be offered to the parents if the diagnosis is confirmed prior to 24 weeks' gestation, since these kidneys are irreversibly compromised, and there is a high mortality rate in the newborn period.[13]

REFERENCES

1. Hewer EE. Secretion by the human fetal kidney. *Q J Exp Physiol.* 1924;14:49–56.
2. Wladimiroff JW, Campbell S. Fetal urine production rates in normal and complicated pregnancy. *Lancet.* 1974;1;151–154.
3. Grannum P, Bracken M, Silverman R, et al. Assessment of fetal kidney size in normal gestation by comparison of ratio of kidney circumference to abdominal circumference. *Am J Obstet Gynecol.* 1980;136:249–254.

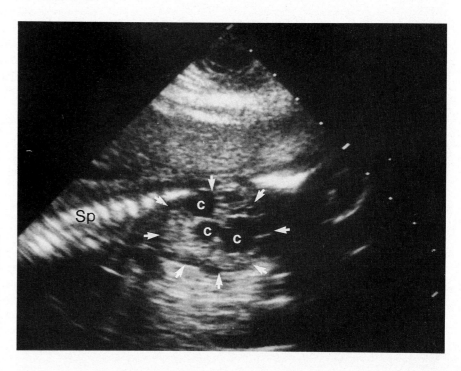

Figure 10–7. Transverse scan of the kidneys of a fetus in the second trimester, demonstrating multiple cystic echolucent areas. These findings are consistent with a diagnosis of multicystic kidney disease. It should be noted, however, that these cysts have echodense borders that form complete circles and do not empty into a central renal pelvis, as can be seen in dilated calyces. Sp = spine; C = cysts

4. Green JJ, Hobbins JC. Abdominal ultrasound examination of the first-trimester fetus. *Am J Obstet Gynecol.* 1988;159:165–175.

5. Bowie JD, Rosenberg ER, Andreotti RF, et al. The changing sonographic appearance of fetal kidneys during pregnancy. *J Ultrasound Med.* 1983;2:505–507.

6. Blyth H, Ockenden BG. Polycystic disease of kidneys and liver presenting in childhood. *J Med Genet.* 1971;8:257–284.

7. Hobbins JC, Romero R, Grannum P, et al. Antenatal diagnosis of renal anomalies with ultrasound, III: bilateral renal agenesis. *Am J Obstet Gynecol.* 1985;151:38–43.

8. Potter EL. Bilateral renal agenesis. *J Pediatr.* 1946;29:68–79.

9. Beck AD: The effect of intrauterine urinary obstruction upon the development of the fetal kidney. *J Urol.* 1971;105:784–789.

10. Mahony BS, Callen PW, Filly RA: Fetal urethral obstruction: ultrasound evaluation. *Radiology.* 1985;157:221–224.

11. Hayden SA, Russ PD, Pretorious DH, et al. Posterior urethral obstruction: prenatal sonographic findings and clinical outcome in fourteen cases. *J Ultrasound Med.* 1988;371–375.

12. Dalton M, Romero R, Grannum P, et al. Antenatal diagnosis of renal anomalies with ultrasound. *Am J Obstet Gynecol.* 1986;154:532–537.

13. Potter EL. *Normal and Abnormal Development of the Kidney.* Chicago, Ill: Year Book Medical Publishers; 1972.

11

The Limb Bones

The Fetal Upper and Lower Limb Bones

EMBRYOLOGY

The upper and lower limb bones of the fetus appear initially as mesenchymal condensation in the limb buds. The limbs begin to appear toward the end of the fourth week of gestation. The tissues of the limb buds are derived from mesoderm and ectoderm. During the sixth week, the mesenchymal primordia of bones in the limb buds undergo chondroossification to form the appendicular skeleton. Ossification begins in the long bones by the end of the embryonic period. It initially occurs in the diaphysis of the long bones, from the primary center of ossification. The primary centers have appeared in nearly all bones of the limbs by 12 weeks' gestation.

The clavicle begins to ossify before any other bones in the body. It initially develops by intramembranous ossification, but it later develops growth cartilages at both ends.[1] The relationship between the fetal clavicular development and gestational age was studied sonographically. Its length determines the shoulder width; measuring the clavicle may provide information on the risk of shoulder dystocia during delivery. In late gestation, however, it is difficult to image the clavicle in its entirety because it is most often shadowed.

The femurs are the next bones to show ossification. The primary ossification centers appear at different times in different developing bones, but most of them appear between the 7th and 12th weeks of gestation. The part of a bone ossified from a primary center is the *diaphysis*.[1]

SONOANATOMY

Queenan et al[2] in 1980 studied the ultrasound measurement of the fetal limb bones. The authors reported that the femur was first identified at 8 weeks' gestation and could be measured accurately from the 10th week of gestation and beyond. They also substantiated the validity of the sonographic technique by using roentgenograms of aborted fetuses from 15 to 23 weeks of gestation for confirmation. The ultrasound measurements were 1 mm larger than the x-ray value. The suboptimum lateral resolution, however, is a possible explanation for this discrepancy.

BIOMETRY

Femur

The technique for measuring the femur length involves an initial determination of the fetal position. The transducer is then placed at a right angle to the fetal spine and passed down the fetus, maintaining this angle, to the caudal end. Because the fetal femur is usually flexed, the transducer is then rotated from this position through 30 to 45 degrees toward the fetal abdomen until the full length of the femur is visualized. Alternatively, the transducer may be aligned along the caudal end of the fetal spine so that it gives the typical "tram-line" appearance described by Campbell,[3] and again the transducer is rotated—this time through 45 to 60 degrees and away from the fetal abdomen. An attempt is made to define both ends of the calcified portion once the femur has been located. This can be done most accurately if both the soft tissue of the buttock and knee joint can be seen, a view that usually avoids the tangential section of the bone.[4] The optimal position for measuring the femur or any other long bones should be:

1. The femur is a position horizontal to the transducer and not in a position oblique or vertical to the transducer.
2. The femur parallel to the transducer, with equal echo brightness throughout the entire length of the image; the proximal edge of the femur closer to the transducer, and the distal edge of the femur distant from the transducer.
3. The two edges of the femur—the greater trochanter

(proximal end) and the lateral condyle (distal end)—should be visualized.

4. The femur should be seen closest to the transducer.
5. Both ends of the image should be sharply demarcated.
6. Only the long axis of the diaphysis should be measured; the measurement should not include the thin pointed structure that represents the surface of the condyles.
7. Measurements should be made from one end to the other (Fig. 11–1).

The measurement of the femur length usually has been used as an indicator of gestational age. Investigators have demonstrated, however, that they were measuring the ossified diaphysis and not the length of the femur.[5,6] The bright linear echo is produced only by the surface of the ossified diaphysis of the bone.

The crown–heel lengths of aborted fetuses increase proportionally with the diaphyseal length of long bones throughout gestation. Since long bone measurements are relatively easy, particularly the femur length, Vintzileos et al[7] have constructed a nomogram correlating femur length to fetal length.

The growth of the fetus in length is a subject of interest to both parents and physician. Peak growth velocity in length occurs between 16 and 20 weeks and appears to result from peak mitotic activity[8] (Table 11–1).

Humerus

The technique for measuring the length of the humerus involves determining the fetal position. The transducer is then placed at a plane axial to the fetal head and passed down the fetus, maintaining this angle until the shoulder and the upper portion of the humeral bone are observed. Because the fetal humerus is usually parallel to the chest cavity, the transducer is then rotated 30 to 45 degrees, while the head of the humerus is visualized during the rotation. This maneuver is like opening a door that has one side fixed to an axis and the other side movable; the same maneuver is applied with the transducer. At the same time the fetal heartbeat is identified; the transducer is in a cross-sectional plane to the fetal chest. Finally, the transducer is passed toward the fetal head until the head of the humerus is seen. The transducer is then rotated 45 to 60 degrees. Once the humerus has been located, an attempt is made to define both ends of the calcified portion. This can be done most accurately if both the soft tissue of the shoulder and the elbow can be seen. Again, the humerus should be horizontal and parallel to the transducer (Fig. 11–2 and Table 11–2).

Tibia

After the femur is measured, pass the transducer toward the lower part of the limb. The tibia may be flexed, extended, or in between the latter positions. The transducer is passed toward the knee. When the tibia is located, attempt to define both ends of the bone. The fibula may be measured in the same way.

Ulna

The ulna and radius can be measured after the humerus is identified. The transducer is passed toward the lower part of the hand. The limbs may be flexed, extended, or in between. Pass the transducer toward the lower part of the hand and try to define both ends of the ulna or the radius. Although this ultrasound

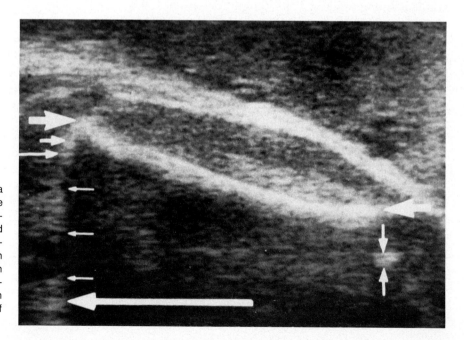

Figure 11–1. Ultrasound view of the femur of a fetus in the third trimester demonstrating the length of the femur as outlined by the thick arrows, the curved head of the femur as outlined by two smaller arrows, and the shadow cast below the bone as outlined by multiple arrows. On the right lower border of the picture there is an isolated echodense structure outlined by two opposing arrows, the distal femoral epiphysis, with arrows indicating the points of measurement of these epiphyses.

TABLE 11–1. SONOGRAPHIC MEASUREMENTS OF THE LONG BONES OF THE LEG IN THE FETUS

Gestational Age (wk)	Tibia (mm) Percentile			Fibula (mm) Percentile			Femur (mm) Percentile		
	5th	50th	95th	5th	50th	95th	5th	50th	95th
15	9	15	20	9	15	21	12	17	21
16	12	17	22	13	18	23	15	20	24
17	15	20	25	13	21	28	18	23	27
18	17	22	27	15	23	31	21	25	30
19	20	25	30	19	26	33	24	28	33
20	22	27	33	21	28	36	26	31	36
21	25	30	35	24	31	37	29	34	38
22	27	32	38	27	33	39	32	36	41
23	30	35	40	28	35	42	35	39	44
24	32	37	42	29	37	45	37	42	46
25	34	40	45	34	40	45	40	44	49
26	37	42	47	36	42	47	42	47	51
27	39	44	49	37	44	50	45	49	54
28	41	46	51	38	45	53	47	52	56
29	43	48	53	41	47	54	50	54	59
30	45	50	55	43	49	56	52	56	61
31	47	52	57	42	51	59	54	59	63
32	48	54	59	42	52	63	56	61	65
33	50	55	60	46	54	62	58	63	67
34	52	57	62	46	55	65	60	65	69
35	53	58	64	51	57	62	62	67	71
36	55	60	65	54	58	63	64	68	73
37	56	61	67	54	59	65	65	71	74
38	58	63	68	56	61	65	67	71	76
39	59	64	69	56	62	67	68	73	77
40	61	66	71	59	63	67	70	74	79

From Jeanty P, Romero R. Obstetrical Ultrasound. New York, NY: McGraw-Hill; 1983, 324, with permission.

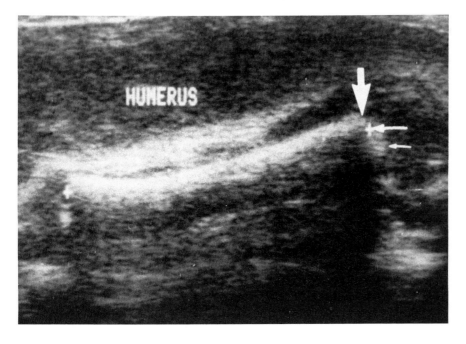

Figure 11–2. Ultrasound picture of the fetal humerus in the early third trimester depicting the length of the humerus as outlined by calipers(+'s). The three arrows indicate the various points that some investigators have used in measuring the humerus length.

TABLE 11–2. SONOGRAPHIC MEASUREMENT OF THE LONG BONES OF THE ARM IN THE FETUS

Gestational Age (wk)	Humerus (mm) Percentile			Ulna (mm) Percentile			Radius (mm) Percentile		
	5th	50th	95th	5th	50th	95th	5th	50th	95th
15	12	17	22	11	16	21	11	15	20
16	15	20	25	13	18	23	13	18	22
17	18	22	27	16	21	26	14	20	26
18	20	25	30	19	24	29	15	22	29
19	23	28	33	21	26	31	20	24	29
20	25	30	35	24	29	34	22	27	32
21	28	33	38	26	31	36	24	29	33
22	30	35	40	28	33	38	27	31	34
23	33	38	42	31	36	41	26	32	39
24	35	40	45	33	38	43	26	34	42
25	37	42	47	35	40	45	31	36	41
26	39	44	49	37	42	47	32	37	43
27	41	46	51	39	44	49	33	39	45
28	43	48	53	41	46	51	33	40	48
29	45	50	55	43	48	53	36	42	47
30	47	51	56	44	49	54	36	43	49
31	48	53	58	46	51	56	38	44	50
32	50	55	60	48	53	58	37	45	53
33	51	56	61	49	54	59	41	46	51
34	53	58	63	51	56	61	40	47	53
35	54	59	64	52	57	62	41	48	54
36	56	61	65	53	58	63	39	48	57
37	57	62	67	55	60	65	45	49	53
38	59	63	68	56	61	66	45	49	54
39	60	65	70	57	62	67	45	50	54
40	61	66	71	58	63	68	46	50	55

From Jeanty P, Romero R. Obstetrical Ultrasound. New York, NY: McGraw-Hill; 1983, 323, with permission.

technique is not difficult to use, it requires practice and persistence to obtain a clear image of the full calcified long bone lengths that is reproducible within a 2-mm range.[4]

Clavicle

The growth of the fetal clavicle during pregnancy is linear, as is clavicular growth, biparietal diameter (BPD), and femur length (Fig. 11–3, Table 11–3, and Table 11–4).

The more biologic parameters used in estimating gestational age, the greater the reliability of these predictions. Since real-time equipment allows easy measurement of long limb bone lengths, these parameters can be added to the list already in use.

Queenan et al[2] demonstrated that the growth of all limb bones was linear between 12 and 22 weeks' gestation. O'Brien and Queenan[9] found a linear relationship between the gestational age and the femur length growth between 12 and 40 weeks' gestation, with variability of approximately 1 week between 12 and 23 weeks.[4] Hadlock et al[10] studied the fetal femur length growth in relationship to the gestational age from 12 to 40 weeks' gestation. They demonstrated that the femur growth curve is nonlinear. Variability is ± 9.5 days between 12 and 23 weeks; between 23 and 40 weeks variability is ± 22 days.

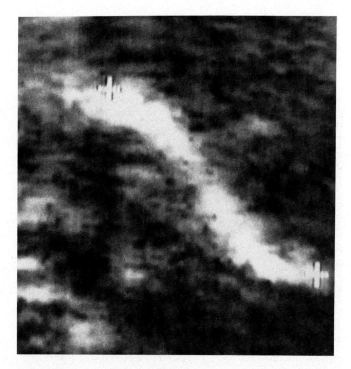

Figure 11–3. Ultrasound picture of a fetal clavicle showing the straight middle portion and the curved ends with the calipers(+'s) measuring the length of the clavicle.

TABLE 11-3. GESTATIONAL AGE AS OBTAINED FROM CLAVICLE LENGTH

Clavicle Length (mm)	Gestational Age (wk and days) Percentile		
	5th	*50th*	*95th*
11	8 + 3	13 + 6	17 + 2
12	9 + 1	14 + 4	18 + 1
13	10 + 0	14 + 3	19 + 6
14	11 + 6	15 + 2	20 + 5
15	12 + 5	16 + 1	21 + 4
16	12 + 3	18 + 0	21 + 3
17	13 + 2	18 + 5	22 + 2
18	14 + 1	19 + 4	23 + 0
19	16 + 0	19 + 3	24 + 6
20	16 + 6	20 + 2	25 + 5
21	17 + 4	21 + 1	26 + 4
22	17 + 3	22 + 6	26 + 2
23	18 + 2	23 + 5	27 + 1
24	19 + 1	24 + 4	28 + 0
25	21 + 0	24 + 3	29 + 6
26	21 + 5	25 + 1	30 + 5
27	22 + 4	26 + 0	30 + 3
28	22 + 3	27 + 6	31 + 2
29	23 + 2	28 + 5	32 + 1
30	24 + 0	29 + 4	34 + 0
31	25 + 6	29 + 2	34 + 6
32	26 + 5	30 + 1	35 + 4
33	27 + 4	31 + 0	35 + 3
34	27 + 3	32 + 6	36 + 2
35	28 + 1	33 + 5	37 + 1
36	29 + 0	33 + 3	39 + 0
37	30 + 6	34 + 2	39 + 5
38	31 + 5	35 + 1	40 + 4
39	32 + 4	37 + 0	40 + 3
40	32 + 2	37 + 6	41 + 2
41	33 + 1	38 + 4	42 + 0
42	35 + 0	38 + 3	43 + 6
43	35 + 6	39 + 2	44 + 5
44	36 + 5	40 + 1	45 + 4
45	36 + 3	41 + 6	45 + 3

From Yarkoni S, Schmidt W, Jeanty P, et al. Clavicular measurement: a new biometric parameter for fetal evaluation. J Ultrasound Med. 1985; 4:467–470, with permission.

TABLE 11-4. CLAVICLE LENGTH AS OBTAINED FROM GESTATIONAL AGE

Gestational Age (wk)	Clavicle Length (mm) Percentile		
	5th	*50th*	*95th*
15	11	16	21
16	12	17	22
17	13	18	23
18	14	19	24
19	15	20	25
20	16	21	26
21	17	22	27
22	18	23	28
23	19	24	29
24	20	25	30
25	21	26	31
26	22	27	32
27	23	28	33
28	24	29	34
29	25	30	35
30	26	31	36
31	27	32	37
32	28	33	38
33	29	34	39
34	30	35	40
35	31	36	41
36	32	37	42
37	33	38	43
38	34	39	44
39	35	40	45
40	36	41	46

From Yarkoni S, Schmidt W, Jeanty P, et al. Clavicular measurement: a new biometric parameter for fetal evaluation. J Ultrasound Med. 1985; 4:467–470, with permission.

Jeanty et al[11] studied long bone measurements in predicting gestational age. The authors demonstrated that the mean standard deviations in weeks for femur, humerus, tibia, and ulna were 1.3, 1.6, 1.7, and 1.8, respectively.

Queenan et al[2] also demonstrated that the growth rate of fetal limb bones (femur, humerus, radius, ulna, tibia, and fibula) between 12 and 22 weeks' gestation ranged between 2.5 and 3 mm per week. O'Brien and Queenan[9] calculated the growth rate of the femur throughout gestation; femur growth began at 3.15 mm per week and slowly decreased to 1.55 mm per week at 40 weeks' gestation. This summary of various studies on long bone growth demonstrates the linearity and semi-linearity between bone growth and gesta-

tional age, with slight discrepancy in findings relating to standard deviations (Table 11–5).

THE FETAL FOOT

The use of ultrasonography in obstetrics has significantly improved our evaluation of fetal growth and development. Studies involving fetal long bones have established a characteristic pattern of growth for these bones. Presumably, the fetal foot also has a characteristic growth pattern and therefore can be used to estimate gestational age or identifying pathologic conditions when there is deviation from the normal growth profile. In addition, some of these measurements may also be useful in prenatal diagnosis of certain skeletal syndromes.

Embryology

Bones appear initially as mesenchymal condensation in limb buds. Ossification begins by the end of the embryonic period. Most of the primary centers appear

TABLE 11–5. GESTATIONAL AGES AS OBTAINED FROM THE LONG BONES (IN WEEKS + DAYS)

Bone Length (mm)	Femur Percentile			Humerus Percentile			Ulna Percentile			Tibia Percentile		
	5th	50th	95th	5th	50th	95th	5th	50th	95th	5th	50th	95th
10	10 + 3	12 + 4	14 + 6	9 + 6	12 + 4	15 + 2	10 + 1	13 + 1	16 + 1	10 + 4	13 + 3	16 + 2
11	10 + 5	12 + 6	15 + 1	10 + 1	12 + 6	15 + 4	10 + 4	13 + 4	16 + 4	10 + 6	13 + 5	16 + 4
12	11 + 1	13 + 2	15 + 4	10 + 3	13 + 1	15 + 6	10 + 6	13 + 6	16 + 6	11 + 1	14 + 1	17
13	11 + 3	13 + 4	15 + 6	10 + 6	13 + 4	16 + 1	11 + 1	14 + 1	17 + 2	11 + 4	14 + 3	17 + 2
14	11 + 5	13 + 6	16 + 1	11 + 1	13 + 6	16 + 4	11 + 4	14 + 4	17 + 5	11 + 6	14 + 6	17 + 5
15	12	14 + 1	16 + 3	11 + 3	14 + 1	16 + 6	11 + 6	15	18	12 + 1	15 + 1	18
16	12 + 3	14 + 4	16 + 6	11 + 6	14 + 4	17 + 2	12 + 2	15 + 3	18 + 3	12 + 4	15 + 4	18 + 3
17	12 + 5	14 + 6	17 + 1	12 + 1	14 + 6	17 + 4	12 + 5	15 + 5	18 + 6	13	15 + 6	18 + 6
18	13	15 + 1	17 + 3	12 + 4	15 + 1	18	13 + 1	16 + 1	19 + 1	13 + 2	16 + 1	19 + 1
19	13 + 3	15 + 4	17 + 6	12 + 6	15 + 4	18 + 2	13 + 4	16 + 4	19 + 4	13 + 5	16 + 4	19 + 4
20	13 + 5	15 + 6	18 + 1	13 + 1	15 + 6	18 + 5	13 + 6	16 + 6	20	14 + 1	17	19 + 6
21	14 + 1	16 + 2	18 + 4	13 + 4	16 + 2	19 + 1	14 + 2	17 + 2	20 + 3	14 + 4	17 + 3	20 + 2
22	14 + 3	16 + 4	18 + 6	13 + 6	16 + 5	19 + 3	14 + 5	17 + 5	20 + 6	14 + 6	17 + 6	20 + 5
23	14 + 5	16 + 6	19 + 1	14 + 2	17 + 1	19 + 6	15 + 1	18 + 1	21 + 1	15 + 1	18 + 1	21 + 1
24	15 + 1	17 + 2	19 + 4	14 + 5	17 + 3	20 + 1	15 + 4	18 + 4	21 + 4	15 + 4	18 + 4	21 + 3
25	15 + 3	17 + 4	19 + 6	15 + 1	17 + 6	20 + 4	16	19	22 + 1	16	18 + 6	21 + 6
26	15 + 6	18	20 + 1	15 + 4	18 + 1	21	16 + 3	19 + 3	22 + 4	16 + 3	19 + 2	22 + 1
27	16 + 1	18 + 2	20 + 4	15 + 6	18 + 4	21 + 3	16 + 6	19 + 6	22 + 6	16 + 6	19 + 5	22 + 4
28	16 + 4	18 + 5	20 + 6	16 + 2	19	21 + 6	17 + 2	20 + 2	23 + 3	17 + 1	20 + 1	23
29	16 + 6	19	21 + 1	16 + 5	19 + 3	22 + 1	17 + 5	20 + 6	23 + 6	17 + 4	20 + 4	23 + 4
30	17 + 1	19 + 3	21 + 4	17 + 1	19 + 6	22 + 4	18 + 1	21 + 1	24 + 2	18 + 1	21	23 + 6
31	17 + 4	19 + 6	22	17 + 4	20 + 2	23	18 + 4	21 + 5	24 + 6	18 + 4	21 + 3	24 + 2
32	17 + 6	20 + 1	22 + 2	18	20 + 5	23 + 4	19 + 1	22 + 1	25 + 1	18 + 6	21 + 6	24 + 5
33	18 + 2	20 + 4	22 + 5	18 + 3	21 + 1	23 + 6	19 + 4	22 + 5	25 + 5	19 + 2	22 + 1	25 + 1
34	18 + 5	20 + 6	23 + 1	18 + 6	21 + 4	24 + 2	20 + 1	23 + 1	26 + 1	19 + 5	22 + 4	25 + 4
35	19	21 + 1	23 + 3	19 + 2	22	24 + 6	20 + 4	34 + 4	26 + 5	20 + 1	23 + 1	26
36	19 + 3	21 + 4	23 + 6	19 + 5	22 + 4	25 + 1	21 + 1	24 + 1	27 + 1	20 + 4	23 + 4	26 + 3
37	19 + 6	22	24 + 1	20 + 1	22 + 6	25 + 5	21 + 4	24 + 4	27 + 5	21	23 + 6	26 + 6
38	20 + 1	22 + 3	24 + 4	20 + 4	23 + 3	26 + 1	22 + 1	25 + 1	28 + 1	21 + 4	24 + 3	27 + 2
39	20 + 4	22 + 5	24 + 6	21 + 1	23 + 6	26 + 4	22 + 4	25 + 4	28 + 5	21 + 6	24 + 6	27 + 5
40	20 + 6	23 + 1	25 + 2	21 + 4	24 + 2	27 + 1	23 + 1	26 + 1	29 + 1	22 + 3	25 + 2	28 + 1
41	21 + 2	23 + 4	25 + 5	22	24 + 6	27 + 4	23 + 4	26 + 5	29 + 5	22 + 6	25 + 5	28 + 4
42	21 + 5	23 + 6	26 + 1	22 + 4	25 + 2	28	24 + 1	27 + 1	30 + 2	23 + 2	26 + 1	29 + 1
43	22 + 1	24 + 2	26 + 4	23	25 + 5	28 + 4	24 + 5	27 + 5	30 + 6	23 + 5	26 + 4	29 + 4
44	22 + 4	24 + 5	26 + 6	23 + 4	26 + 1	29	25 + 1	28 + 2	31 + 2	24 + 1	27 + 1	30
45	22 + 6	25	27 + 1	24	26 + 5	29 + 4	25 + 6	28 + 6	31 + 6	24 + 4	27 + 4	30 + 4

between the 7th and 12th weeks of gestation, after which the primary center will appear in nearly all bones. The development of the calcaneus in the foot is derived from a secondary center of ossification.

Biometry

The fetal foot can be visualized sonographically by the end of the first trimester of pregnancy. The measurement of the fetal foot is obtained from the outer margin of the posterior heel to the outer margin of the big toe. There are two planes in which the foot can be measured: plantar and longitudinal (Fig. 11–4, Fig. 11–5, and Fig. 11–6). A linear relationship was found between fetal foot length and gestational age; it is also found between foot length and biparietal diameter[11,12,13] (Fig. 11–7 and Table 11–6). A linear relationship was also found between fetal femur and foot lengths, with the femur to foot length ratio remain-

ing approximately constant throughout gestation (Fig. 11–8).[12]

FETAL LENGTH

The growth of the fetus in length is a subject of interest to both parents and physician. Peak length growth velocity occurs between 16 and 20 weeks and appears to result from peak mitotic activity.[1–3]

Embryology

During the third and early fourth weeks of gestation embryos are nearly straight, and measurements indicate the greatest growth in length. The sitting height, or crown–rump length, is used for older embryos and is considered one of the most accurate means of as-

TABLE 11–5. (CONTINUED)

Bone Length (mm)	Femur Percentile			Humerus Percentile			Ulna Percentile			Tibia Percentile		
	5th	50th	95th	5th	50th	95th	5th	50th	95th	5th	50th	95th
46	23 + 1	25 + 3	27 + 4	24 + 4	27 + 1	30	26 + 2	29 + 3	32 + 3	25 + 1	28	30 + 6
47	23 + 4	25 + 6	28	25	27 + 5	30 + 4	26 + 6	29 + 6	33	25 + 4	28 + 4	31 + 3
48	24	26 + 1	28 + 3	25 + 4	28 + 1	31	27 + 3	30 + 4	33 + 4	26 + 1	29	31 + 6
49	24 + 3	26 + 4	28 + 6	26	28 + 6	31 + 4	28	31 + 1	34 + 1	26 + 4	29 + 3	32 + 2
50	24 + 6	27	29 + 1	26 + 4	29 + 2	32	28 + 4	31 + 4	34 + 5	27	29 + 6	32 + 6
51	25 + 1	27 + 3	29 + 4	27 + 1	29 + 6	32 + 4	29 + 1	32 + 1	35 + 2	27 + 4	30 + 3	33 + 2
52	25 + 4	27 + 6	30	27 + 4	30 + 2	33 + 1	29 + 5	32 + 6	35 + 6	28	30 + 6	33 + 6
53	26	28 + 1	30 + 3	28 + 1	30 + 6	33 + 4	30 + 2	33 + 3	36 + 3	28 + 4	31 + 3	34 + 2
54	26 + 3	28 + 4	30 + 6	28 + 5	31 + 3	34 + 1	30 + 6	34	37	29	31 + 6	34 + 6
55	26 + 6	29 + 1	31 + 2	29 + 1	32	34 + 5	31 + 4	34 + 4	37 + 5	29 + 4	32 + 3	35 + 2
56	27 + 2	29 + 4	31 + 5	29 + 6	32 + 4	35 + 2	32 + 1	35 + 1	38 + 2	30	32 + 6	35 + 6
57	27 + 5	29 + 6	32 + 1	30 + 2	33 + 1	35 + 6	32 + 6	35 + 6	38 + 6	30 + 4	33 + 3	36 + 2
58	28 + 1	30 + 2	32 + 4	30 + 6	33 + 4	36 + 3	33 + 3	36 + 3	39 + 4	31	33 + 6	36 + 6
59	28 + 4	30 + 5	32 + 6	31 + 3	34 + 1	36 + 6	34	37 + 1	40 + 1	31 + 4	34 + 3	37 + 2
60	28 + 6	31 + 1	33 + 2	32	34 + 6	37 + 4	34 + 4	37 + 5	40 + 6	32	34 + 6	37 + 6
61	29 + 3	31 + 4	33 + 6	32 + 4	35 + 2	38 + 1	35 + 2	38 + 2	41 + 3	32 + 4	35 + 3	38 + 2
62	29 + 6	32	34 + 1	33 + 1	35 + 6	38 + 5	35 + 6	39	42	33	35 + 6	38 + 6
63	30 + 1	32 + 3	34 + 4	33 + 6	36 + 4	39 + 2	36 + 4	39 + 4	42 + 5	33 + 4	36 + 4	39 + 3
64	30 + 5	32 + 6	35 + 1	34 + 3	37 + 1	39 + 6	37 + 1	40 + 2	43 + 2	34 + 1	37	39 + 6
65	31 + 1	33 + 2	35 + 4	35	37 + 5	40 + 4				34 + 4	37 + 4	40 + 3
66	31 + 4	33 + 5	35 + 6	35 + 4	38 + 2	41 + 1				35 + 1	38	41
67	32	34 + 1	36 + 3	36 + 1	38 + 6	41 + 5				35 + 5	38 + 4	41 + 4
68	32 + 3	34 + 4	36 + 6	36 + 6	39 + 4	42 + 2				36 + 1	39 + 1	42
69	32 + 6	35	37 + 1	37 + 3	40 + 1	42 + 6				36 + 6	39 + 5	42 + 4
70	33 + 2	35 + 4	37 + 5									
71	33 + 5	35 + 6	38 + 1									
72	34 + 1	36 + 3	38 + 4									
73	34 + 4	36 + 6	39									
74	35 + 1	37 + 2	39 + 4									
75	35 + 4	37 + 5	39 + 6									
76	36	38 + 1	40 + 3									
77	36 + 3	38 + 4	40 + 6									
78	36 + 6	39 + 1	41 + 2									
79	37 + 2	39 + 4	41 + 5									
80	37 + 6	40	42 + 1									

From Jeanty P, Rodesch F, Delbeke D, et al. Estimation of gestational age from measurements of fetal long bones. J Ultrasound Med. 1984; 3:75–79, with permission.

sessing fetal growth. The embryo, the amnion, and the yolk sac form a structure over 5-mm long at 6 weeks after the last menstrual period, and subsequent growth follows a semisigmoid curve.

Biometry

The crown–heel lengths of aborted fetuses show an increase, proportionate with the diaphyseal length of long bones throughout gestation. Since long bone measurements, particularly femur length, are relatively easy to make, Vintzileos et al[7] have constructed a nomogram correlating fetal length to femur length (Table 11–7).

Pathology and Prenatal Diagnosis

Major skeletal disorders affecting only the foot are very uncommon. Deformities of the foot are usually part of a syndrome of skeletal disorders described in detail in the following section.

SKELETAL DEFORMITIES

The fetal skeleton can be sonographically evaluated as early as the second trimester. The ossified diaphysis of the long bones is easily identified and measured with current real-time equipment. Measurement of the femur length is commonly included in routine examination and assessment of both gestational age and fetal growth. In selected cases at risk, however, the various types of skeletal deformities, as outlined in Table 11–1, require detailed visualization and measurement of all long bones as well as a qualitative and quantitative evaluation of skull, chest, and spine (Table 11–5). The visualization of hands, feet, and digits is

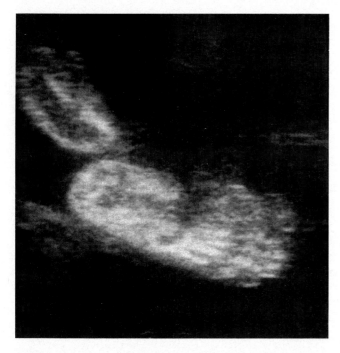

Figure 11–4. This figure demonstrates the sole of the foot shown by ultrasound and the measurements taken from the toe to the heel.

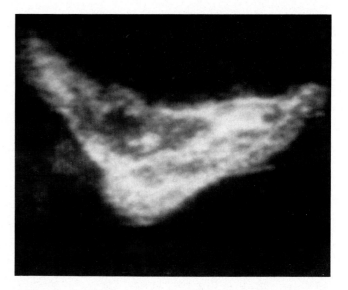

Figure 11–5. Ultrasound picture of the profile of the fetal foot.

important as well. The evaluation of fetal motion is also important, to observe flexion and abduction of the limbs. The most relevant sonographic features for the diagnosis of fetal skeletal dysplasias are reported in Table 11–8).

Ultrasound has several limitations for assessing the fetal skeleton. Measurement of the long bones is easily obtained, but it is difficult to assess bone density and the degree of mineralization. Evaluation of acoustic shadowing cast by the bones has been suggested as an indirect sign of the degree of mineralization, but this has limited value. Conversely, extreme demineralization, manifested as fractures and caput membranaceum, are easily detected. Gross bowing of the long bones and scoliosis can be rapidly demonstrated, but subtle alterations are probably undetectable. Measurement of the chest is essential, as thoracic hypoplasia is not only an important diagnostic clue but also because it is one of the most important determinants of postnatal survival. Further hints can be provided by demonstrating the number of digits, the presence or absence of associated visceral anomalies, and the age of onset of the findings. Evaluation of amniotic fluid volume is also relevant. Polyhydramnios is found in many types of skeletal dysplasias, particularly in those cases with hypoplasia of the thorax. Triangulation is obtained by identifying the major findings of an anom-

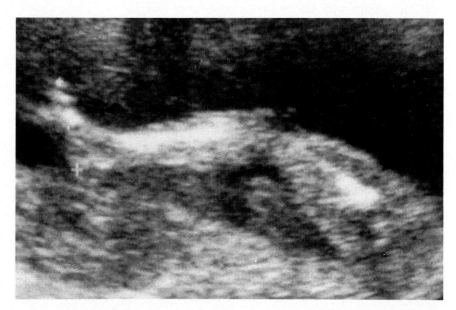

Figure 11–6. An ultrasound of a fetal foot showing the leg as well as the foot. The calipers(+'s) are placed at the tip of the toe and the heel.

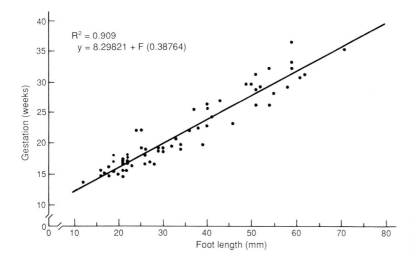

Figure 11–7. Scatter plot with a regression line demonstrating a linear relationship between foot length and gestational age.

aly and comparing different lists of defects that have the same findings in common.[14]

The type of shortening of long bones is relevant. Micromelia indicates a condition characterized by extreme shortness of all segments of the limbs. Rhizomelic and mesomelic shortening indicates conditions characterized by a reduction in the size of the proximal segments (femur, humerus) and median segments (ulna and radius, tibia and fibula), respectively. Useful hints derive also from the search of findings that are invariably associated with a specific entity.[14]

TABLE 11–6. NOMOGRAM OF FETAL FOOT SIZE THROUGHOUT GESTATION

Gestational age	Length (cm)		Percentile		
(wk)	Mean	± 2 SD	10th	50th	90th
14	1.8	2.5	1.6	1.8	2.1
15	1.9	2.3	1.6	1.9	2.2
16	2.3	2.3	1.8	2.2	2.8
17	2.1	1.3	1.9	2.2	2.2
18	2.6	2.5	1.9	2.7	3.0
19	3.1	2.6	2.5	3.0	3.9
20	3.3	2.5	3.3	3.3	3.3
21	3.4	2.6	2.4	2.4	2.4
22	3.5	2.8	2.5	3.6	4.0
23	4.1	2.6	4.1	4.1	4.0
24	4.6	2.5	4.6	4.6	4.6
25	4.7	2.1	4.0	4.7	5.3
26	4.7	2.5	4.0	4.7	5.4
27	5.0	2.6	4.5	5.0	5.6
28	5.3	2.8	5.1	5.3	5.5
29	5.2	2.9	4.9	5.4	5.8
30	6.1	2.8	6.1	6.1	6.1
31	5.6	3.5	5.1	5.6	5.2
32	5.6	3.5	5.4	5.7	6.2
33	5.9	2.9	5.9	5.9	5.9
34	6.5	3.1	6.0	6.5	7.1
35	7.1	2.9	7.1	7.1	7.1

From Goldstein I, Reece EA, Hobbins JC. Sonographic appearance of the fetal heel ossification centers and foot length measurements provide independent markers for gestational age estimation. Am J Obstet Gynecol. 1988; 159:923–926, with permission.

Despite the use of triangulation it is often impossible to identify the precise nature of a fetal bone abnormality. Sonography allows the formulation of a rather accurate prognostic judgment about the severity of a fetal skeletal dysplasia. Micromelia, that is, gross reduction of the length of the long bones of all segments of the limbs; thoracic hypoplasia; and gross demineralization, manifested as either multiple fractures or caput membranaceum, are usually associated with a very poor prognosis.

Skeletal anomalies can be divided into two broad categories (Table 11–9 and Table 11–10): osteochondrodysplasias and dysostoses.

OSTEOCHONDRODYSPLASIAS

Achondrogenesis

This is a lethal form of skeletal dysplasia featured by extreme micromelia, demineralization, and a very short trunk. Two varieties are presently recognized: type I (Parenti–Fraccaro) is associated with severe demineralization of both calvarium and spine and multiple rib fractures; type II (Langer–Saldino) is characterized by a lesser extent of demineralization. Both types are transmitted as autosomal recessive traits.

Prenatal diagnosis of achondrogenesis is feasibly based on characteristic in utero sonographic findings, including micromelia and extreme thoracic hypoplasia. The simultaneous demonstration of absence of ossification of the vertebral bodies and normal to decreased calvarial mineralization allows for a specific diagnosis of this condition.[14,15] (Fig. 11–9).

Thanatophoric Dysplasia

Thanatophoric dysplasia is one of the most commonly encountered forms of skeletal dysplasias. This condition is lethal and is characterized by micromelia, marked bowing of femurs, thoracic hypoplasia, and

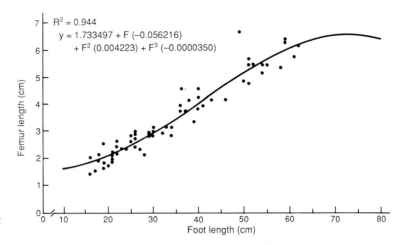

Figure 11–8. This figure demonstrates the curvilinear, or third-degree, relationship between the growth in foot length and femur length throughout pregnancy.

macrocrania. The most typical radiographic finding in newborns is the presence of flat vertebral bodies with wide spaces between them (H-shaped vertebrae). Although an autosomal recessive transmission has been suggested, the etiology is probably multifactorial, with a suggested recurrence risk of 2%.[14,16]

Prenatal diagnosis is feasible and is usually not difficult due to the marked shortening of long bones, bowed femurs (Fig. 11–10), severe thoracic hypoplasia (Fig. 11–11), redundant soft tissues, and usually polyhydramnios. A large head with a prominent forehead is also commonly found. Cloverleaf skull (Fig. 11–12) is found in 14% of cases.[17] Demonstration of this peculiar type of craniosynostosis in a fetus with short-limbed dwarfism allows for a prenatal diagnosis of thanatophoric dysplasia (Table 11–10).[18]

Asphyxiating Thoracic Dysplasia (Jeune Syndrome)

This condition characteristically presents with a narrow bell-shaped thorax, mildly to moderately shortened long bones with polydactyly, and visceral anomalies such as polycystic kidneys. Jeune syndrome is transmitted as an autosomal recessive trait. Most affected infants die from respiratory failure and infections in the neonatal period. Long-term survivors have been reported, however.

Prenatal diagnosis is aided by the striking finding of thoracic hypoplasia and a foreshortened femur greater than 2 standard deviations below the mean. In addition, the overall appearance of the chest cavity or the presence of visceromegaly will enhance the confidence in prenatal diagnosis.

Chondroectodermal Dysplasia (Ellis–van Creveld Syndrome)

The main findings include a long and narrow thorax, foreshortened forearm and leg, postaxial polydactyly,

hypoplastic nails, and congenital heart disease (atrial septal defect or common atrium). Thirty percent of affected infants die in the neonatal period because of cardiopulmonary complications. The recurrence risk is 25%, based on its autosomal recessive inheritance pattern. Prenatal diagnosis is based on the demonstration of short limbs, small thorax, polydactyly, and congenital heart disease.[14]

Short Rib–Polydactyly Syndromes

Short rib–polydactyly syndromes (SRP) include a group of similar types of lethal skeletal dysplasias transmitted as autosomal recessive traits. This syndrome is characterized by thoracic hypoplasia, short limbs, polydactyly, and multiple visceral anomalies. Three different types of SRP have been described: type I, or Saldino–Noonan syndrome; type II, or Majewski type; type III, or Naumoff type.

Prenatal diagnosis of all three types are based on the similarity of sonographic criteria between these different types. The main features of SRP include short limbs and thoracic hypoplasia. The easiest way to assess rib length is to image the thorax in cross section at the level of a four-chamber view of the heart. Under normal circumstances, the ribs should encircle between 50% and 66% of the chest cavity. Dysplasias of the ribs (and spine) only cover about one third of the chest perimeter. Other sonographic features include polydactyly associated with visceral anomalies, such as congenital heart disease, intestinal atresia, and polycystic kidneys.[19–21]

Diastrophic Dysplasia

This form of skeletal dysplasia with autosomal recessive transmission is characterized by rhizomelic shortening of the long bones, contractures, kyphoscoliosis, and clubfoot. Cleft palate may be found. The thumb

TABLE 11–7. CALCULATED FETAL LENGTHS*

Ultrasound femur length (mm)	Mean fetal length (cm)	SE (cm)	5th percentile (cm)	95th percentile (cm)
30	23.880	0.636	22.634	25.126
31	24.470	0.616	23.263	25.677
32	25.060	0.596	23.892	26.228
33	25.650	0.576	24.521	26.779
34	26.240	0.556	25.150	27.330
35	26.830	0.536	25.779	27.881
36	27.420	0.517	26.407	28.433
37	28.010	0.497	27.035	28.985
38	28.600	0.478	27.664	29.536
39	29.190	0.458	28.292	30.088
40	29.780	0.439	28.919	30.641
41	30.370	0.420	29.547	31.193
42	30.960	0.401	30.174	31.746
43	31.550	0.382	30.801	32.299
44	32.140	0.364	31.427	32.853
45	32.730	0.345	32.053	33.407
46	33.320	0.327	32.679	33.961
47	33.910	0.309	33.304	34.516
48	34.500	0.292	33.928	35.072
49	35.090	0.275	34.551	35.629
50	35.680	0.258	35.173	36.187
51	36.270	0.243	35.794	36.746
52	36.860	0.228	36.414	37.306
53	37.450	0.214	37.031	37.869
54	38.040	0.201	37.646	38.434
55	38.630	0.189	38.259	39.001
56	39.220	0.179	38.868	39.572
57	39.810	0.171	39.474	40.146
58	40.400	0.166	40.075	40.725
59	40.990	0.162	40.672	41.308
60	41.580	0.162	41.263	41.897
61	42.170	0.164	41.849	42.491
62	42.760	0.168	42.431	43.089
63	43.350	0.175	43.007	43.693
64	43.940	0.184	43.580	44.300
65	44.530	0.194	44.149	44.911
66	45.120	0.207	44.715	45.525
67	45.710	0.220	45.279	46.141
68	46.300	0.235	45.840	46.760
69	46.890	0.250	46.400	47.380
70	47.480	0.266	46.959	48.001
71	48.070	0.283	47.516	48.624
72	48.660	0.300	48.072	49.248
73	49.250	0.317	48.628	49.872
74	49.840	0.335	49.183	50.497
75	50.430	0.354	49.737	51.123
76	51.020	0.372	50.291	51.749
77	51.610	0.391	50.844	52.376
78	52.200	0.410	51.397	53.003
79	52.790	0.429	51.950	53.630
80	53.380	0.448	52.502	54.258
81	53.970	0.467	53.054	54.886
82	54.560	0.487	53.606	55.514
83	55.150	0.506	54.158	56.142
84	55.740	0.526	54.709	56.771
85	56.330	0.546	55.261	57.399
86	56.920	0.565	55.812	58.028
87	57.510	0.585	56.363	58.657
88	58.100	0.605	56.914	59.286
89	58.690	0.625	57.465	59.915
90	59.280	0.645	58.016	60.544

* Confidence intervals and standard error (SE) based on the regression line. *From Vintzileos AM, Campbell WA, Neckles S, et al. The ultrasound femur length as a predictor of fetal length. Obstet Gynecol. 1984; 64:779–782, with permission.*

TABLE 11–8. ASSESSMENT OF FETAL SKELETAL DYSPLASIAS

Bone length
Bone density
  Head
  Spine
  Long bones
Bowing of long bones
Small chest size
Polydactyly
Associated malformations
Age at presentation

projects laterally, in some cases, with a peculiar configuration ("hitchhiker" thumb) (Fig. 11–13).

Prenatal diagnosis of diastrophic dysplasia has been reported on several occasions.[22] Diastrophic dysplasia can be suspected when short-limbed dwarfism is found in association with clubfoot. Sonographic recognition of the hitchhiker thumb is possible and may allow certain diagnosis, although less benign forms of this disorder can go undetected. Although progressive scoliosis may lead in time to respiratory compromise, diastrophic dysplasia is compatible with long survival.[14,22]

Achondroplasia

This is a condition transmitted via an autosomal dominant pattern of inheritance and is the most common osteochrondrodysplasia found at birth. Most cases, however, are believed to be new mutations, as evidenced by the sporadic occurrence of this disorder in the offspring of normal parents. Although the homozygous form is lethal, heterozygous achondroplasia is compatible with a normal life expectancy and normal intelligence.

Prenatal diagnosis of achondroplasia is based on typical sonographic features of rhizomelic shortening of the long bones (Fig. 11–14), lumbar lordosis, large skull (Fig. 11–15), increased prominent forehead, depressed nasal bridge, and a large mandible. The base of the skull is small, and there is frequently a reduction in size of the foramen magnum. This may lead in time to impairment of cerebrospinal fluid circulation and hydrocephalus.[23]

The most relevant sonographic finding in utero is the demonstration of shortened long bones. It has been reported by several investigators, however, that measurement of the femur may be within the normal range in the second trimester.[14,24,25] The relationship between femur and biparietal diameter or head perimeter seems to be more predictive than femur length alone,[24] as achondroplasia is usually associated with macrocrania.

TABLE 11–9. INTERNATIONAL NOMENCLATURE OF CONSTITUTIONAL BONE DISEASE (1983)

Osteochondrodysplasias

Abnormalities of Cartilage and/or Bone Growth and Development

Defects of Growth of Tubular Bones, Spine, or Both

	Transmission
Identifiable at birth	
Usually lethal before or shortly after birth	
1. Achondrogenesis type I (Parenti–Fraccaro)	AR
2. Achondrogenesis type II (Langer–Saldino)	
3. Hypochondrogenesis	
4. Fibrochondrogenesis	AR
5. Thanatophoric dysplasia	
6. Thanatophoric dysplasia with cloverleaf skull	
7. Atelosteogenesis	
8. Short rib syndrome (with or without polydactyly)	
a. Type I (Saldino–Noonan)	AR
b. Type II (Majewski)	AR
c. Type III (lethal thoracic dysplasia)	AR
Usually nonlethal dysplasia	
9. Chondrodysplasia punctata	
a. Rhizomelic form autosomal recessive	AR
b. Dominant X-linked form	XLD Lethal in male
c. Common mild form (Sheffield) Exclude: symptomatic stippling (warfarin, chromosomal aberration . . .)	
10. Campomelic dysplasia	
11. Kyphomelic dysplasia	AR
12. Achondroplasia	AD
13. Diastrophic dysplasia	AR
14. Metatropic dysplasia (several forms)	AR, AD
15. Chondroectodermal dysplasia (Ellis–van Creveld)	AR
16. Asphyxiating thoracic dysplasia (Jeune)	AR
17. Spondyloepiphyseal dysplasia congenita	
a. Autosomal dominant form	AD
b. Autosomal recessive form	AR
18. Kniest dysplasia	AD
19. Dyssegmental dysplasia	AR
20. Mesomelic dysplasia	
a. Type Nievergelt	AD
b. Type Langer (probable homozygous dyschondrosteosis)	AR
c. Type Robinow	
d. Type Rheinardt	AD
e. Others	
21. Acromesomelic dysplasia	AR
22. Cleidocranial dysplasia	AD
23. Otopalatodigital syndrome	
a. Type I (Langer)	XLSD
b. Type II (André)	XLR
24. Larsen's syndrome	AR, AD
25. Other multiple dislocation syndromes	AR
Identifiable in later life	
1. Hypochodroplasia	AD
2. Dyschondrosteosis	AD
3. Metaphyseal chondrodysplasia type Jansen	AD
4. Metaphyseal chondrodysplasia type Schmid	AD
5. Metaphyseal chondrodysplasia type McKusick	AR

TABLE 11–9. (*CONTINUED*)

6. Metaphyseal chondrodysplasia with exocrine pancreatic insufficiency and cyclic neutropenia	AR
7. Spondylometaphyseal dysplasia	
a. Type Kozlowski	AD
b. Other forms	
8. Multiple epiphyseal dysplasia	
a. Type Fairbank	AD
b. Other forms	
9. Multiple epiphyseal dysplasia with early diabetes (Wolcott-Rallisson)	AR
10. Arthro-ophthalmopathy (Stickler)	AR
11. Pseudoachondroplasia	
a. Dominant	AD
b. Recessive	AR
12. Spondyloepiphyseal dysplasia tarda (X-linked recessive)	XLR
13. Progressive pseudorheumatoid chondrodysplasia	AR
14. Spondyloepiphyseal dysplasia—other forms	
15. Brachyolmia	
a. Autosomal recessive	AR
b. Autosomal dominant	AD
16. Dyggve–Melchior–Clausen dysplasia	AR
17. Spondyloepimetaphyseal dysplasia (several forms)	
18. Spondyloepimetaphyseal dysplasia with joint laxity	AR
19. Otospondylometaphyseal dysplasia (OSMED)	AR
20 Myotonic chondrodysplasia (Catel–Schwartz–Jampel)	AR
21. Parastremmatic dysplasia	AD
22. Trichorhinophalangeal dysplasia	AD
23. Acrodysplasia with retinitis pigmentosa and nephropathy (Saldino–Mainzer)	AR

Disorganized Development of Cartilage and Fibrous Component of Skeleton

1. Dysplasia epiphyseal hemimelica	
2. Multiple cartilaginous exostoses	AD
3. Acrodysplasia with exostoses (Giedion–Langer)	
4. Enchondromatosis (Ollier)	
5. Enchondromatosis with hemangioma (Maffucci)	
6. Metachondromatosis	AD
7. Spondyloenchondroplasia	AR
8. Osteoglophonic dysplasia	
9. Fibrous dysplasia (Jaffe–Lichtenstein)	
10. Fibrous dysplasia with skin pigmentation and precocious puberty (McCune–Albright)	
11. Cherubism (familial fibrous dysplasia of the jaws)	AD

Abnormalities of Density of Cortical Diaphyseal Structure, Metaphyseal Modeling, or Both

1. Osteogenesis imperfecta (several forms)	AR, AD
2. Juvenile idiopathic osteoporosis	
3. Osteoporosis with pseudoglioma	AR
4. Osteopetrosis	
a. Autosomal recessive lethal	AR
b. Intermediate recessive	AR
c. Autosomal dominant	AD
d. Recessive with tubular acidosis	AR
5. Pyknodysostosis	AR
6. Dominant osteosclerosis type Stanescu	AD

TABLE 11–9. (*CONTINUED*)

7. Osteomesopycnosis	AD
8. Osteopoikilosis	AD
9. Osteopathia striata	AD
10. Osteopathia striata with cranial sclerosis	AD
11. Melorheostosis	
12. Diaphyseal dysplasia (Camurati–Engelmann)	AD
13. Craniodiaphyseal dysplasia	AR
14. Endosteal hyperostosis	
a. Autosomal dominant (Worth)	AD
b. Autosomal recessive (van Buchem)	AR
c. Autosomal recessive (sclerosteosis)	AR
15. Tubular stenosis (Kenny–Caffey)	AD
16. Pachydermoperiostosis	AD
17. Osteodysplasty (Melnick–Needles)	AD
18. Frontometaphyseal dysplasia	XLR
19. Craniomethaphyseal dysplasia (several forms)	AD
20. Metaphyseal dysplasia (Pyle)	AR or AD
21. Dysosteosclerosis	AR or XLR
22. Osteoectasia with hyperphosphatasia	AR
23. Oculodento-osseous dysplasia	
a. Mild type	AD
b. Severe type	AR
24. Infantile cortical hyperostosis (Caffey disease, familial type)	

DYSOSTOSES

Malformation of Individual Bones, Singly or in Combination

Dystostoses with Cranial and Facial Malformations

1. Craniosynostosis (several forms)	
2. Craniofacial dysostosis (Crouzon)	
3. Acrocephalosyndactyly	
a. Type Apert	AD
b. Type Chotzen	AD
c. Type Pfeiffer	AD
d. Other types	
4. Acrocephalopolysyndactyly (Carpenter and others)	AR
5. Cephalopolysyndactyly (Greig)	AD
6. First and second branchial arch syndromes	
a. Mandibulofacial dysostosis (Treacher–Collins–Franceschetti)	AD
b. Acrofacial dysostosis (Nager)	
c. Oculoauricolovertebral dysostosis (Goldenhar)	AR
d. Hemifacial microsomia	
e. Others (probably parts of a large spectrum)	
7. Oculomandibulofacial syndrome (Hallermann–Streiff–François)	

Dysostoses with Predominant Axial Involvement

1. Vertebral segmentation defects (including Klippel-Feil)	
2. Cervico-oculoacoustic syndrome (Wildervanck)	
3. Sprengel anomaly	
4. Spondylocostal dysostosis	
a. Dominant form	AD
b. Recessive form	AR
5. Oculovertebral syndrome (Weyers)	
6. Osteo-onychodysostosis	AD
7. Cerebrocostomandibular syndrome	AR

TABLE 11–9. (*CONTINUED*)

Dysostoses with Predominant Involvement of Extremities

1. Acheiria	
2. Apodia	
3. Tetraphocomelic syndrome (Robert) (SC pseudothalidomide syndrome)	AR
4. Ectrodactyly	
a. Isolated	
b. Ectrodactyly–ectodermal dysplasia–cleft palate syndrome	AD
c. Ectrodactyly with scalp defects	AD
5. Oroacral syndrome (aglossia syndrome, Hanhart syndrome)	
6. Familial radioulnar synostosis	
7. Brachydactyly, types A, B, C, D, E (Bell's classification)	AD
8. Symphalangism	AD
9. Polydactyly (several forms)	
10. Syndactyly (several forms)	
11. Polysyndactyly (several forms)	
12. Camptodactyly	
13. Manzke syndrome	
14. Poland syndrome	
15. Rubinstein–Taybi syndrome	
16. Coffin–Siris syndrome	
17. Pancytopenia–dysmelia syndrome (Fanconi)	AR
18. Blackfan–Diamond anemia with thumb anomalies (Aase syndrome)	AR
19. Thrombocytopenia–radial aplasia syndrome	AR
20. Orodigitofacial syndrome	
a. Type Papillon–Leage	XLD Lethal in male
b. Type Mohr	AR
21. Cardiomelic syndromes (Holt–Oram and others)	AD
22. Femoral focal deficiency (with or without facial anomalies)	
23. Multiple synostoses (includes some forms of symphalangism)	AD
24. Scapuloiliac dysostosis (Kosenow–Sinios)	AD
25. Hand–foot–genital syndrome	AD
26. Focal dermal hypoplasia (Goltz)	Lethal in male

Idiopathic Osteolysis

1. Phanlangeal (several forms)	
2. Tarsocarpal	
a. Including François form and others	AR
b. With nephropathy	AD
3. Multicentric	
a. Hajdu-Cheney form	AD
b. Winchester form	AR
c. Torg form	AR
d. Other forms	

Miscellaneous Disorders with Osseous Involvement

1. Early acceleration of skeletal maturation	
a. Marshall–Smith syndrome	
b. Weaver syndrome	
c. Other types	
2. Marfan syndromes	AD
3. Congenital contractural arachnodactyly	AD
4. Cerebrohepatorenal syndrome (Zellweger)	
5. Coffin–Lowry syndrome	XLR
6. Cockayne's syndrome	AR
7. Fibrodysplasia ossificans congenita	AD

TABLE 11–9. (CONTINUED)

8. Epidermal nevus syndrome (Solomon)	
9. Nevois basal cell carcinoma syndrome	
10. Multiple congenital fibromatosis	
11. Neurofibromatosis	AD

Chromosomal Aberrations

Primary Metabolic Abnormalities

Calcium, Phosphorus, or Both

1. Hypophosphatemic rickets	XLD
2. Vitamin D dependency or pseudodeficiency rickets	
a. Type I with probable deficiency in 25-hydroxy vitamin D-1-alpha-hydroxylase	AR
b. Type II with target-organ resistance	AR
3. Late rickets (McCance)	
4. Idiopathic hypercalciuria	
5. Hypophosphatasia (several forms)	AR
6. Pseudohypoparathyroidism (normocalcemic and hypocalcemic forms, includes acrodysostosis)	AD

Complex Carbohydrates

1. Mucopolysaccaridosis type I (alpha-L-iduronidase deficiency)	
a. Hurler form	AR
b. Scheie form	AR
c. Other forms	AR
2. Mucopolysaccharidosis type II (Hunter) (sulfoiduronate sulfatase deficiency)	XLR
3. Mucopolysaccharidosis type III (Sanfilippo)	
a. Type III A (heparin sulfamidase deficiency)	AR
b. Type III B (*N*-acetyl-alpha-glucosaminidase deficiency)	AR
c. Type III C (alpha-glucosaminide-*N*-acetyl transferase deficiency)	AR
d. Type III D (*N*-acetyl-glucosamine-6-sulfate deficiency)	
4. Mucopolysaccharidosis type IV	
a. Type IV A (Morquio) (*N*-acetyl-galactosamine-6-sulfate sulfatase deficiency)	AR
b. Type IV B (beta-galactosidase deficiency)	AR
5. Mucopolysaccharidosis type VI (Maroteaux–Lamy) (aryl-sulfatase B deficiency)	AR
6. Mucopolysaccharidosis type VII (beta-glucuronidase deficiency)	AR
7. Aspartylglycosaminuria (aspartyl-glucosaminidase deficiency)	AR
8. Mannosidosis (alpha-mannosidase deficiency)	AR
9. Fucosidosis (alpha-fucosidase deficiency)	AR
10. GMI-gangliosidosis (beta-galactosidase deficiency) (several forms)	AR
11. Multiple sulfatases deficiency (Austin-Thieffry)	AR
12. Isolated neuraminidase deficiency, several forms	
a. Mucolipidosis I	AR
b. Nephrosialidosis	AR
c. Cherry red spot myoclonia syndrome	AR
13. Phosphotransferase deficiency, several forms	
a. Muclipidosis II (I-cell disease)	AR
b. Mucolipidosis III (pseudopolydystrophy)	AR

TABLE 11–9. (CONTINUED)

14. Combined neuraminidase beta-galactosidase deficiency	AR
15. Salla disease	AR
Lipids	
1. Niemann–Pick disease (sphingomyelinase deficiency) (several forms)	AR
2. Gaucher disease (beta-glucosidase deficiency) (several forms)	AR
3. Farber disease lipogranulomatosis (ceraminidase deficiency)	AR
Nucleic Acids	
1. Adenosine deaminase deficiency and others	AR
Aminoacids	
1. Homocystinuria and others	AR
Metals	
1. Menkes' syndrome (kinky hair syndrome and others)	AR

AD = autosomal dominant transmission, AR = autosomal recessive transmission, XLR = X-linked recessive transmission, XLD = X-linked dominant transmission.

From Beighton P, Cremin B, Faure C, et al. International nomenclature of constitutional diseases' of bones: Revision, May, 1983. Ann Radiol (Paris). 1983; 26:452–457, with permission.

TABLE 11–10. SKELETAL DEFORMITIES ASSOCIATED WITH SONOGRAPHIC FINDINGS

Bone Length–Micromelia
   Achondrogenesis
   Thanatophoric dysplasia
   Fibrochondrogenesis
   Short rib–polydactyly syndromes
   Diastrophic dysplasia

Bone Density
   Achondrogenesis
   Osteogenesis imperfecta
   Hypophosphatasia

Bowing of Long Bones
   Campomelic syndrome
   Osteogenesis imperfecta
   Dyssegmental dysplasia
   Otopalatodigital syndrome
   Thanatophoric dysplasia
   Hypophosphatasia

Small Chest Size
   Achondrogenesis
   Thanatophoric dysplasia
   Short rib–polydactyly syndromes
   Asphyxiating thoracic dysplasia
   Chondroectodermal dysplasia
   Metatropic dysplasia
   Fibrochondrogenesis
   Campomelic dysplasia

Polydactyly
   Chondroectodermal dysplasia
   Short rib–polydactyly syndromes
   Asphyxiating thoracic dysplasia

Associated Malformations Present
   Cloverleaf skull (thanatophoric dysplasia)
   Hitchhiker thumb (diastrophic dysplasia)

Courtesy of Dr. Gianluigi Pilu. Table modified for our purposes.

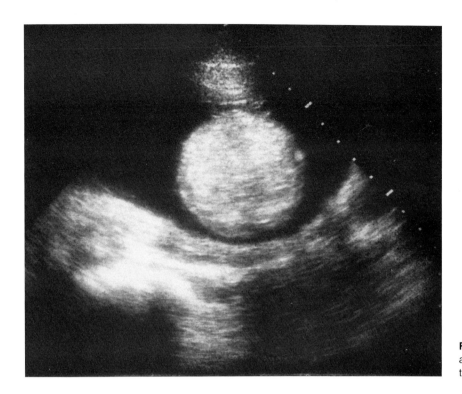

Figure 11–9. Ultrasound picture of a fetus with achondrogenesis depicting absence of ossification of vertebral bodies.

Osteogenesis Imperfecta

Osteogenesis imperfecta (OI) includes a group of osteochondrodysplasias characterized by bone demineralization that are invariably transmitted as mendelian traits. Four different types have been recognized: OI type I is transmitted in an autosomal dominant fashion. Affected individuals are normal at birth, but they have blue sclerae and bone fragility that may lead in time to fractures. OI type II is transmitted as an autosomal recessive condition. Neonates and fetuses have short limbs, multiple fractures of the long bones and ribs, and demineralization of the skull. This condition is uniformly lethal. OI type III may be transmitted either as an autosomal dominant or autosomal recessive trait. The sclerae are blue, and fractures are found usually at birth. This condition is not lethal but carries significant disability. OI type IV is the mildest form of the disease. Patients have blue sclerae, but fractures and deformities are quite uncommon. OI type IV is transmitted as an autosomal dominant trait.[14]

Prenatal sonographic diagnosis of OI type II is possible, even in early gestation. The limbs are usually quite short. The long bones and the thorax are severely deformed due to multiple fractures.[26] Demineralization of the skull leads to an unusual resolution of intracranial anatomy, and the outline of the head can be significantly molded even by slight pressure. Polyhydramnios is frequently found.

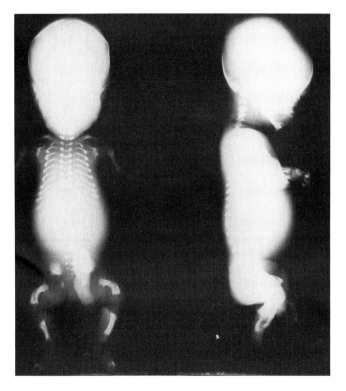

Figure 11–10. Radiogram of a fetus with thanatophoric dysplasia depicting extreme curvature of the limb referred to as "telephone-receiver" femur.

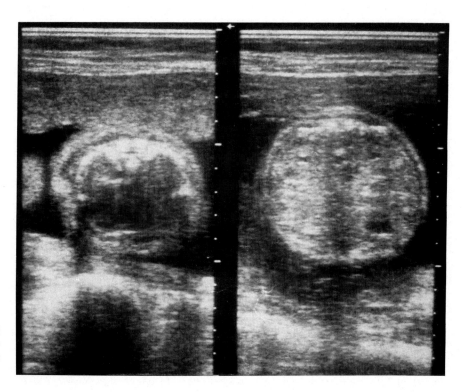

Figure 11–11. Ultrasound picture of a fetus with thanatophoric dysplasia demonstrating hypoplastic chest (left) compared with abdomen (right).

Both OI type I and type III have been diagnosed in utero, with sonographic demonstration of long bonedeformities (Fig. 11–16).[27–30] As fractures do not necessarily occur early in pregnancy, sonographic prenatal diagnosis has obvious limitations. Diagnosis using DNA analysis is also feasible in some cases and should be favored when possible.

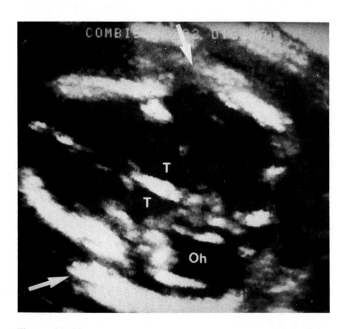

Figure 11–12. Ultrasound picture of fetus with thanatophoric dysplasia demonstrating cloverleaf skull. (T=thalami; Oh=occipital horn; arrows=areas of synotosis).

TABLE 11–11. FETAL THORACIC CIRCUMFERENCE MEASUREMENTS

Gestational Age (wk)	Thoracic circumference (mm) Percentile		
	5th	*50th*	*95th*
16	64	91	119
17	73	100	128
18	82	110	137
19	91	119	146
20	100	128	155
21	110	137	164
22	119	146	173
23	128	155	182
24	137	164	191
25	146	173	200
26	155	182	210
27	164	191	219
28	168	200	228
29	182	210	237
30	191	219	246
31	200	228	255
32	209	237	264
33	218	246	273
34	228	255	282
35	237	264	291
36	246	273	300
37	255	282	309
38	264	291	319
39	273	300	328
40	282	309	337

From Chitkara U, Rosenberg J, Chervenak F, et al. Prenatal sonographic assessment of the fetal thorax: normal values. Am J Obstet Gynecol. 1987; 156:1069, with permission.

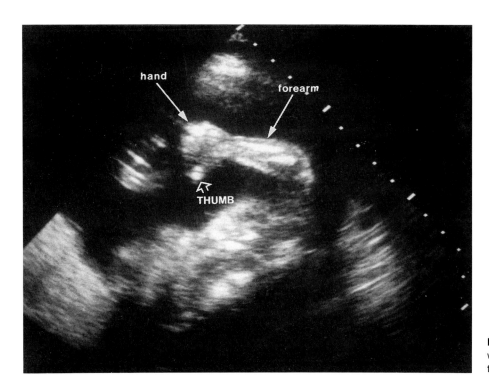

Figure 11–13. Ultrasound picture of a fetus with diastrophic dysplasia depicting hitchhiker thumb.

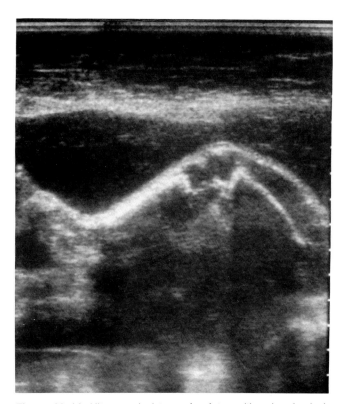

Figure 11–14. Ultrasound picture of a fetus with achondroplasia demonstrating rhizomelic shortening of the leg.

DYSOSTOSES

Dysostoses with Predominant Involvement of the Extremities

Robert's syndrome is transmitted as an autosomal recessive condition. Tetraphocomelia is associated with cleft lip–palate, hypotelorism, and microcephaly. Hydrocephalus, spina bifida, and encephalocele have also been described. Early prenatal diagnosis of this condition is possible by demonstrating severe limb reductions. Most affected infants die in the neonatal period.

Holt–Oram syndrome is typically characterized by the association of abnormalities of the forearm and congenital heart disease (atrial or ventricular septal defects). The radius and the thumb may be absent or hypoplastic. This condition is transmitted as an autosomal dominant trait with variable degrees of penetrance.

Thrombocytopenia–absent radius (TAR) syndrome is featured by the absence of the radius in the presence of a small or even normal thumb and thrombocytopenia that is usually manifested at birth. It is inherited with an autosomal recessive pattern.

Clubfoot

This condition is characterized by medial deviation and inversion of the sole of the foot, usually resulting

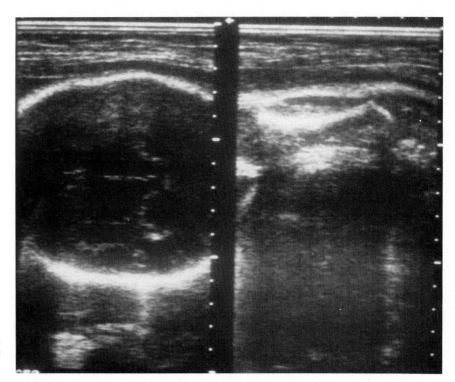

Figure 11–15. Ultrasound picture of a fetus with achondroplasia depicting a large head (left) and small femur (right).

from restriction of fetal movements, as in oligohydramnios, uterine tumors, and paralysis secondary to neurologic abnormalities such as spina bifida. It is also commonly found in many syndromes and malformation clusters. The navicular bones are closely related to the medical aspect of the calcaneus.

Prenatal diagnosis with ultrasound is possible,[31] and it relies on demonstration of an abnormal relationship between the lower leg and the foot (Fig. 11–17). The recognition of the clubfoot deformity in a fetus should immediately prompt a careful search for associated anomalies, including fetal karyotyping.

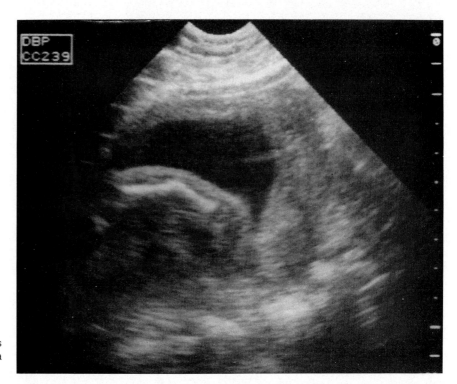

Figure 11–16. An ultrasound picture of a fetus with osteogenesis imperfecta depicting a bowed, fractured femur.

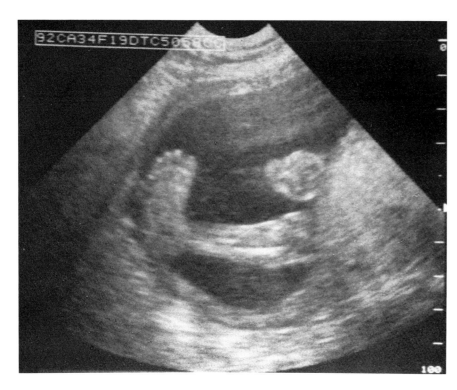

Figure 11–17. Simultaneous demonstration of the leg and of the sole of the foot allow the diagnosis of clubfoot in this fetus.

REFERENCES

1. Moore KL. The articular and skeletal systems. In: *The Developing Human: Clinically Oriented Embryology.* 3rd ed. Philadelphia, Pa: WB Saunders Co; 1982:356–357.

2. Queenan JT, O'Brien GD, Campbell S. Ultrasound measurement of the fetal limb bones. *Am J Obstet Gynecol.* 1988;138:297–302.

3. Campbell S. Early prenatal diagnosis of neural tube defects by ultrasound. *Clin Obstet Gynecol.* 1977;20:351–359.

4. O'Brien GD, Queenan JT, Campbell S. Assessment of gestational age in the second trimester by real-time ultrasound measurement of the femur length. *Am J Obstet Gynecol.* 1981;139:540–545.

5. Mahony BS, Filly RA. High-resolution sonographic assessment of the fetal extremities. *J Ultrasound Med.* 1984;3:489–498.

6. Deter RL, Rossavik I, Hill RM, et al. Longitudinal studies of femur growth in normal fetuses. *J Clin Ultrasound.* 1987;15:299–305.

7. Vintzileos AM, Campbell WA, Neckels S, et al. The ultrasound femur length as a predictor of fetal length. *Obstet Gynecol.* 1984;64:779–782.

8. Streeter G. Weight, sitting height, head size, foot length, and menstrual age of the human embryo. *Contrib Embryol.* 1920;11:143–147.

9. O'Brien GD, Queenan JT. Growth of the ultrasound fetal femur length during normal pregnancy, part I. *Am J Obstet Gynecol.* 1981;141:833–837.

10. Hadlock FP, Harrist RB, Deter RL, et al. Fetal femur length as a predictor of menstrual age: sonographically measured. *AJR.* 1982;138:875–878.

11. Jeanty P, Rodesch F, Delbeke D, et al. Estimation of gestational age from measurements of fetal long bones. *J Ultrasound Med.* 1984;3:75–79.

12. Goldstein I, Reece EA, Hobbins JC. Sonographic appearance of the fetal heel ossification centers and foot length measurements provide independent markers for gestational age estimation. *Am J Obstet Gynecol.* 1988;159:923–926.

13. Platt L, Medearias AL, DeVore GR, et al. Fetal foot length: relationship to menstrual age and fetal measurements in the second trimester. *Obstet Gynecol.* 1988;71:526–531.

14. Pilu G, Rizzo N, Perolo A. Anomalies of the skeletal system. In: Chervenak F, Isaacson GC, Campbell S (eds). *Ultrasound in Obstetrics and Gynecology.* Boston: Little Brown and Co; 1993:981–997.

15. Mahony BS, Filly RA, Cooperberg PL. Antenatal sonographic diagnosis of achondrogenesis. *J Ultrasound Med.* 1984;3:277–279.

16. Pena SDJ, Goodman HO. The genetics of thanatophoric dwarfism. *Pediatrics.* 1973;51:104–109.

17. Isaacson G, Blakemore KJ, Chervenak FA. Thanatophoric dysplasia with cloverleaf skull. *Am J Dis Child.* 1983;137:896–898.

18. Mahony BS, Filly RA, Callen PW, et al. Thanatophoric dwarfism with the cloverleaf skull: a specific antenatal sonographic diagnosis. *J Ultrasound Med.* 1985;4:151–154.

19. Grote W, Weisner D, Jaenig U, et al. Prenatal diagnosis of short rib–polydactyly syndrome type Saldino–Noonan at 17 weeks gestation. *Eur J Pediatr.* 1983;140:63–66.

20. Gembruch U, Hansmann M, Foedisch HJ. Early prenatal diagnosis of short rib polydactyly syndrome type I (Majewski) by ultrasound in a case at risk. *Prenatal Diagn.* 1985;5:357–362.

21. Thomson GS, Reynolds P, Cruikshank J. Antenatal detection of recurrence of Majewski dwarf (short–rib poly-

dactyly syndrome type II Majewski). *Clin Radiol.* 1982;33:509–511.

22. Walker BA, Scott CI, Hall JG, et al. Diastrophic dwarfism. *Medicine.* 1972;51:41–59.

23. Dennis JP, Rosenberg HS, Ellsworth CA. Megalencephaly, internal hydrocephalus and other neurological aspects of achondroplasia. *Brain.* 1961;84:427–433.

24. Filly RA, Golbus MS, Carey JC, et al. Short-limbed dwarfism: ultrasonographic diagnosis by mensuration of fetal femoral length. *Radiology.* 1981;138:653–656.

25. Kurtz AB, Filly RA, Wapner RJ, et al. In utero analysis of heterozygous achondroplasia: variable time of onset as detected by femur length measurements. *J Ultrasound Med.* 1986;5:137–140.

26. Beluffi G, Fraccaro M. Genetical and clinical aspects of campomelic dysplasia. *Prog Clin Biol Res.* 1982;104:53–68.

27. Hobbins JC, Bracken MB, Mahoney MJ. Diagnosis of fetal skeletal dysplasias with ultrasound. *Am J Obstet Gynecol.* 1982;142:306–312.

28. Fryns JP, van der Berghe K, van Assche A, et al. Prenatal diagnosis of campomelic dwarfism. *Clin Genet.* 1981;19:199–201.

29. Winter R, Rosenkranz W, Hofmann, et al. Prenatal diagnosis of campomelic dysplasia by ultrasonography. *Prenatal Diagn.* 1985;5:1–8.

30. Aylsworth AS, Seeds JW, Bonner-Guilford W, et al. Prenatal diagnosis of a severe deforming type of osteogenesis imperfecta. *Am J Med Genet.* 1984;19:707–714.

31. Jeanty P, Romero R, d'Alton M, et al. In utero sonographic detection of hand and foot deformities. *J Ultrasound Med.* 1985;4:595–601.

12

Ultrasound and Fetal Dysmorphology Syndromes

INTRODUCTION

Improved resolution in ultrasound technology has led to the detection of even subtle fetal anomalies, including mild deformities of the face and extremities.[1-4] Experienced sonologists can now perform physical examinations of fetuses, even in early gestation, similar, in terms of the information obtainable, to those performed on neonates. Growing attention is given to the use of ultrasound in the detection of fetal dysmorphology syndromes.[5,6] This ability to detect penatal features of fetuses at risk for malformations will enable sonologists to better target fetuses for detailed examinations. More than one half of fetuses who possess chromosomal anomalies will go undiagnosed until birth. Current karyotypic examination criteria include pregnant women of age 35 years and older (which will only identify 20% of Down syndrome fetuses) and low maternal serum alpha-fetoprotein (MSAFP). Ultrasound thus may be useful in expanding the population of at-risk fetuses.

The study of certain sonographically detectable malformations and their frequency of occurrence, especially as part of syndromes, is also useful in counseling patients regarding their risk of occurrence, recurrence, significance, and in recommending the most appropriate obstetric management. Selected dysmorphology syndromes will be presented along with the identifiable ultrasound features.

experienced sonologist may obtain valuable information, however, simply by views of the fetal profile (Fig. 12–1). Interorbital measurements, for example, are a classic tool of the postnatal dysmorphologists which can be easily and rapidly performed on the fetus as well.[7] Hypotelorism, decreased interorbital distance, has a striking association with several severe conditions, especially the holoprosencephalic sequence and trisomy 13. Although increased interorbital distance, hypertelorism, may be a benign finding, it is recognized as a part of an extremely long list of syndromes.[8] Ocular biometry also permits the recognition of microphthalmia, which often serves as a marker for many chromosomal and other malformation syndromes.

Other facial abnormalities recognized sonographically include cataract[9] and clefting. Facial clefting occurs as a component of a well-defined malformation syndrome in 3% of cases.[10] Approximately 1% of cases are of the median cleft type which can be associated with either the holoprosencephalic sequence or the median cleft face syndrome, also known as the frontonasal dysplasia sequence.[11] Ultrasound evaluation of the extremities can allow the demonstration of relevant findings such as clubhand, clubfoot, and polydactyly. Specific publications on this subject give detailed lists of potentially associated syndromes.[12] Using these sonographic clues, the sonologist can consider potential fetal dysmorphology syndromes when a constellation of features is detected.

SONOGRAPHIC CLUES IN THE FETUS AT RISK FOR DYSMORPHOLOGY SYNDROME

The obstetric sonologist is faced with the problem of a fetal dysmorphology syndrome in two different clinical settings: examination of a pregnant patient at risk either because of a positive familial history or exposure to teratogens, or because a fetal anomaly was serendipitously encountered during a routine scan. An

SONOGRAPHIC FEATURES IN THE FETUS WITH OVERT DYSMORPHOLOGY SYNDROME

Selected dysmorphology syndromes and their relevant sonographic features are presented in this section. Most of these data were derived from targeted ultrasound examinations performed on pregnancies at risk, or in pregnancies for which a suspicion of a fetal

159

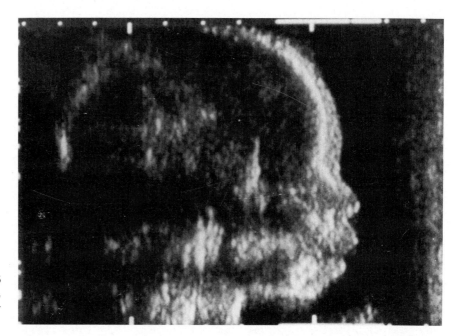

Figure 12–1. A normal profile of the fetus at 25 weeks' gestation. Normal structures (calvarium, nose, mouth, lips, chin, and neck) and the normal contours of the fetal head can be seen.

anomaly was formulated during a routine scan. As a result, there is a possibility that these data are biased toward the inclusion of greater numbers of sonographically detectable anomalies.

Trisomy 21

Trisomy 21 is the most frequent chromosomal aberration found at birth, with an overall incidence of 1 in 600 births. Infants with Down syndrome have typical stigmata that include flattened facial features, oblique palpebral fissures, epicanthal folds, brachycephaly with a flat occiput, and redundant skin in the neck.

The birth weight is usually toward the lower limits of normal, and the limbs tend to be short. A large number of these infants are affected by major malformations. Congenital heart disease occurs in at least 50% of cases, with atrioventricular septal defects the most common anomaly (Fig 12–2). Gastrointestinal anomalies such as duodenal atresia and omphalocele are also reported to occur, although less frequently.

The largest available series of ultrasound antenatal diagnosis of Down syndrome cases includes 91 consecutive cases prospectively examined at a single institution.[13] One or more abnormalities could be detected sonographically in 33% of these fetuses. Pos-

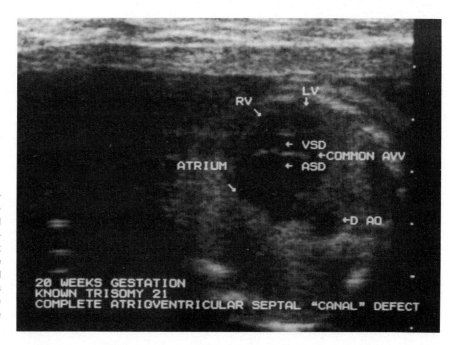

Figure 12–2. (A) Transabdominal view of a fetus with trisomy 21 at 20 weeks gestation depicting a complete atriolventricular (AV) septal defect, sometimes referred to as AV canal defect. In this sagittal view of the heart the apex points anteriorly with a right and left ventricle (RV, LV), and the atrium is located inferiorly and to the right. The common AV valve (AVV) as well as the septal defects (ASD, VSD) can be seen. A small descending aorta (D Ao) can be seen in the lower right of this picture.

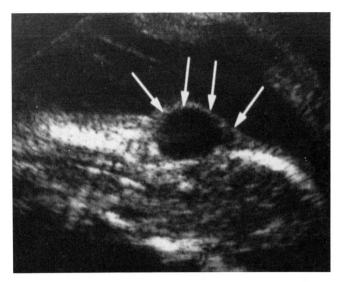

Figure 12–3. Fetus with echolucent mass (arrows) in the neck representing a cystic hygroma.

itive findings were closely related to the gestational age in which the scan was performed. Prior to 14 weeks, the most frequent anomaly was cystic hygroma (Fig. 12–3); in later gestation cardiovascular anomalies, hydrops, duodenal atresia, and omphalocele were seen. Although a considerable proportion of fetuses were found postnatally to have congenital heart disease, these lesions were missed by antenatal sonography in over 60% of cases. These false-negative diagnoses occurred mainly in fetuses examined early in pregnancy. Duodenal atresia was correctly identified in four cases seen after the 24th week but missed in one case examined at 17 weeks. Two cases of omphalocele were identified, and in both only bowel loops were seen inside the amnioperitoneal sac. This sup-

ports a report that small omphaloceles, without external herniation of the liver, carry the highest risk of association with chromosomal aberrations.[14] Mild enlargement of cerebral ventricles, presumably dependent upon brain atrophy, has also been reported in fetuses with trisomy 21.[13,15]

Demonstration of a thick nuchal fold increases the risk of Down syndrome (Fig. 12–4). In a suboccipitobregmatic scan of the fetal head, also referred to as a transcerebellar view, the soft tissues of the neck should have a diameter of less than 6 mm. The positive predictive value of this finding has been reported to vary between 8% and 69%.[13–17] The threshold of 6 mm has been established in fetuses between 15 and 20 weeks.[18] It is unclear whether this threshold applies to older fetuses as well.

In a recent report by Crane and Gray[19] using the 6-mm skin fold thickness as the upper limit of normal, 12 of 16 (75%) Down syndrome cases were identifiable, with a positive predictive value of 1 in 13. These findings are even more remarkable than those of Benecerraf et al.[16] The nuchal skin fold thickness, for example, was significantly more predictive of Down syndrome than advanced maternal age or low MSAFP, allowing identification of 75% of Down syndrome fetuses compared with only 20% using maternal age of 35 or over, and 33% for low MSAFP.[20,21] In addition, the false-positive rate was only 1% compared with 5% when maternal age of 35 or over or low MSAFP were used to recommend amniocentesis. A previous study by Benacerraf et al.[18] had only a 39% sensitivity, but a positive predictive value of 1 in 5 and a false-positive rate of 0.1%. Other reports have refuted the claims of the 6-mm skin fold having such a high prenatal diagnostic accuracy.[17,22]

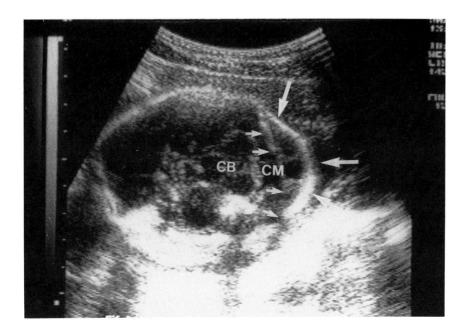

Figure 12–4. Down syndrome fetus with thickened nuchal fold obtained at the transcerebellar level. CB = cerebellum; CM = cepterna magna; small arrows = posterior skull table; large arrows = skin fold.

Infants with Down syndrome have short limbs, and several reports have recently addressed the problem of measuring femur length in the second trimester as a screening tool for Down syndrome. Different results have been reported thus far.

Fizsimmons et al.[23] have shown that long bone measurements of affected fetuses fall below the normal regression life for that bone. Benacerraf et al[18] have reported that if a measured-to-expected femur length ratio of 0.91 is used as a limit, the sensitivity for identifying Down syndrome fetuses was 68%, with 2% false-positive rate. This same group showed how the addition of the positive nuchal fold to the femur length criterion increased their predictive value from 3.1% to 4.3% in a population with a 1 in 250 risk for Down syndrome.[23-25] These data have been corroborated by some researchers[15,26-28] and refuted by others.[29-32]

Benacerraf et al[18] have also shown that the length of the humerus of Down syndrome fetuses is foreshortened as well. Once again, using a measured-to-expected humeral length ratio of less than 0.90, 12 of 24 fetuses (50%) with Down syndrome and 25 of 400 normal fetuses (6.25%) were identified. In addition, 12 of the 24 Down syndrome fetuses had a nuchal fold measuring 6 mm or more. Combining nuchal skin-fold findings with humeral length criteria, 18 of 24 affected fetuses (75%) were identified, yielding a positive predictive value of 4.6% for women with a 1 in 250 risk for delivering a fetus with Down syndrome.

The association between nonimmune fetal hydrops and Down syndrome has been established.[33] In many cases, hydrops is probably the final result of congestive heart failure secondary to one of the cardiac lesions frequently associated with trisomy 21.[34] Cardiac malformations are not found in 50% of cases, however, and the etiology of hydrops is unknown.[33]

Although there is not unequivocal agreement on the association and prediction of Down syndrome by fetal biometry, there are sufficient data to suggest that when clearly abnormal biometric measurements are obtained, including excess skinfold, foreshortened humerus and femur, and altered ratios, further evaluation is needed.

Hyperechogenic bowel has been noted in fetuses with Down syndrome.[33] The pathophysiology is unknown. Echogenic bowel has also been documented in fetuses with cystic fibrosis[35] and may be seen occasionally in normal fetuses as well.[36] At present, the relative risks are therefore uncertain.

Growth retardation is a common finding in chromosomal aberrations. There was sonographic evidence of this condition in 6 of 94 fetuses (6.3%) in the series reported by Nyberg and coworkers.[13] In two of these cases, growth retardation could be detected prior to 26 weeks. Hypoplasia of the middle phalanx of the fifth digit, a typical sign associated with Down syn-

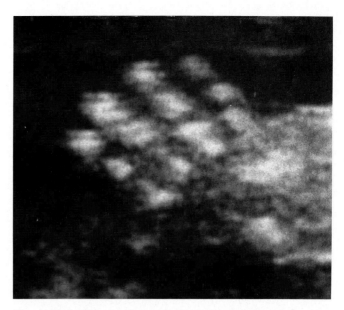

Figure 12–5. Ultrasound scan depicting normal fetal hand.

drome, has been recently demonstrated by ultrasound in the second trimester. (Fig. 12–5, Fig. 12–6, and Fig. 12–7).[37] A possible association between renal pyelectasis and Down syndrome has also been suggested.[38] Table 12–1 summarizes the most common sonographic features.

Trisomy 18

The incidence of trisomy 18 (Edwards syndrome) is 1 in 3,000 to 6,000 births. Severe growth retardation is the rule, with birth weights usually below the fifth

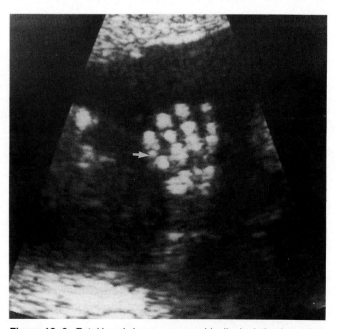

Figure 12–6. Fetal hand shown sonographically depicting hypoplastic middle phalanx of fifth digit (arrow).

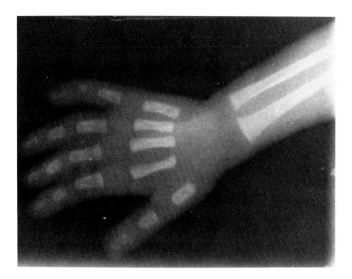

Figure 12–7. X-ray picture of fetal hand shown in Figure 12–6.

percentile. Major anomalies are consistently seen at birth. Congenital heart disease, mostly ventricular septal defects, is reported to occur in more than 95% of cases. Omphalocele (Fig 9–23 and Fig. 9–35), esophageal atresia (Fig. 9–15), and rockerbottom foot (Fig. 12–8) are seen frequently, as well as a variety of skeletal deformities, including an elongated skull with a prominent occiput, micrognathia, overlapping digits, and clubhand, with or without mesomelic shortening of the upper extremities.

The sonographic findings in trisomy 18 have been the object of many reports.[39] There is a consensus that a careful survey of fetal anatomy will almost always demonstrate sonographic anomalies, usually in the setting of a small-for-gestational-age fetus with associated polyhydramnios.

Several reports have recently explored the association between choroid plexus cysts and trisomy 18. It is now clear that choroid plexus cysts can be identified in 2% of all fetuses examined sonographically during the second trimester (Fig. 12–9).[40] Usually the cysts disappear by the third trimester, and thus far at birth these infants have been reported to be neurologically normal. The frequency of trisomy 18 in fetuses with choroid plexus cysts varies tremendously in the reported series due to the small number of cases. An incidence of 4.8% was found in the largest available series, which includes 82 fetuses.[41] This was a heterogeneous series, including cases referred both from level 1 facilities and from routine studies of the general population. A bias is expected, as the concomitance of choroid plexus cysts and other anomalies is probably the indication for most referrals.

One series now includes 103 fetuses with choroid plexus cysts that were prospectively identified in low-risk second-trimester pregnancies. Five fetuses (4.8%) with trisomy 18 were detected in this group. Three of these fetuses had other characteristic anomalies that were identified by ultrasound. No associated malformations, however, could be clearly recognized in one fetus examined at 16 weeks and in another fetus of an obese mother. One fetus with trisomy 21 was also identified in this series, but this was thought to be coincidental. Clearly fetal chromosomal analysis should be offered when a choroid plexus cyst is seen in association with an anatomic abnormality, since the incidence of aneuploidy appears high by various reports. It is still uncertain whether or not isolated choroid plexus cysts represent an indication for fetal karyotyping. Benacerraf and coworkers[42] strongly oppose the need for karyotypic analysis in this setting, assuming that most fetuses with trisomy 18 will have other anatomic anomalies that can be detected with ultrasound. The anomalies associated with trisomy 18 are often subtle. The most typical lesions associated with trisomy 18 include ventricular septal defects and anomalies of the extremities (Fig. 12–10). In midtrimes-

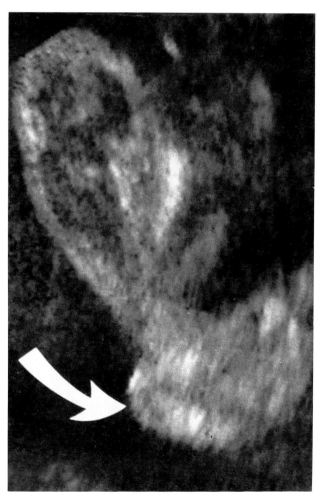

Figure 12–8. Rockerbottom foot (arrow) and clubfoot are seen in a fetus with trisomy 18.

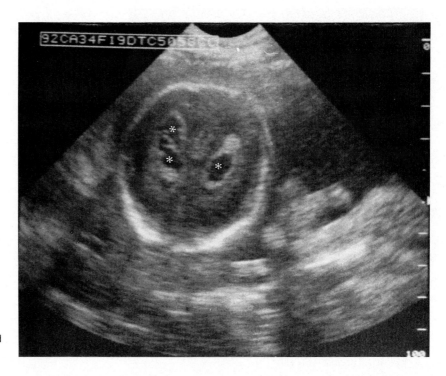

Figure 12–9. Choroid plexus cysts (*) depicted in a fetus with trisomy 18.

ter, these sonographic findings are frequently overlooked. The sonologist's level of expertise and diagnostic accuracy is a critical issue in counseling patients.

Some malformation complexes are invariably associated with trisomy 18. The concomitance of a choroid plexus cyst with either congenital heart disease, clubfoot, (Fig. 12–11 and Fig. 12–12) or both represent one of the malformation complexes associated with

trisomy 18. The other one is the association between spina bifida and congenital heart disease, omphalocele, or both. Examination of the fetal profile may offer further information, as micrognathia and a small nose are almost the rule in these cases (Fig. 12–13). A single umbilical artery is found in from 10% to 50% of cases.

In 10 consecutive cases seen in the third trimester, severe growth retardation of the symmetric type was

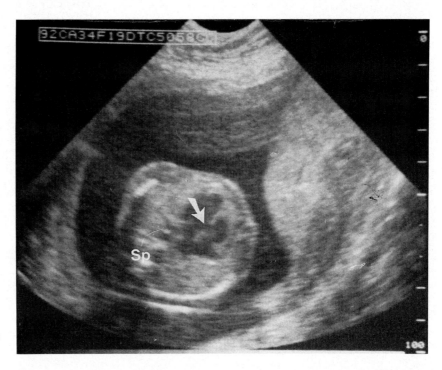

Figure 12–10. Ventricular septal defect (arrow) in a fetus with trisomy 18. SP = spine.

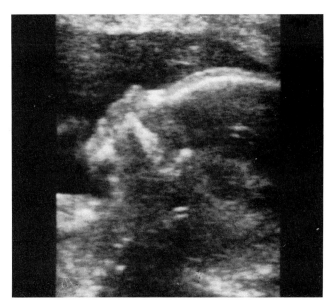

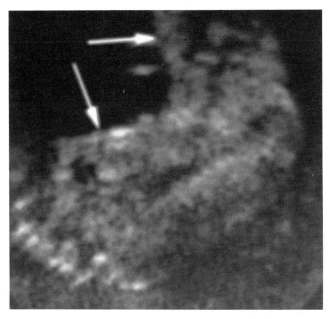

Figure 12–11. Ultrasound picture showing a fetal leg (top arrow) and fetal foot and toes (bottom arrow). Note that both the profile of the leg and the sole of the foot can be easily visualized. These findings are typical of a clubfoot. It should be noted that the heel is not excessively prominent, nor is there an exaggerated curvature of the heel or sole. Therefore, a diagnosis of rockerbottom foot is ruled out.

Figure 12–13. Abnormal fetal profile showing a small nose and chin and elongated skull in a fetus with trisomy 18.

usually found in association with very abnormal Doppler waveforms in the umbilical arteries. (See Table 12–1 for a summary of the common sonographic features.)

Trisomy 13

The incidence of trisomy 13 (Patau syndrome) is about 1 in 6,000 births. This condition is characterized by multiple major anomalies, most of which involve the

central nervous system and the heart. The most typical anomaly is certainly the allobar form of the holoprosencephalic sequence, a malformation complex involving the brain and face. This malformation complex is readily detectable with ultrasound in the second trimester[43] and can be recognized by the 14th week of pregnancy.[6] Allobar holoprosencephaly oc-

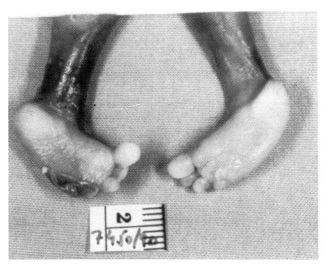

Figure 12–12. Abortus showing clubbing with leg profile and sole in the same view.

TABLE 12–1. COMMON SONOGRAPHIC FINDINGS ASSOCIATED WITH FETUSES WITH CHROMOSOMAL ANOMALIES

Trisomy 21	Trisomy 18
1. Cystic hygroma	1. CHD especially VSD
2. CHD	2. Choroid plexus cyst especially with CHD or clubfoot
3. Hydrops	
4. Duodenal atresia	3. NTD especially with CHD or omphalocele
5. Omphalocele	
6. Mild ventriculomegaly	4. Single umbilical artery
7. Nuchal skin fold (>6mm)	5. Micrognathia
8. Hyperechogenic bowel	6. Early IUGR
9. Early IUGR	
10. Hypoplasia of middle phalanx of fifth digit	
11. Renal pyelectasis	
12. Short femur and humerus	

Trisomy 13	Turner Syndrome
1. Alobar holoprosencephaly and craniofacial malformations	1. Coarctation
	2. Cystic hygroma
2. CHD	3. Hydrops
3. NTD	4. First-trimester nuchal bleb
4. Polydactyly	

CHD = congenital heart disease, NTD = Neural tube defect, IUGR = Intrauterine growth retardation, VSD = Ventricular septal defect.

curs in 60% to 70% of cases of trisomy 13.[44] Conversely, trisomy 13 has been found in 3 of 24 (12.5%) of holoprosencephalic fetuses. There is also a constellation of malformations associated with trisomy 13.[39] Researchers have found heterogenous cardiac malformations, including one case each of ventricular septal defect, atrioventricular septal defect, hypoplastic left heart syndrome, and truncus arteriosus. Spina bifida, Potter type II dysplastic kidneys, and megaureters due to vesicourinary reflux have also been documented. Polydactyly of hands and feet, as well as a single umbilical artery, is another frequent finding. There is a less stringent association with growth retardation than in trisomy 18. Abnormal Doppler waveforms in the umbilical artery have been documented in at least one case in the third trimester (see Table 12–3).

Turner Syndrome

Turner syndrome is reported to occur in 1 in 10,000 live females and is mainly featured by short stature, sexual infantilism, primary amenorrhea, atypical facies, and webbed neck. Congenital heart disease is found in 20% of cases, with left-sided lesions clearly predominant. Coarctation of the aorta is the most frequent anomaly. The karyotype is 45,X in over 50% of cases. Mosaicism accounts for the remaining cases; 45,X/46,XX is the most frequent finding. In these cases, the coexistence of normal 46,XX cell line may reduce the phenotypic and functional manifestations of the syndrome.

The 45,X karyotype is associated with a very high rate of spontaneous abortion. Approximately 20% of chromosomally abnormal first-trimester abortuses are

TABLE 12–2. ABNORMALITIES ASSOCIATED WITH AMNIOTIC BAND SYNDROME

Limb defects, multiple, asymmetric
   Constriction rings of limbs or digits
   Amputation of limbs or digits
   Pseudosyndactyly
   Abnormal dermal ridge pattern
   Simian crease
   Clubfoot
Craniofacial defects
   Encephalocele, multiple, asymmetric
   Anencephaly
   Facial clefting—lip, palate
      Embryologically appropriate
      Embryologically inappropriate
   Severe nasal deformity
   Asymmetric microphthalmia
   Incomplete or absent cranial calcification
Visceral defects
   Omphalocele

45,X. Turner syndrome is associated with a specific fetal anomaly, cystic hygroma colli resulting from lymphatic obstruction (Fig. 12–14). At one time, this malformation was considered pathognomonic of Turner syndrome.

It is now clear that cystic hygroma may be associated with other aneuploidies, including autosomal trisomies,[45] and rarely with nonchromosomal disorders such as Noonan syndrome, multiple pterygium syndrome, Robert syndrome, distichiasis–lymphedema syndrome, and the hereditary lethal nuchal cyst.[46] Hydrops is present in most cases recognized in the midtrimester, and intrauterine demise is almost always the rule.[47] More recently, cystic hygromas were identified

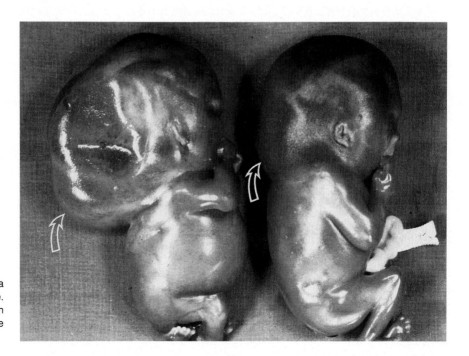

Figure 12–14. Cystic hygroma colli in a monozygotic twin gestation with 45,X karyotype. Thus different expressions of the malformation of cystic hygroma (arrows) are shown in these two monozygotic fetuses.

in first-trimester fetuses with the use of transvaginal sonography. It is estimated that 40% of normal embryos prior to 10 weeks have small accumulations of fluid in the posterior cervical region, commonly referred to as "nuchal blebs."[48] Initially there was concern that these nuchal blebs would be misdiagnosed as cystic hygroma colli during this period of pregnancy. The largest available series, however, indicates that first-trimester sonographic demonstration of cervical fluid collections larger than 5 mm were associated with chromosomal abnormalities in 15 of 29 (52%) fetuses.[49] The list of karyotypic abnormalities was heterogeneous, with a markedly different distribution than described in midtrimester fetuses. Trisomy 21 accounted for 6 of the 15 detected abnormalities, while 45,X was present in only one case. In six of the fetuses with normal chromosomes, including two with hydrops, remission of cystic hygromas was documented in the following weeks, and normal infants were delivered. These data support the importance of chromosomal analysis when cystic hygromas are detected in utero independent of gestational age. First-trimester hygromas may represent a different clinical entity from those classically identified in the midtrimester. (See Table 12–1 for a summary of common sonographic features.)

Triploidy

Polyploidy is one of the most frequent chromosomal anomalies identified in spontaneous abortions. Triploidy is invariably present in partial hydatidiform moles. A pregnancy with a triploid conceptus will continue beyond the first trimester only in rare cases. The sonographic findings in this condition have been extensively described.[50,51]

In the most typical case, a large placenta is seen in association with a severely growth-retarded fetus that has a dramatic head-to-body disproportion (Fig. 12–15). Major malformations are the rule and include holoprosencephaly, porencephaly, spina bifida, and congenital heart disease. Triploidy is a uniformly lethal condition. It frequently coexists with a partial hydatidiform mole that can result in maternal complications such as pregnancy-induced hypertension. Under these circumstances therapeutic termination can be offered to patients.

Meckel Syndrome

Meckel syndrome is a lethal anomaly transmitted as an autosomal recessive trait. It is featured by multiple anomalies, the most relevant of which are bilateral polycystic dysplastic kidney, microcephaly, and congenital heart disease.[52] Pathologic studies indicate that the renal cystic dysplasia is of the Potter III type, although cases with Potter II features have been described.[53] Potter facies, polydactyly, occipital encephalocele, allobar holoprosencephaly, polycystic liver, and facial clefting are also frequently found.

The most striking sonographic finding is bilateral renal enlargement. The ultrasound appearance of kidneys, despite the pathologic type, is very similar to the one that is found with Potter type I infantile polycystic kidney disease. Several pregnancies at risk for this condition were studied; five affected fetuses were diagnosed prospectively. The presence of enlarged echogenic kidneys were the most useful as well as the earliest sign to appear in all cases. Renal sonographic abnormalities could always be identified by the midtrimester, and in one fetus as early as the 15th week. This limited experience seems to suggest that, unlike other forms of renal dysplasia, the one associated with Meckel syndrome can be consistently recognized in early gestation.

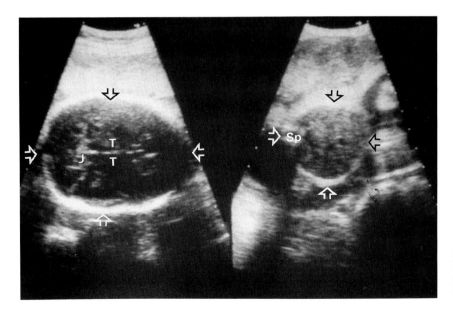

Figure 12–15. Severe discrepancy between head circumference and abdominal circumference, T = thalami, SP = spine; open arrows = borders of head and abdomen.

Amniotic Band Syndrome

Amniotic band syndrome is a sporadic condition with a frequency that varies in different surveys from 1 in 12,000 to 1 in 15,000 live births (Fig. 12–16 and Fig. 19–1). Although several theories have been proposed to explain the genesis of amniotic band syndrome, the most widely accepted view is that early rupture of the amnion results in mesodermic bands that emanate from the chorionic side of the amnion and insert on the fetal body, leading to amputations, constrictions, and postural deformities secondary to immobilization.[54] The earlier the insult occurs, the more severe the lesion.

Amniotic rupture in the first weeks of pregnancy results in craniofacial and visceral defects, whereas during the second trimester it may lead to limb and digital constriction and amputations.[55] An alternative view is that amniotic band syndrome is the consequence of an insult that results in typical malformations, as well as ectodermal and mesenchymal disrup-

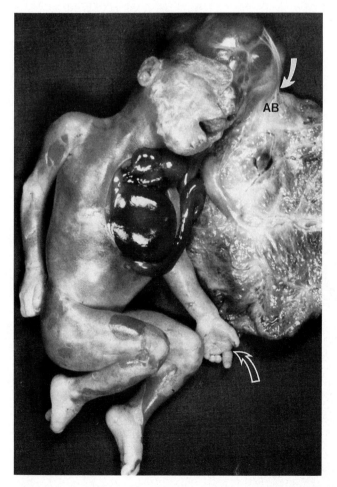

Figure 12–16. Documented case of amniotic band syndrome depicting a large encephalocele with facial clefting, abdominal wall defect, and finger with ring constrictions (arrow). AB = analytic band.

tion. Vascular compromise may have a pathogenic role in the genesis of external defects.

Amniotic band syndrome has been reported after amniocentesis.[56] The pathologic findings of amniotic band syndrome have been extensively reviewed.[57] Table 12–2 illustrates the abnormalities most commonly associated with this condition. A diagnosis is made when one or more of these defects are found. An example of a documented case of amniotic band syndrome is demonstrated in Figure 12–10. Fibrous strings originating from the surface of the placenta are frequently seen inserting into the fetal body at the level of the defects, but their presence is not necessary for the diagnosis.

Amniotic band syndrome has been identified in utero with sonography.[58,59] This condition encompasses a broad constellation of anomalies that differ in each case. This syndrome should be suspected when one or more of the anomalies indicated in Table 12–2 are encountered. Asymmetric or multiple encephaloceles in combination with amputations, ventral wall defects, and postural deformities should strongly raise the index of suspicion. Amniotic bands are sometimes seen as linear echoes floating in the amniotic cavity and entangling the fetal body. These bands may be confused with three other conditions that may cause linear echoes crossing the amniotic cavity: chorioamniotic separation, intrauterine synechiae, and a septate uterus. Meticulous scanning will demonstrate that these structures do not insert into the fetal body and that they are not associated with fetal structural anomalies.

Syndromes with Callosal Agenesis

Agenesis of the corpus callosum can be found in association with chromosomal aberrations (trisomy 13 and 18), mostly as a part of the holoprosencephalic malformation sequence. The familial occurrence of this condition is well established. Marked genetic heterogeneity has been documented, with evidence supporting autosomal dominant, autosomal recessive, and X-linked forms of inheritance.[60]

Agenesis of the corpus callosum may also be one component of a genetically determined malformation syndrome, such as 1) Aicardi syndrome (seizures, chorioretinal lacunae, mental retardation, microcephaly, and vertebral anomalies; X-linked dominant transmission)[61]; 2) Andermann syndrome (mental retardation and progressive motor neuropathy; autosomal recessive transmission);[62] 3) acrocallosal syndrome (mental retardation, macrocephaly, and polydactyly; autosomal recessive transmission);[63] 4) FG syndrome (mental retardation, macrocephaly, and hypotonia; X-linked recessive transmission).[64]

It has been demonstrated that the traditional radiologic criteria for recognition of agenesis of the corpus callosum (enlargement of posterior horns and increased separation between the bodies of lateral ventricles, superior displacement of third ventricle) can be identified by ultrasound at the midtrimester (Fig. 5–72, Fig. 5–73, and Fig. 12–17).[65] Couples at risk for familial syndromes associated with callosal agenesis can now be offered the possibility of prenatal diagnosis.

Pierre Robin Syndrome (Robin Anomalad)

The Pierre Robin syndrome is featured by the association of micrognathia and glossoptosis. A posterior cleft palate or a high arched palate is frequently present.[66] These elements are possibly related (hypoplasia of the mandible would lead to posterior displacement of the tongue and abnormal closure of the posterior palatine processes); this condition should be regarded as a malformation sequence rather than a syndrome.

According to Cohen,[67] Pierre Robin syndrome is found as an isolated lesion in 39% of patients. In 36%, one or more associated anomalies are present but do not conform to a well-established syndrome. In 25% of patients, a known syndrome is found (Table 12–3). The Pierre Robin syndrome per se is, in many cases, a neonatal emergency. Glossoptosis may lead to obstruction of the airways and suffocation. Many cases of sudden death have been described. Infants have

TABLE 12–3. SYNDROMES ASSOCIATED WITH THE ROBIN ANOMALAD

Genetic syndromes
  Monogenic
    Diastrophic dysplasia
    Stickler syndrome
    Spondyloepiphyseal dysplasia
    Beckwith–Wiedemann syndrome
    Myotonic dystrophy
    Campomelic syndrome
Chromosomal
  Trisomy 11q+
Nongenetic syndromes
  Fetal alcohol syndrome
  Fetal hydantoin syndrome
  Fetal trimethadione syndrome

Adapted from Cohen MM Jr. The Robin anomalad: its nonspecificity and associated syndromes. J Oral Surg. 1976;34:587–593.

had difficulty feeding because of the ball–valve effect of the tongue in the oropharynx and because of vomiting, which frequently leads to failure to thrive. With proper assistance these infants may overcome the difficulties of this anomaly. With time there is some growth of the mandible.

Pierre Robin syndrome has been recognized in utero with ultrasound. Prenatal diagnosis was once possible only late in gestation by identification of a small mandible in a profile view of the fetal face.[68] More recently, this condition has been recognized, us-

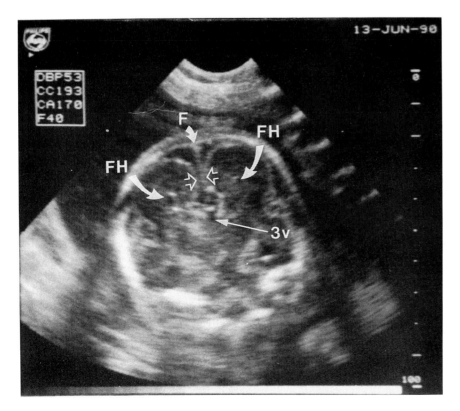

Figure 12–17. Agenesis of the corpus callosum in a coronal scan demonstrating wide separation of the frontal horns (FH); wide separation of hemispheric fissures (open arrow heads). F = falx cerebri, 3V = third ventricle.

ing the same approach, in several midtrimester fetuses (Fig. 12–18). Qualitative evaluation obviously carries some subjectivity. Measurements of the mandible in a transverse plane have recently been reported; these measurements may allow a more certain diagnosis on a quantitative basis.[69]

Noonan Syndrome

This condition is featured by short stature, mental retardation, hypertelorism, epicanthal folds, dental malocclusion, pectus excavatum, and congenital heart disease (mainly ventricular septal defects and pulmonic stenosis). The phenotype has some similarities with Turner syndrome, but the karyotype is normal and both sexes are affected. Noonan syndrome is mostly sporadic, but autosomal dominant transmission has been documented. The intrauterine sonographic findings have been described in a few cases.[70] The most relevant sign is cystic hygroma colli; these defects were reported to be small and bilateral (Fig. 12–3). This sign is, however, atypical; it is probably shared in common by all conditions that are associated at birth with webbed neck. A high index of suspicion for Noonan syndrome is suggested when a male fetus or a female fetus with normal chromosomes is found to have small bilateral cervical hygromas in association with congenital heart disease.

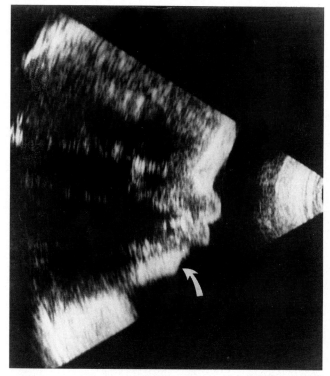

Figure 12–18. An abnormal profile of fetus with Pierre Robin anomalad and with micrognathia (arrow).

SONOGRAPHIC CRITERIA FOR KARYOTYPIC ANALYSIS

Documented Fetal Anomalies

The routine use of sonography in pregnancy results in an increasingly high rate of detection of fetal malformations. These diagnoses, once extremely rare, have become a part of everyday practice, but still raise concerns for both patients and physicians. An accurate diagnosis is required to counsel a couple with appropriate prognostic data and to enable sensible obstetric management. The association between structural anomalies and chromosomal aberrations is an issue of major concern. Because a combination of chromosomal and anatomic anomalies carries a major influence on the final outcome of pregnancy, several authorities have suggested that fetal karyotyping be offered in all cases of documented structural anomalies.

This attitude is further supported by several reports indicating a much higher incidence of chromosome abnormalities among fetuses with ultrasound-detected structural anomalies than among newborns with malformations recognized after birth, with figures ranging from 20% to 45%.[71–73] The discrepancy between fetal and neonatal studies seems to be due to the high intrauterine fetal death rate among pregnancies complicated by abnormal karyotype and fetal malformations.

The risk of chromosomal aberrations is heavily influenced by sonographic findings. In a series of 237 consecutive cases seen at several institutions, the incidence of an abnormal karyotype was only 10.6% when one malformation was seen but increased to 35.6% when two or more malformations were present.[74] In those with a single malformation, the malformation that led to an abnormal karyotype most often was cystic hygroma. Similar figures were found when the series was updated to 451 cases (Fig. 12–19).

A targeted examination is indicated when a fetal anomaly is suspected on ultrasound. An experienced sonologist can identify subtle defects, such as cardiac lesions, and may be able to infer the presence of an underlying syndrome from a cluster of findings. Multiple fetal anomalies are associated with a high risk of chromosomal aberrations, and a cytogenetic examination is strongly recommended. The consensus is that fetal karyotyping should be offered to a couple, even when only a single anomaly is found (Fig. 12–20).

Suspicious Fetal Developmental Aberrations

At present, the main indications for fetal karyotyping include advanced maternal age, family history, and abnormal biochemical screening (alpha-fetoprotein, human chorionic gonadotropin, [HCG], estriol).

Suspicious fetal developmental aberrations

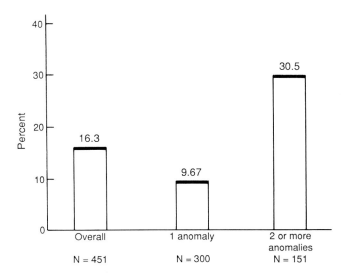

Figure 12–19. Ultrasound diagnosis of fetal malformations and aneuploids. With one anomaly, the incidence of aneuploidy is about 9.67%, whereas with two or more anomalies, the incidence is 30.5%, with an overall rate of 16.3%.

readily identifiable with sonography are probably present in most fetuses with trisomy 13 and 18, but they can be found in only about 30% of Down syndrome fetuses.[13] Furthermore, some of these aberrations (duodenal atresia, congenital heart defects) usually go undetected in the second trimester. Special attention recently has been given to the issue of sonographic identification of two main findings commonly associated with trisomy 21 (increased nuchal fold thickness and short limbs), which might lead the sonologist to a more detailed examination.

Benaceraff and coworkers first reported in 1985 measurements of the nuchal fold in Down syndrome fetuses.[75] They used a suboccipito-bregmatic view of the fetal head (which has been referred to as a transcerebellar view) between 15 and 20 weeks and measured the thickness of the soft tissues at the level of the occiput. Using a 6-mm threshold (Fig. 12–20), these authors later reported a sensitivity of 38%, a positive

predictive value of 69%, and a false positive rate of 0.1%.[18] Other reports have documented sensitivities ranging between 9% and 21%.[15,17] Nyberg and co-workers[13] reported a sensitivity of 16% and a positive predictive value of 8%. Although the diagnostic indices vary considerably among reports, there seems to be a strong association between the sonographic demonstration of a thickened nuchal fold and Down syndrome. Fetal karyotyping is currently considered for indications that carry a significantly lower risk than the presence of a thickened nuchal fold. A maternal age of 35 and 38, for example, are associated with Down syndrome in 0.35% and 0.81% of cases, respectively. Decreased maternal serum alpha-fetoprotein carries similar risks. Present experience thus supports offering fetal karyotyping when excess nuchal fold is detected in the second trimester.

Infants with Down syndrome have short limbs. Several reports have recently addressed the issue of measuring femur length in the second trimester as a screening tool for Down syndrome, with differing results and conclusions. Individual variability in femur length measurement probably accounts for some of these discrepancies; it is now clear that each center should establish its own nomograms.[17,29,31,76,77] A measured-to-predicted femur length ratio equal to or less than 0.91, however, may result in a positive predictive value ranging between 3% and 12% in a high-risk population (estimated risk of Down syndrome 1 in 250), while in a low risk population (estimated prevalence of Down syndrome 1 in 600), a positive predictive value of only 0.33% would result. In the latter group, only 14% of fetuses with Down syndrome would be identified, requiring amniocentesis to be performed in 6% of normal fetuses. Further experience is probably required with regard to femur length measurement in predicting Down syndrome. Because, however, a maternal age of 35 is associated with a 0.35% risk of fetal Down syndrome, it does seem that femur length measurements or foreshortened humerus may find a role among the indications for fetal karyotyping.

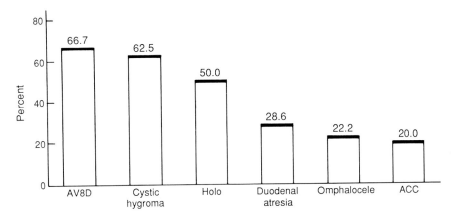

Figure 12–20. Histogram depicts the associated incidence of chromosome anomalies in the presence of single fetal malformations. Chromosome anomalies are identified in 66.7% of cases of atrioventricular septal defects. Other examples are shown on figure.

Hyperechogenic bowel has been noted in fetuses with Down syndrome.[13] The pathophysiology is unknown. Echogenic bowel has also been documented in fetuses with cystic fibrosis[35] and may occasionally be seen in normal fetuses as well.[36] The relative risks are uncertain at present.

A variety of sonographic findings have been reported for the identification of fetuses with Down syndrome. Demonstration of hypoplasia of the middle phalanx of the fifth digit, a typical sign associated with Down syndrome, has been made in the second trimester fetus.[37] The fetal cisterna magna can be consistently visualized from the early second trimester to the 29th week.[78] The distance between the posterior aspect of the cerebellum and the inner calvarium is less than 1 cm in a normal condition. This measurement has been proposed to identify posterior fossa abnormalities such as the Dandy–Walker malformation and the Arnold–Chiari malformation.[79] Later a strong association between an abnormally large cisterna magna with aneuploidies, mostly trisomy 13 and 18, was reported. A large cisterna magna with cerebral ventricles of normal size carries the highest risk, with chromosomal aberrations in 17 of 22 fetuses (77%).[80] The possible association between choroid plexus cysts and aneuploidies was described in the section on trisomy 18.

Growth retardation is a common finding in fetuses with chromosomal aberrations. The prevalence of aneuploidies in small-for-gestational-age infants is quoted as 2% to 20%, depending on the severity of the growth retardation and the gestational age at which such reduced growth became manifest.[81] Many infants with moderate-to-severe growth delay have major malformations readily detectable with sonography. It is uncertain whether the sonographic detection of a mild-to-moderate degree of growth delay is an indication for karyotyping. In a study of 137 consecutive cases of growth-regarded fetuses in otherwise uncomplicated pregnancies—without sonographic evidence of abnormalities—detected between 26 and 37 weeks, there were five aneuploidies (3.6% including two with trisomy 21). There is a consensus on the need to offer karyotyping at least in those cases in which growth retardation is found in the second trimester, in the absence of maternal disease, and in cases of moderate-to-severe growth delay. Analysis of the fetal circulation with Doppler ultrasound may prove useful in distinguishing the types and causes of growth retardation. A relevant proportion of third-trimester fetuses with trisomy 21 and most cases of trisomy 18 have very abnormal Doppler waveforms. More work is needed in this area, however, before routine clinical utility of these modalities can be recommended.

Although experience is still limited, the available studies suggest that sonography is useful in identifying pregnancies at increased risk for fetal aneuploidies. More detailed sonographic examinations will permit prenatal detection of greater numbers of dysmorphic infants.

REFERENCES

1. Benacerraf BR, Frigoletto FD, Bieber FD. The fetal face: ultrasound examination. *Radiology.* 1984;153:495–497.
2. Jeanty P, Romero R, d'Alton M, et al. In utero sonographic detection of hand and foot deformities. *J Ultrasound Med.* 1985;4:595–601.
3. Mahony BS, Filly RA. High-resolution sonographic assessment of the fetal extremities. *J Ultrasound Med.* 1984;3:489–498.
4. Pilu G, Reece EA, Romero R, et al. Prenatal diagnosis of cranio-facial malformations with sonography. *Am J Obstet Gynecol.* 1986;155:45–50.
5. Benacerraf BR. The antenatal sonographic diagnosis of syndromes. In: Fleisher AC, Romero R, Manning FA, et al, eds: *The Principles and Practice of Ultrasonography in Obstetrics and Gynecology.* 4th ed. Norwalk, Conn: Appleton & Lange; 1991:307–329.
6. Birnholz JC. Fetal syndromes. In: Benacerraf BR, Hobbins JC, eds. *Diagnosis and Therapy of Fetal Anomalies: Clinics in Diagnostic Ultrasound 5.* New York, NY: Churchill Livingstone; 1989:1–20.
7. Jeanty P, Dramaix-Wilmet M, Van Gansbeke D, et al. Fetal ocular biometry by ultrasound. *Radiology.* 1982; 143:513–516.
8. DeMyer W. Orbital hypertelorism. In: Vinken PJ, Bruyn GW, eds. *Handbook of Clinical Neurology.* vol 30. Amsterdam: Elsevier/North Holland; 1977:235–255.
9. Bronshtein M, Zimmer E, Gershoni-Baruch R, et al. First and second trimester diagnosis of fetal ocular defects and associated anomalies: report of 8 cases. *Obstet Gynecol.* 1991;77:443–449.
10. Gorlin RJ, Cervenka J, Prusanky S. Facial clefting and its syndromes. *Birth Defects Original Article Series* 1971;7:3.
11. DeMyer W. The median cleft face syndrome. *Neurology.* 1967;17:961–967.
12. Smith DW, Jones KL. *Recognizable Patterns of Human Malformation: Genetic Embryology and Clinical Aspects.* 3rd ed. WB Saunders Co, Philadelphia, Pa; 1982.
13. Nyberg DA, Resta RG, Luthy DA, et al. Prenatal sonographic findings of Down syndrome: review of 94 cases. *Obstet Gynecol.* 1990;76:370–377.
14. Nyberg DA, Fitzsimmons J, Mack LA, et al. Chromosomal abnormalities in fetuses with omphalocele: significance of omphalocele contents. *J Ultrasound Med.* 1989;8:299–308.
15. Hill LM, Guzick D, Belfar HI, et al. The current role of sonography in the detection of Down syndrome. *Obstet Gynecol.* 1989;74:620–623.
16. Benacerraf BR, Gelman R, Frigoletto D. Sonographic identification of second-trimester fetuses with Down's syndrome. *N Engl J Med.* 1987;317:1371–1376.
17. Perrella R, Duerinckx AJ, Grant EG, et al. Second-trimester sonographic diagnosis of Down syndrome: role of femur-length shortening and nuchal fold thickening. *AJR* 1988;151:981–985.

18. Benacerraf BR, Frigoletto FD. Soft tissue nuchal fold in the second trimester fetus: standards for normal measurements compared with those in Down syndrome. *Am J Obstet Gynecol.* 1987;157:1146–1149.

19. Crane JP, Gray DL. Sonographically measured nuchal skin fold thickness as a screening tool for Down syndrome: results of a perspective clinical trial. *Obstet Gynecol.* 1991;77:4:533–536.

20. DiMaio MS, Baumgarten A, Greenstein RM, et al. Screening for fetal Down's syndrome in pregnancy by measuring maternal serum alpha-fetoprotein levels. *N Engl J Med.* 1987;317:342–346.

21. Schreinemachers DM, Cross PK, Hook EB. Rates of trisomies 21, 18, 13 and other chromosome abnormalities in about 20,000 prenatal studies compared with estimated rates in live births. *Hum Genet.* 1982;61:318–324.

22. Toi A, Simpson GF, Filly RA. Ultrasonically evident fetal nuchal skin thickening: is it specific for Down syndrome? *Am J Obstet Gynecol.* 1987;156:150–153.

23. Fitzsimmons J, Droste S, Shepard TH, et al. Long-bone growth in fetuses with Down syndrome. *Am J Obstet Gynecol.* 1989;161:1174–1177.

24. Benacerraf, BR, Gelman R, Frigoletto FD. Sonographic identification of second-trimester fetuses with Down's syndrome. *N Engl J Med.* 1987;317:1371–1376.

25. Benacerraf BR, Cnann A, Gelman R, et al. Can sonographers reliably identify anatomy features associated with Down syndrome? *Radiology.* 1989;173:377–380.

26. Brumfield, CG, Hauth JC, Cloud, GA, et al. Sonographic measurements and ratios in fetuses with Down syndrome. *Obstet Gynecol.* 1989;73:644–646.

27. Dicke JM, Gray DL, Songster GS, et al. Fetal biometry as a screening tool for the detection of chromosomally abnormal pregnancies. *Obstet Gynecol.* 1980;74:726–729.

28. Grist TM, Fuller RW, Albiez KL, et al. Femur length in the ultrasound prediction of trisomy 21 and other chromosomal abnormalities. *Radiology.* 1989;174:837–839.

29. LaFollette L, Filly RA, Anderson R, et al. Fetal femur length to detect trisomy 21: a reappraisal. *J Ultrasound Med.* 1989;8:657–660.

30. Lynch L, Berkowitz GS, Chitkara U, et al. Ultrasound detection of Down syndrome: is it really possible? *Obstet Gynecol.* 1989;73:267–270.

31. Nyberg DA, Resta RG, Hickok DE, et al. Femur length shortening in the detection of Down syndrome: is prenatal screening feasible? *Am J Obstet Gynecol.* 1990;162:1247–1252.

32. Shah YG, Eckl CJ, Stinson SK, et al. Biparietal diameter/femur length ratio, cephalic index and femur length measurements: not reliable screening techniques for Down syndrome. *Obstet Gynecol.* 1990;75:186–188.

33. Fujimoto A, Broom DL, Shinno NW, et al. Nonimmune fetal hydrops and Down syndrome. *Am J Med Genet.* 1983;14:533–537.

34. Allan LD, Crawford DC, Sheridan R, et al. Aetiology of nonimmune hydrops: the value of echocardiography. *Br J Obstet Gynaecol.* 1986;93:223–225.

35. Muller F, Aubry MC, Gasser B, et al. Prenatal diagnosis of cystic fibrosis, II: meconium ileus in affected fetuses. *Prenat Diagn.* 1985;5:109–117.

36. Fakhry J, Reiser M, Shapiro LR, et al. Increased echogenicity in the lower fetal abdomen: a common variant in the second trimester. *J Ultrasound Med.* 1986;5:489–492.

37. Benacerraf BR, Harlow BL, Frigoletto FD. Hypoplasia of the middle phalanx of the fifth digit: a feature of the second trimester fetus with Down syndrome. *J Ultrasound Med.* 1990;9:389–394.

38. Benacerraf BR, Mandell J, Estroff JA, et al. Fetal pyelectasis: a possible association with Down syndrome. *Obstet Gynecol.* 1990;76:58–60.

39. Benacerraf BR, Miller WA, Frigoletto FD. Sonographic detection of fetuses with trisomy 13 and 18: accuracy and limitations. *Am J Obstet Gynecol.* 1988;158:404–409.

40. Chudleigh P, Pearce JM, Campbell S. The prenatal diagnosis of transient cysts of the fetal choroid plexus. *Prenat Diagn.* 1984;4:135–137.

41. Gabrielli S, Reece EA, Pilu G, et al. The clinical significance of prenatally diagnosed choroid plexus cysts. *Am J Obstet Gynecol.* 1989;160:1207–1210.

42. Benacerraf BR, Harlow B, Frigoletto FD. Are choroid plexus cysts an indication for second trimester amniocentesis? *Am J Obstet Gynecol.* 1990;162:1001–1006.

43. Pilu G, Romero R, Rizzo N, et al. Criteria for the prenatal diagnosis of holoprosencephaly. *Am J Perinatol.* 1987; 4:41–49.

44. Battin JJ. Congenital malformations and chromosomal aberrations. *Fetal Therap.* 1986;1:68–72.

45. Romero R, Pilu G, Jeanty P, et al. Cystic hygroma. In: *Prenatal Diagnosis of Congenital Anomalies.* Norwalk, Conn: Appleton & Lange, 1987.

46. Elejalde BR, Elejalde NM, Leno J. Nuchal cysts syndromes: etiology, pathogenesis and prenatal diagnosis. *Am J Med Genet.* 1985;21:417–432.

47. Chervenak FA, Isaacson G, Blakemore KJ, et al. Fetal cystic hygroma: cause and natural history. *N Engl J Med.* 1983;309:822–825.

48. Nishimura H, Okamoto N. *Sequential Analysis of Human Congenital Malformations: Observations of Embryos, Fetuses, and Newborns.* Baltimore, Md: University Park Press; 1976.

49. Cullen MT, Gabrielli S, Green JJ, et al. Diagnosis and significance of cystic hygroma in the first trimester. *Prenat Diagn.* 1990;10:643–651.

50. Crane JP, Beaver HA, Cheung SW. Antenatal ultrasound findings in fetal triploidy syndrome. *J Ultrasound Med.* 1985;4:519–524.

51. Lockwood CJ, Scioscia A, Stiller R, et al. Sonographic features of the triploid fetus. *Am J Obstet Gynecol.* 1987;157:285–287.

52. Opitz JM, Howe JJ. The Meckel syndrome (dysencephalia splanchnocystica, the Gruber syndrome). *Birth Defects Original Article Series.* 1969;5:167.

53. Zerres K, Volpel LC, Weiss H. Cystic kidneys: genetics, pathologic anatomy, clinical picture and prenatal diagnosis. *Hum Genet.* 1984;68:104–135.

54. Torpin R. Amniochorionic mesoblastic fibrous strings and amniotic bands: associated constricting fetal malformation or fetal death. *Am J Obstet Gynecol.* 1965;91:65.

55. Higginbottom MC, Jones K, Hall BD, et al. The amniotic band disruption complex: timing of amniotic rupture and variable spectra of consequent defects. *J Pediatr.* 1979;95:544–549.

56. Moessinger AC, Blanc WA, Byrne J, et al. Amniotic band syndrome associated with amniocentesis. *Am J Obstet Gynecol.* 1981;141:588–591.

57. Seeds JW, Cefalo RC, Herbert WN. Amniotic band syndrome. *Am J Obstet Gynecol.* 1982;144:243–248.

58. Fiske CE, Filly RA, Golbus MS. Prenatal ultrasound diagnosis of amniotic band syndrome. *J Ultrasound Med.* 1982;1:45–49.

59. Mahony BS, Filly RA, Callen PW, et al. The amniotic band syndrome: antenatal sonographic diagnosis and potential pitfalls. *Am J Obstet Gynecol.* 1985;152:63–68.

60. Young ID, Trunce JQ, Levene MI, et al. Agenesis of the corpus callosum and macrocephaly in siblings. *Clin Genet.* 1985;28:225–230.

61. Aicardi J, Lefebvre J, Lerique-Koechlin A. A new syndrome: spasms in flexion, callosal agenesis, ocular abnormalities. *Electroencephalographic Clin Neurophysiol.* 1965;19:609–615.

62. Andermann F, Andermann E, Joubert M, et al. Familial agenesis of the corpus callosum with anterior horn cell disease: A syndrome of mental retardation, areflexia and paraplegia. *Trans Am Neurol Assn.* 1972;97:242–247.

63. Schinzel A. Four patients including two sisters with the acrocallosal syndrome (agenesis of the corpus callosum in combination with preaxial hexadactyly). *Hum Genet.* 1982;62:328.

64. Opitz JM, Kaveggia EG. The FG syndrome: an X-linked recessive syndrome of multiple congenital anomalies and mental retardation. *Z Kinderheilk.* 1974;117:1–18.

65. Sandri F, Pilu G, Cerisoli M, et al. Sonographic diagnosis of agenesis of the corpus callosum in the fetus and newborn infant. *Am J Perinatol.* 1988;5:226–231.

66. Dennison WM. The Pierre Robin syndrome. *Pediatrics.* 1965;36:336–339.

67. Cohen MM Jr.. The Robin anomalad: its nonspecificity and associated syndromes. *J Oral Surg.* 1976;34:587–593.

68. Pilu G, Romero R, Reece EA, et al. Prenatal diagnosis of Robin anomalad. *Am J Obstet Gynecol.* 1986;154:630–632.

69. Otto C, Platt LD. The fetal mandible measurement: an objective determination of fetal jaw size. *Ultrasound Obstet Gynecol.* 1991;1:12–17.

70. Benacerraf BR, Greene MF, Holmes LB. The prenatal sonographic features of Noonan's syndrome. *J Ultrasound Med.* 1989;8:59–63.

71. Nicolaides KH, Rodeck CH, Gosden C. Rapid karyotyping in nonlethal fetal malformations. *Lancet.* 1986;1:283–287.

72. Palmer CG, Miles JH, Howard-Peebles PN, et al. Fetal karyotype following ascertainment of fetal anomalies by ultrasound. *Prenat Diagn.* 1987;7:551–555.

73. Wladimiroff JW, Sachs ES, Reuss A, et al. Prenatal diagnosis of chromosomal abnormalities in the presence of fetal structural defects. *Am J Med Genet.* 1988;29:289–291.

74. Rizzo N, Pittalis MC, Pilu G, et al. Prenatal karyotype in malformed fetuses. *Prenat Diagn.* 1990;10:17–23.

75. Benacerraf BR, Frigoletto FD, Laboda LA. Sonographic diagnosis of Down syndrome in the second trimester. *Am J Obstet Gynecol.* 1985;153:49–52.

76. Cuckle H, Wald N, Quinn J, et al. Ultrasound fetal femur length measurement in the screening for Down syndrome. *Br J Obstet Gynaecol.* 1989;96:1373–1378.

77. Lockwood C, Benacerraf BR, Krinsky A, et al. A sonographic screening method for Down syndrome. *Am J Obstet Gynecol.* 1987;157:803–808.

78. Mahony BS, Callen PW, Filly RA, et al. The fetal cisterna magna. *Radiology.* 1984;153:773–776.

79. Pilu G, DePalma L, Romero R, et al. The fetal subarachnoid cisterns: an ultrasound study with report of a case of congenital communicating hydrocephalus. *J Ultrasound Med.* 1986;5:365–372.

80. Nyberg DA, Mahony BS, Hegge FN, et al. Enlarged cisterna magna and the Dandy-Walker malformation: factors associated with chromosome abnormalities. *Obstet Gynecol.* 1991;77:436–442.

81. Chen AT, Falek A. Chromosome aberrations in full term low birthweight neonates. *Hum Genet.* 1974;21:13–16.

13

Estimation of Gestational Age

INTRODUCTION

Assessment of gestational age is a cornerstone in the delivery of optimum obstetrical care. The ability to diagnose and treat conditions, such as premature labor, premature rupture of the membranes, intrauterine growth retardation, and postdatism, depends on knowing precisely the gestational age. The timing of certain prenatal diagnostic procedures, for example, early amniocentesis, chorionic villous sampling, or maternal serum alpha-fetoprotein testing, is also influenced by the accurate dating of the pregnancy.

Human gestation lasts for 266 to 294 days, averaging 280 days, or 40 weeks, from the last menstrual period (LMP). Usually in cases of planned pregnancies the information relating to gestational age is available to the physician. There may be documentation of basal body temperature charting, evidence of menstrual cyclicity, and the exact date of the last menses and ovulation. When the gestational age or last menstrual period is unknown, however, or there is a history of irregular menstrual cycles, irregular bleeding, or intrauterine growth retardation, alternative means for the estimation of gestational age should be sought.

An assessment of gestational age is possible if uterine size is examined by an experienced practitioner before 12 weeks' gestation. After the first trimester, factors, such as maternal obesity or the presence of uterine fibromas or malformations, can confuse the determination of gestational age.

From about 20 to 36 weeks' gestation, the fundal height from the pubic symphysis to the top of the uterine fundus approximates the gestational age, ie, this distance in centimeters is approximately equal to the gestational age in weeks. Fetal heart tones should be audible no earlier than 12 weeks. Quickening, the mother's first perception of fetal movement, is also valuable for pregnancy dating.

Some women are unable to provide a reliable date for their LMP. Wenner and Young[1] reported that one third of their patients had a nonspecific date of LMP. Grennert et al[2] reported that 4.8% of 5468 women were unable to provide the date of their LMP; 9.8% had irregular cycles or oligomenorrhea; 3.2% had been on

oral contraceptives; and 7.2% had bleeding in the first trimester. Johnson and coworkers[3] proposed a graphic method of recording gestational estimators and suggested that it might be possible to predict the LMP by the best fit straight line through several clinical methods of estimating gestational age.

Ultrasound is one of the main tools used in obstetrics, and its principal function still remains the estimation of gestational age.

ULTRASOUND ASSESSMENT OF GESTATIONAL AGE BIOMETRIC MEASUREMENTS

First trimester
   Gestational sac GS
   Crown–rump length CRL
   Yolk sac YS
Second and third trimesters
   The head
      Biparietal diameter BPD
      Occipitofrontal diameter OFD
      Head circumference HC
      Transverse cerebellar diameter TCD
      Outer orbital diameter OOD
      Inner orbital diameter IOD
   The neck
      Neck
      Clavicle
   The chest
      Thoracic circumference TC
   The abdomen: internal organs
      Abdominal circumference AC
      Kidneys
      Heart
      Liver
   The long bones
      Femur length FL
      Humerus length HL
      Tibia length TL
      Ulna length UL
Third trimester: Nonbiometric measurements
Ossification centers: 1) Calcaneus 2) Talus 3) Distal femoral epiphysis (DFE) 4) Proximal tibial epiphysis (PTE) 5) Proximal humeral epiphysis (PHE)
Organ maturity: 1) Small intestine 2) Colon 3) Placenta

FIRST-TRIMESTER BIOMETRY

Sonoanatomy

First-trimester ultrasound evaluations of the GS, CRL, and YS are detailed in Chapter 4.

SECOND-TRIMESTER BIOMETRY

The Head

Biparietal Diameter

The BPD can be measured by ultrasound from the end of the first trimester and throughout the second and third trimesters. This measurement, although the most popular, can be one of the most problematic measurements. Hadlock et al[4] determined that the sagittal section for BPD measurement was the most appropriate sonographic choice because the transverse diameter of the fetal head was maximal at that level, specific anatomic landmarks were present making BPD measurement technically easy and reproducible, and other intracranial structures could be measured and assessed in the process of performing the BPD measurement.

The fetal head should be visualized in an axial plane at an angle of 15 to 20 degrees from the horizontal plane. The sonographic image must include the entire calvarium, which appears ellipsoidlike on the screen. Survey of the intracranial anatomy should include the falx cerebri and structures in the anterior and posterior fossae. The thalami appear as two triangular echo-free areas in the midportion, and in the anterior portion of the head the septum cavi pellucidi appear as two short parallel lines. The third ventricle should be visualized between the thalami by a slitlike appearance. It is also possible to identify a cross section of the aqueduct of Sylvius. The hippocampal gyri appear as a circular space delineated medially by the ambient cistern, on both sides of the thalami; laterally it is delineated by the atrium of the lateral ventricles. It is also possible to visualize the frontal horn of the lateral ventricles, which is separated by the septum cavum pellucidum. Pulsation of the middle cerebral artery in the sylvian fissure can also be seen.

The BPD can be obtained by measuring from the outer margin of the parietal bone (proximal to the transducer) to the inner margin of the parallel parietal bone (distal to the transducer). The variables in the sonographic examination depend on parameters, such as fetal position, fetal movement, amount of amniotic fluid present, the resolution of the ultrasound equipment, and the experience of the sonographer.

In 1969 Campbell[5] studied the BPD measurement and showed that there was a linear relationship between the fetal BPD and the gestational age between 20 and 30 weeks' gestation. From his findings, he was able to predict the correct gestational age ± 9 days in 95% of pregnancies studied. These results reflect the reduced biologic variability at this time of gestation.

Sabbagha et al[6] studied the differences in predicting gestational age from the sonographic measurement of the BPD. Single BPD measurements performed after 26 weeks' gestation should be interpreted with caution because, at best, the predictive accuracy is within a range of 2 weeks in approximately 80% of normal pregnancies.[7] In the remaining 20% of such pregnancies gestational age will vary by as much as ± 3 weeks.

Kurtz et al[8] reviewed 17 studies concerning the accurate estimation of the gestational age using the BPD. The authors included six A-mode, seven B-mode, and four studies combining both methods. Their analysis revealed enlargement in the BPD as the gestational age increased, with variation only 2 weeks prior to 35 mm, from 36 to 80 mm or from 17 to 32 weeks, a variation of as much as 3 weeks was observed. Beyond 81 mm the variation was as great as 4 weeks. This observation made more than a decade ago remains generally true, even with improved technology and greater experience with ultrasound.

Hadlock et al[9] examined the relationship between fetal BPD and menstrual age using a linear array real-time (dynamic image) scanner. The variability associated with predicting menstrual age from BPD increased progressively throughout gestation, with the maximal variability noted between 36 and 42 weeks ± 3.6 weeks (Table 5–5).

Shepard and Filly[10] postulated that the variability of BPD measurements is due predominantly to biologic variation in fetal growth rates rather than to technical errors. Campbell et al[11] suggested that BPD appeared to be the best single parameter for predicting gestational age when obtained before 18 weeks' gestation. These researchers found that BPD measurements performed between 12 and 18 weeks' gestation were significantly more accurate in gestational age predictions (89.4%) than those based on menstrual history (69.7%). The study established that the best time to apply ultrasonic cephalometry is between 12 and 18 weeks' gestation.

BPD is a reliable indicator of gestational age. In the second trimester of pregnancy it is accurate to within ± 1 to 1.5 weeks (± 2 SD), but in the third trimester the reported accuracy is considerably less. A BPD obtained after 28 weeks is accurate only within ± 3 weeks (± 2 SD). The observed variation in the third trimester is undoubtedly multifactorial in etiology, related only in part to technical errors in imaging.

Occipitofrontal Diameter (OFD)

The OFD should be obtained in the same plane used for the BPD. An axial plane of the head is obtained at

15 to 20 degrees from the horizontal plane. The thalami, septum cavum pellucidum, and the third ventricle are identified; the distance from the midechogenic plane of the occipital bone to the midechogenic plane of the frontal bone should be measured (Table 5–6). While most ultrasound equipment have similar axial resolutions, they may vary in their lateral resolutions. The anteroposterior resolution is less than 2 mm in most ultrasound machines; the lateral resolution, however, is from 3 to 5 mm.

Cephalic Index

Fetuses in the breech presentation have been shown to have a smaller mean BPD. Neonatal measurements were compared with those of a matched group of newborns delivered in the vertex presentation.[12] This reduction in mean BPD measurements was due to a mild skull deformation called the breech head shape. Features of skull deformation include dolichocephaly, a prominent occiput, an elongated face, and a parallel-sided head. The small BPD was consistent with the skull deformation that occurred in a proportion of breech-presenting fetuses.[13] A cephalic index was calculated using the ratio of the BPD to the OFD to determine whether the BPD was normal or affected by deformation of the skull.

Variation in BPD is multifactorial in etiology. Assuming a technically adequate BPD image and an accurate measurement—and eliminating pathologic causes of variation in the fetal head size, such as microcephaly, hydrocephaly, and intrauterine growth retardation—there remain three obvious reasons that women with the same LMP may have different BPD measurements: 1) genetic variation in the head size in fetuses of the same conceptual age; 2) differences in the time of ovulation and fertilization with respect to the first day of the LMP; and 3) variation in the shape of the fetal head.

The cephalic index is the ratio of the short axis (BPD) to the long axis (OFD) × 100. The average value of the cephalic index in utero is 78%. Values 1 standard deviation from the mean (less than 74% or greater than 83%) may be associated with significant changes in the BPD measurement for any given gestational age. Dolichocephaly can be defined essentially by a cephalic index below 74%, while brachycephaly is defined when the cephalic index is greater than 83%.[4,14] Therefore, when the shape of the fetal skull may adversely affect the accuracy of the BPD, the sonologist or sonographer must resort to other fetal parameters for estimating the gestational age.

Head Perimeter

Head circumference is an important measurement for assessing head growth in newborns; it has also gained importance for in utero evaluation of fetal head size.

Head circumference measurement can assist in predicting the gestational age when an abnormal cephalic index is calculated. Measurement of the head circumference is essential, especially in cases of microcephaly or intrauterine growth retardation.

The ideal anatomic plane for obtaining head circumference measurement is the axial plane of the fetal head, obtained at 15 to 20 degrees from the horizontal plane. The anatomic features observed at this level are the thalami, septum cavum pellucidum, and the third ventricle. Head circumference measurement is calculated using both the short diameter (BPD) and the long diameter (OFD)

$$(BPD + OFD)/2 \times 3.14$$

or it can be measured by tracing the sonographic image directly on the screen (Fig. 13–1 and Table 13–1).

Transverse Cerebellar Diameter

Transverse cerebellar diameter (TCD) has become a standard measurement for evaluating the fetal head and somatic growth. The cerebellum, an intracranial organ, is located in the posterior fossa of the fetal head. Morphologically, it has a butterflylike shape and is easy to identify sonographically.

Measurements of the TCD are independent of the shape of the fetal head, and thus they should remain an accurate method of estimating gestational age, even in cases of dolichocephaly or brachycephaly.[15] It has been suggested that the posterior fossa is not affected by external pressure; therefore measurements of the TCD may convey more precise information about fetal growth than would bony measurements of the fetal head. The TCD, moreover, seems to be relatively unaffected in either growth-retarded[16] or macrosomic fetuses. These findings indicate that the growth of the TCD may serve as a useful marker of gestational age against which potential deviations in growth may be compared. However, in cases of abnormal fetal intercerebellar structure, such as Arnold–Chiari type II or Dandy–Walker syndrome, the TCD measurement may deviate from the norm, reflecting a size larger than the gestational age would predict. This is presumably due to expansion of the cerebellar hemispheres.

The TCD measurement is obtained in an axial plane of the fetal head at an angle slightly inferior to the BPD level. The measurements are obtained by placing the ultrasound calipers at the outer-to-outer margins of the cerebellum.[15] From 15 weeks to about 24 weeks, the TCD in millimeters is equivalent to the gestational age in weeks; beyond this gestational age, the growth rate becomes nonlinear, and a TCD growth curve should be consulted to estimate gestational age from obtained measurements (Table 5–4, Table 5–5).

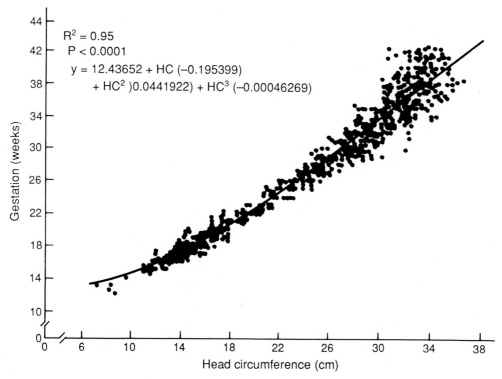

Figure 13–1. Scattergram with regression line depicting the growth profile of head circumference (HC) throughout gestation.

Fetal Orbits

The ability to identify the fetal orbits sonographically should permit the diagnosis of conditions associated with hypotelorism (eg, holoprosencephaly) and hypertelorism (eg, the fetal hydantoin syndrome), since they affect the inner and outer orbital diameters.

The standard measurement for dating pregnancies, the BPD, is virtually impossible when the fetal head is facing directly up or down. The orbits, however, can be identified and measured when the head is in an occiput posterior position, in lieu of BPD measurements.[17]

The inner orbital diameter and the outer orbital diameter can be measured by using electronic calipers. The outer orbital diameter is measured from the lateral border of the orbit to the opposite lateral border. The inner orbital diameter is measured from the medial border of the orbit to the opposite medial border (Fig. 6–1).

There are two different planes for measuring the orbits in the frontal view with an occipitotransverse position: 1) the coronal plane and 2) the orbito-mental plane (below the level of the BPD). The gestational age is easily determined by applying the measurements to the nomogram (Table 6–1).

The Abdomen

The Abdominal Circumference

The ultrasonically derived fetal abdominal circumference is one of the essential parameters used to predict birth weight, to assess fetal growth, and to follow the evolution of fetal ascites. Certain maternal disease states may influence the abdominal circumference, for example, maternal diabetes, pregnancy-induced hypertension, or maternal vasculopathy. The fetal abdominal perimeter measurement adds another dimension to the interpretation of cephalic growth, and is particularly useful in identifying either macrosomic or growth-retarded fetuses. The abdominal perimeter can be a difficult measurement since fetal body and breathing movements occur during the course of an ultrasound examination. An accurate abdominal circumference measurement is, nevertheless, necessary since it is used as part of various formulas in the estimated fetal weight.

To obtain the fetal abdominal circumference, the position of the fetus is determined. The fetal spine is localized in a longitudinal plane, and the transducer is rotated perpendicularly to that plane. The transducer passes caudally in a cross-sectional plane, using the fetal heart as a marker, until the fetal liver, the umbilical vein bifurcation (the "hook" sign), and the stomach are visualized in the same plane (Fig. 13–2 and Fig. 13–3). An effort is also made to visualize the entire fetal abdomen on the screen. The fetal liver is considered to be the organ most affected by variations in fetal nutrition; therefore it seems reasonable that the level of the fetal liver was chosen by many investigators as the plane for the abdominal circumference measurement (Fig. 13–4A and Fig. 13–4B).

TABLE 13–1. NOMOGRAM OF FETAL HEAD CIRCUMFERENCE

| Gestational Age (Wk) | Mean | 2 SD | Percentile | | | | | | | N |
			5th	10th	25th	50th	75th	90th	95th	
13	7.8	1.4	7.3	7.3	7.3	7.8	8.4	8.4	8.4	2
14	10.9	1.6	9.6	9.6	9.9	11.2	11.5	11.5	11.5	4
15	12.0	1.2	11.0	11.0	11.5	12.0	12.6	13.0	13.1	11
16	13.0	1.2	12.0	12.2	12.5	13.0	13.4	13.8	14.2	72
17	14.2	1.4	13.3	13.4	13.6	14.3	14.7	15.1	15.7	41
18	15.4	2.4	13.9	14.3	14.7	15.6	15.7	16.3	16.7	40
19	16.2	1.8	14.4	14.8	15.6	16.4	17.0	17.2	17.8	37
20	17.2	3.2	14.7	16.4	16.5	17.0	17.5	17.7	23.1	21
21	17.5	3.4	13.9	13.9	16.5	18.3	19.0	19.1	19.2	16
22	19.4	1.6	17.5	18.4	19.0	19.3	20.1	20.6	20.6	18
23	20.6	2.0	19.3	19.3	19.7	20.5	21.1	22.5	22.5	8
24	21.8	2.0	20.6	20.6	21.1	21.5	22.5	23.3	24.5	17
25	22.8	2.6	19.6	20.7	21.9	23.0	23.8	24.5	24.5	18
26	23.5	2.4	20.2	21.9	23.2	23.7	24.3	26.7	25.2	26
27	25.5	4.6	23.5	23.7	24.1	25.0	25.8	29.5	32.5	24
28	25.8	2.2	24.1	24.5	25.3	25.6	26.7	27.6	28.3	23
29	27.1	2.8	24.7	24.9	26.1	27.2	28.0	29.1	29.6	30
30	27.8	2.2	25.7	26.7	27.2	27.9	28.4	29.5	30.2	35
31	28.5	3.0	25.8	26.4	27.4	28.7	29.5	30.9	32.2	25
32	29.4	2.2	27.3	27.9	28.5	29.4	30.4	30.8	31.6	28
33	30.0	2.4	27.9	28.2	29.2	30.0	30.9	31.8	32.2	31
34	31.3	2.8	28.2	29.5	30.4	31.6	32.1	33.7	34.1	30
35	31.2	3.4	27.9	28.7	30.3	31.3	32.6	33.2	33.5	39
36	32.2	2.6	30.3	30.5	31.3	32.1	32.8	34.7	35.0	37
37	32.5	2.6	30.3	30.5	31.6	32.7	33.4	34.3	34.7	37
38	33.1	3.0	30.5	31.2	32.2	33.2	33.9	35.6	36.0	37
39	32.1	4.0	25.5	31.1	31.3	32.1	33.2	34.1	35.0	23
40	33.6	2.2	31.6	31.8	32.8	33.6	34.8	35.1	35.3	14
41	33.3	2.4	30.6	31.1	32.5	33.5	34.1	34.8	35.2	22
42	32.9	2.4	30.6	30.6	32.0	32.9	33.9	34.7	34.7	9

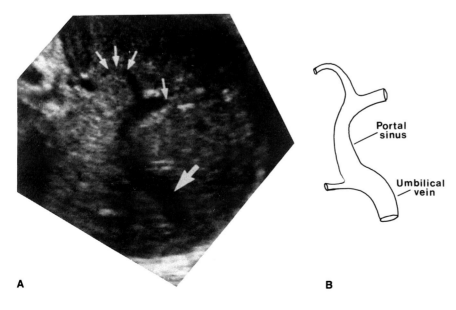

A   **B**

Figure 13–2. (A) Ultrasound picture of fetal abdominal circumference at the level of the umbilical vein bifurcation (arrows). **(B)** Schematic diagram of umbilical vein leading into the portal sinus, then bifurcating.

Portal sinus

Umbilical vein

Figure 13–3. (A) Ultrasound picture of the cross-section of the fetal abdomen at the level necessary to obtain the optimal abdominal circumference (AC) measurement. Arrows indicate umbilical vein, and stomach is annotated. **(B)** Schematic representation of the view in **(A)** showing the various structures. (UV = umbilical vein, stomach) and the appropriate orientations (anterior, posterior, right, and left).

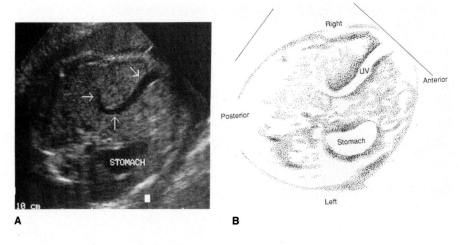

A   B

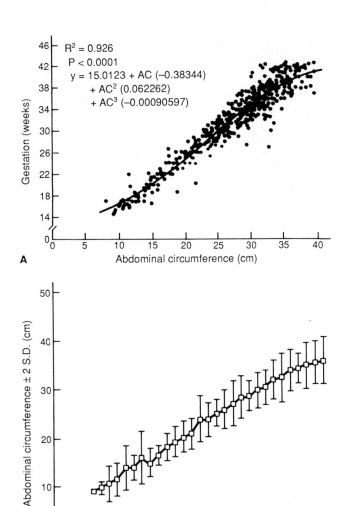

A

B

Figure 13–4. (A) Scattergram with regression line depicting growth of the AC throughout gestation. **(B)** Mean ± 2 SD (in cm) of the AC throughout gestation.

Sonographic biometry should be obtained when neither body nor breathing movements are present. The image of the fetal abdomen will not be well visualized because of the vertebral shadowing when the fetal spine is in an anterior position. Scanning can be deferred for a few minutes in this situation until the fetus changes its position; sometimes only the fetal stomach is used as the sonographic marker, since the umbilical vessel is shadowed. Ideally, the biometric measurements of the abdominal circumference is obtained when the fetal abdomen forms a circle and the anteroposterior and the transverse diameters are close to each other in dimension.

There are two main techniques for measuring the abdominal circumference: 1) by using the anterioposterior and the transverse dimensions and 2) by tracing the abdominal circumference with a map reader or directly on the screen using the electronic calipers. Each measurement should include the soft tissue of the fetal abdomen.

The former method was described by Ott[18] in which he computed the abdominal circumference with the formula:

Abdominal circumference = anterioposterior diameter + transverse diameter × 1.57.

Tamura and Sabbagha[19] found the abdominal circumference to be highly reproducible (2%); the accuracy of the measurements fell within 5.2% of the actual anatomic value. Hadlock et al[20] studied the fetal abdominal circumference as a predictor of gestational age and reported the variability to be wider than that observed using the fetal BPD; they indicated a progressive increase with increasing gestational age. Nomograms were generated, nevertheless, for gestational age estimation according to given abdominal circumference measurements (Table 13–2).

TABLE 13–2. NOMOGRAM OF FETAL ABDOMINAL CIRCUMFERENCE

Gestational Age (Wk)	Mean	2 SD	Percentile 5th	10th	25th	50th	75th	90th	95th	N
13										
14	9.0	0.1	9.0	9.0	9.0	9.1	9.1	9.1	9.1	3
15	9.7	1.2	9.3	9.3	9.3	9.4	10.4	10.4	10.4	3
16	10.6	3.6	4.4	9.3	10.4	10.7	11.3	12.5	14.7	18
17	11.4	3.4	8.0	8.0	10.6	11.5	12.7	13.7	13.7	8
18	13.8	4.6	12.1	12.1	12.3	12.7	14.8	18.7	18.7	7
19	13.8	2.6	11.5	11.5	13.1	13.9	14.6	15.6	15.6	6
20	15.9	5.4	14.1	14.1	14.4	14.0	17.1	21.5	21.5	6
21	14.9	3.0	11.3	11.3	14.5	15.1	16.2	16.7	16.7	9
22	16.3	2.0	14.3	14.5	15.6	16.2	17.4	17.8	17.9	11
23	18.0	2.8	16.0	16.0	16.4	18.3	19.3	19.5	19.5	4
24	19.1	3.0	17.0	17.0	17.9	18.5	20.7	21.3	21.4	10
25	20.2	3.2	17.4	17.5	19.6	20.0	21.0	23.4	23.7	10
26	20.8	3.0	17.3	18.1	19.9	21.0	21.9	22.5	23.4	17
27	23.8	4.8	21.3	21.3	21.8	22.8	24.5	29.7	32.5	17
28	23.7	3.6	20.3	21.2	22.4	24.0	24.7	25.9	27.9	19
29	24.9	2.8	22.6	22.8	23.6	25.0	26.2	26.6	27.1	22
30	25.8	4.0	22.8	23.3	24.6	25.6	26.3	28.9	30.9	30
31	27.0	4.6	23.6	24.3	25.1	27.1	28.9	29.6	32.4	24
32	28.3	4.4	24.8	25.1	26.5	28.1	29.9	32.1	32.6	20
33	28.6	3.0	25.7	26.1	28.2	28.6	29.8	30.8	31.3	30
34	29.7	3.6	26.6	27.0	28.5	29.1	31.1	32.1	33.6	30
35	30.2	3.4	26.7	27.6	29.4	30.5	31.3	32.5	33.4	31
36	31.8	4.0	27.9	28.8	30.5	31.7	33.0	34.7	35.1	35
37	32.4	4.8	28.9	29.7	30.9	32.0	33.6	36.0	37.8	35
38	33.8	4.2	30.9	31.3	32.4	33.6	35.0	37.2	38.9	35
39	34.1	3.0	31.5	32.4	32.6	34.4	35.3	36.0	37.0	25
40	34.8	4.8	29.8	29.9	33.9	34.6	36.6	38.5	38.8	18
41	35.3	4.4	31.9	32.9	33.5	35.0	37.2	38.6	40.1	25
42	35.6	4.8	31.3	31.4	34.6	35.2	37.7	39.1	39.4	12

The Long Bones

Gestational age can also be estimated from measurements of the fetal long bones, such as femur, humerus, tibia, and ulna. The fetal foot length can also be useful especially if there is skeletal dysplasia with or without cranial abnormalities. The approach to measurement and the relative accuracy of these parameters are discussed in detail in Chapter 11.

Nonbiometric Parameters

The use of nonbiometer parameters, such as visualization of bony epiphyses and indices that characterize fetal organ maturity, can provide an adjunct to long bone measurements in assessing gestational age. The sonographic approach in the identification and interpretation of these parameters is described in Chapter 16.

REFERENCES

1. Wenner, WH, Young EB. Nonspecific date of last menstrual period. *Am J Obstet Gynecol.* 1974;120:1071–1079.
2. Grennart L, Persson PH., Gennser G. Benefits of ultrasonic screening of a pregnant population. *Acta Obstet Gynecol Scand.* 1978;78:5–14.
3. Johnson TR, Work BA. A dynamic graph for documentation of gestational age. *Obstet Gynecol.* 1979;54:115–119.
4. Hadlock FP, Deter RL, Harrist RB, et al. Fetal biparietal diameter: rational choice of plane of section for sonographic measurement. *AJR.* 1982;138:871–874.
5. Campbell S. The prediction of fetal maturity by ultrasonic measurement of the biparietal diameter. *J Obstet Gynaecol Br Cwlth.* 1969;76:603–609.
6. Sabbagha RE, Hughey M. Standardization of sonar cephalometry and gestational age. *Obstet Gynecol.* 1978; 52:402–406.
7. Sabbagha RE, Turner JH, Rockette H, et al. Sonar BPD and fetal age: definition of relationship. *Obstet Gynecol.* 1973;43:7–14.
8. Kurtz AB, Wapner RJ, Kurtz RJ, et al. Analysis of biparietal diameter as an accurate indicator of gestational age. *J Clin Ultrasound.* 1980;8:319–326.
9. Hadlock FP, Deter RL, Harrist RB: Fetal biparietal diameter: a critical re-evaluation of the relation to menstrual age by means of real-time ultrasound. *J Ultrasound Med.* 1982;1:97–104.
10. Shepard M, Filly RA. A standardized plane for biparietal diameter measurement. *J Ultrasound Med.* 1982;1:145–150.

11. Campbell S, Warsof SL, Little D, et al. Routine ultrasound screening for prediction of gestational age. *Obstet Gynecol.* 1985;65:613–619.

12. Kasby CB, Poll V. The breech head and its ultrasound significance. *Br J Obstet Gynaecol* 1982;89:106–110.

13. Hadlock FP, Deter RL, Carpenter RJ, et al. Estimating fetal age: effect of head shape on BPD. *AJR.* 1981;137:83–85.

14. Gray DL, Songster GS, Parvin CA, et al. Cephalic index: a gestational age-dependent biometric parameter. *Obstet Gynecol.* 1989;74:600–603.

15. Goldstein I, Reece EA, Pilu G, et al. Cerebellar measurements with ultrasonography in the evaluation of the fetal head growth and development. *Am J Obstet Gynecol.* 1987;156:1056–1059.

16. Reece EA, Goldstein I, Pilu G, et al. Fetal cerebellar growth unaffected by intrauterine growth retardation: a new parameter for prenatal diagnosis. *Am J Obstet Gynecol.* 1987;157:632–638.

17. Mayden KL, Tortora M, Berkowitz RL, et al. Orbital diameters: a new parameter for prenatal diagnosis and dating. *Am J Obstet Gynecol.* 1982;144:289–297.

18. Ott WJ. Clinical application of fetal weight determination by real-time ultrasound measurements. *Obstet Gynecol.* 1981;57:758–762.

19. Tamura RK, Sabbagha RE. Percentile ranks of sonar fetal abdominal circumference measurements. *Am J Obstet Gynecol.* 1980;138:475–479.

20. Hadlock FP, Kent WR, Lloyd JL, et al. An evaluation of two methods for measuring fetal head and body circumferences. *J Ultrasound Med.* 1982;1:359–360.

14

Estimated Fetal Weight

There is no doubt about the necessity and the importance of estimating fetal weight in utero. Alterations in intrauterine growth, both retardation and acceleration, contribute significantly to perinatal morbidity and mortality.[1] Accurate antenatal diagnosis of altered fetal growth enables the obstetrician to evaluate and manage these problems more effectively.

Any method that accurately estimates fetal weight is obviously of benefit to the practicing clinician. The estimation of fetal weight via palpation of the uterine fundus is known to be notoriously inaccurate, especially at the upper and lower ends of the weight spectrum. Past researchers attempted to estimate fetal weight by means of estriol,[2] human placental lactogen,[3] and pregnanediol[4] determinations. These biochemical means gave indirect and inaccurate measurements of fetal mass and were thus of limited value. Birth weight depends on many factors, including maternal size, diseases, smoking habits, parental race, and constitutional and sociodemographic characteristics.[5,6]

Curves depicting intrauterine growth have been under investigation for more than a decade. Usher and McLean[7] studied the intrauterine growth of infants born at sea level in Montreal, Canada. Lubchenco and coworkers[6] studied intrauterine growth as estimated from liveborn infants born at 24 to 42 weeks' gestation in Denver, Colorado. Differences in weight, length, and head circumferences were observed between these two populations. These differences may be due, in part, to the effect of high altitude (Denver is 5,000 feet above sea level) on fetal growth, resulting in smaller infants. Since the introduction of modern ultrasound to obstetrics in the mid-1960s, it has become possible to visualize the fetus and to conduct various biometric measurements.

BIOMETRY

A number of techniques are available for antenatal diagnosis of altered fetal growth. The methods most commonly used rely on antenatal ultrasonic measurements of the developing fetus. Several investigators have reported formulas and nomograms for the esti-

mation of fetal weight using a variety of parameters, including the biparietal diameter (BPD),[8–10] abdominal circumference (AC),[11] femur length (FL),[12–15] head circumference (HC),[10] area of the cross section of the fetal chest or fetal abdomen, and combinations of the above parameters.[10,16]

Investigators have searched for a simple and useful way to predict fetal weight when growth abnormalities are present.

Campbell and Wilkin[11] used the AC as an index of fetal weight and found that 95% of the birth weights were within 160 g per kilogram of the estimations.

Warsof et al[17] assessed 85 patients with fetuses of gestational ages ranging between 17 and 41 weeks' gestation who delivered within 48 hours of their sonographic examination. Their results support the finding of Campbell and Wilkin[15] that AC and the BPD accurately predict fetal weight and the fetal internal organs play a significant role in this measurement. For example, the first organ to be affected by any cause is the liver, which is located at the level of the AC measurements. Using the BPD and AC, the standard deviation was only 106 g per kilogram of fetal weight. Ott[18] used the formula of BPD and AC for estimating the fetal weight. The mean error ranged from 5% to 8.4%.

Timor-Tritsch et al[9] studied the estimation of fetal weight by using a mechanical technique for measuring the AC. The absolute mean error was 228 g, or 8.3% of the mean weight.

Shepard et al[8] used the Warsof study for estimating gestational age. Since the authors thought that fetal weights were underestimated by Warsof's original study, a new nomogram was generated using the BPD and the AC diameter (Table 14–1). The accuracy fell within 10% of the actual weight 85% of the time, and the standard error was 103 g for each 1,000 g in fetal weight estimation.

Hadlock et al[12] used a combination of measurements of the fetal head, abdomen, and femur to generate another nomogram of estimated fetal weight. They demonstrated that the use of AC alone for estimating gestational age would result in an error of almost 12%. They were able to confirm the Warsof's standard deviation of 10.6%, however, by using both

TABLE 14-1. ESTIMATED FETAL WEIGHTS

Bi-parietal diameters	Abdominal Circumferences																									
	15.5	16.0	16.5	17.0	17.5	18.0	18.5	19.0	19.5	20.0	20.5	21.0	21.5	22.0	22.5	23.0	23.5	24.0	24.5	25.0	25.5	26.0	26.5	27.0	27.5	28.0
3.1	224	234	244	255	267	279	291	304	318	332	346	362	378	395	412	431	450	470	491	513	536	559	584	610	638	666
3.2	231	241	251	263	274	286	299	312	326	340	355	371	388	405	423	441	461	481	502	525	548	572	597	624	651	680
3.3	237	248	259	270	282	294	307	321	335	349	365	381	397	415	433	452	472	493	514	537	560	585	611	638	666	695
3.4	244	255	266	278	290	302	316	329	344	359	374	391	408	425	444	463	483	504	526	549	573	598	624	652	680	710
3.5	251	262	274	285	298	311	324	338	353	368	384	401	418	436	455	475	495	517	539	562	587	612	638	666	695	725
3.6	259	270	281	294	306	319	333	347	362	378	394	411	429	447	466	486	507	529	552	575	600	626	653	681	710	740
3.7	266	278	290	302	315	328	342	357	372	388	404	422	440	458	478	498	519	542	565	589	614	640	667	696	725	756
3.8	274	286	298	310	324	337	352	366	382	398	415	432	451	470	490	510	532	554	578	602	628	654	682	711	741	772
3.9	282	294	306	319	333	347	361	376	392	409	426	444	462	482	502	523	545	568	592	616	642	669	697	727	757	789
4.0	290	303	315	328	342	356	371	386	403	419	437	455	474	494	514	536	558	581	606	631	657	684	713	743	773	806
4.1	299	311	324	338	352	366	381	397	413	430	448	467	486	506	527	549	572	595	620	645	672	700	729	759	790	828
4.2	308	320	333	347	361	376	392	408	424	442	460	479	498	519	540	562	585	609	634	660	688	716	743	776	807	841
4.3	317	330	343	357	371	387	402	419	436	453	472	491	511	532	554	576	600	624	649	676	703	732	762	793	825	859
4.4	326	339	353	367	382	397	413	430	447	465	484	504	524	545	567	590	614	639	665	692	719	749	779	810	843	877
4.5	335	349	363	377	393	408	425	442	459	478	497	517	538	559	581	605	629	654	680	708	736	765	796	828	861	896
4.6	345	359	373	388	404	420	436	454	472	490	510	530	551	573	596	620	644	670	696	724	753	783	814	846	880	915
4.7	355	369	384	399	415	431	448	466	484	503	523	544	565	588	611	635	660	686	713	741	770	801	832	865	899	934
4.8	366	380	395	410	426	443	460	478	497	517	537	558	580	602	626	650	676	702	730	758	788	819	851	884	919	954
4.9	376	391	406	422	438	455	473	491	510	530	551	572	594	617	641	666	692	719	747	776	806	837	870	903	938	975
5.0	387	402	418	434	451	468	486	505	524	544	565	587	610	633	657	683	709	736	765	794	824	856	889	923	959	996
5.1	399	414	430	446	463	481	499	518	538	559	580	602	625	649	674	699	726	754	783	812	843	876	909	944	980	1,017
5.2	410	426	442	459	476	494	513	532	552	573	595	618	641	665	690	717	744	772	801	831	863	895	929	964	1,001	1,039
5.3	422	438	455	472	489	508	527	547	567	589	611	634	657	682	708	734	762	790	820	851	883	916	950	986	1,023	1,061
5.4	435	451	468	485	503	522	541	561	582	604	627	650	674	699	725	752	780	809	839	870	903	936	971	1,007	1,045	1,084
5.5	447	464	481	499	517	536	556	577	598	620	643	667	691	717	743	771	799	828	859	891	924	958	993	1,030	1,068	1,107
5.6	461	477	495	513	532	551	571	592	614	636	660	684	709	735	762	789	818	848	879	911	945	979	1,015	1,052	1,091	1,131
5.7	474	491	509	527	547	566	587	608	630	653	677	701	727	753	780	809	838	869	900	933	966	1,001	1,038	1,075	1,114	1,155
5.8	488	505	524	542	562	582	603	625	647	670	695	719	745	772	800	829	858	889	921	954	989	1,024	1,061	1,099	1,139	1,180
5.9	502	520	539	558	578	598	619	642	664	688	713	738	764	792	820	849	879	911	943	977	1,011	1,047	1,085	1,123	1,163	1,205
6.0	517	535	554	573	594	615	636	659	682	706	731	757	784	811	840	870	900	932	965	999	1,035	1,071	1,109	1,148	1,189	1,231
6.1	532	550	570	590	610	632	654	677	700	725	750	777	804	832	861	891	922	955	988	1,023	1,058	1,095	1,134	1,173	1,214	1,257
6.2	547	566	586	606	627	649	672	695	719	744	770	797	824	853	882	913	945	977	1,011	1,046	1,083	1,120	1,159	1,199	1,241	1,284
6.3	563	583	603	624	645	667	690	714	738	764	790	817	845	874	904	935	967	1,001	1,035	1,071	1,107	1,145	1,185	1,226	1,268	1,311
6.4	580	600	620	641	663	686	709	733	758	784	811	838	867	896	927	958	991	1,025	1,059	1,096	1,133	1,171	1,211	1,253	1,295	1,339
6.5	597	617	638	659	682	705	728	753	778	805	832	860	889	919	950	982	1,015	1,049	1,084	1,121	1,159	1,198	1,238	1,280	1,323	1,368

TABLE 14–1. (CONTINUED)

Bi-parietal diameters	Abdominal Circumferences																							
	28.5	29.0	29.5	30.0	30.5	31.0	31.5	32.0	32.5	33.0	33.5	34.0	34.5	35.0	35.5	36.0	36.5	37.0	37.5	38.0	38.5	39.0	39.5	40.0
3.1	696	726	759	793	828	865	903	943	985	1,029	1,075	1,123	1,173	1,225	1,279	1,336	1,396	1,458	1,523	1,591	1,661	1,735	1,812	1,893
3.2	710	742	774	809	844	882	921	961	1,004	1,048	1,094	1,143	1,193	1,246	1,301	1,358	1,418	1,481	1,546	1,615	1,686	1,761	1,838	1,920
3.3	725	757	790	825	861	899	938	979	1,022	1,067	1,114	1,163	1,214	1,267	1,323	1,381	1,441	1,504	1,570	1,639	1,711	1,786	1,865	1,946
3.4	740	773	806	841	878	916	956	998	1,041	1,087	1,134	1,183	1,235	1,289	1,345	1,403	1,464	1,528	1,595	1,664	1,737	1,812	1,891	1,973
3.5	756	789	823	858	896	934	975	1,017	1,061	1,107	1,154	1,204	1,256	1,311	1,367	1,426	1,488	1,552	1,619	1,689	1,762	1,839	1,918	2,001
3.6	772	805	840	876	913	953	993	1,036	1,080	1,127	1,175	1,226	1,278	1,333	1,390	1,450	1,512	1,577	1,645	1,715	1,789	1,865	1,945	2,029
3.7	788	822	857	893	931	971	1,012	1,056	1,101	1,147	1,196	1,247	1,300	1,356	1,413	1,474	1,536	1,602	1,670	1,741	1,815	1,893	1,973	2,057
3.8	805	839	874	911	950	990	1,032	1,076	1,121	1,168	1,218	1,269	1,323	1,379	1,437	1,498	1,561	1,627	1,696	1,768	1,842	1,920	2,001	2,086
3.9	822	856	892	930	969	1,009	1,052	1,096	1,142	1,190	1,240	1,292	1,346	1,402	1,461	1,523	1,586	1,653	1,722	1,794	1,870	1,948	2,030	2,115
4.0	839	874	911	949	988	1,029	1,072	1,117	1,163	1,212	1,262	1,315	1,369	1,426	1,486	1,548	1,612	1,679	1,749	1,822	1,898	1,977	2,059	2,145
4.1	857	892	929	968	1,008	1,049	1,093	1,138	1,185	1,234	1,285	1,338	1,393	1,451	1,511	1,573	1,638	1,706	1,776	1,849	1,926	2,005	2,088	2,174
4.2	875	911	948	987	1,028	1,070	1,114	1,159	1,207	1,256	1,308	1,361	1,417	1,475	1,536	1,599	1,664	1,733	1,804	1,878	1,954	2,035	2,118	2,205
4.3	893	930	968	1,007	1,048	1,091	1,135	1,181	1,229	1,279	1,331	1,385	1,442	1,500	1,562	1,625	1,691	1,760	1,832	1,906	1,984	2,064	2,148	2,236
4.4	912	949	987	1,027	1,069	1,112	1,157	1,204	1,252	1,303	1,355	1,410	1,467	1,526	1,588	1,652	1,718	1,788	1,860	1,935	2,013	2,094	2,179	2,267
4.5	932	969	1,008	1,048	1,090	1,134	1,179	1,226	1,275	1,326	1,380	1,435	1,492	1,552	1,614	1,679	1,746	1,816	1,889	1,964	2,043	2,125	2,210	2,298
4.6	951	989	1,028	1,069	1,112	1,156	1,202	1,249	1,299	1,351	1,404	1,460	1,518	1,579	1,641	1,706	1,774	1,845	1,918	1,994	2,073	2,156	2,241	2,330
4.7	971	1,010	1,049	1,091	1,134	1,178*	1,225	1,273	1,323	1,375	1,430	1,486	1,545	1,605	1,669	1,734	1,803	1,874	1,948	2,024	2,104	2,187	2,273	2,363
4.8	992	1,031	1,071	1,113	1,156	1,201	1,248	1,297	1,348	1,401	1,455	1,512	1,571	1,633	1,697	1,763	1,832	1,904	1,978	2,055	2,136	2,219	2,306	2,396
4.9	1,013	1,052	1,093	1,135	1,179	1,225	1,272	1,322	1,373	1,426	1,482	1,539	1,599	1,661	1,725	1,792	1,861	1,934	2,009	2,086	2,167	2,251	2,339	2,429
5.0	1,034	1,074	1,115	1,158	1,203	1,249	1,297	1,347	1,399	1,452	1,508	1,566	1,626	1,689	1,754	1,821	1,891	1,964	2,040	2,118	2,200	2,284	2,372	2,463
5.1	1,056	1,096	1,138	1,181	1,226	1,273	1,322	1,372	1,425	1,479	1,535	1,594	1,655	1,718	1,783	1,851	1,922	1,995	2,071	2,150	2,232	2,317	2,406	2,498
5.2	1,078	1,119	1,161	1,205	1,251	1,298	1,347	1,398	1,451	1,506	1,563	1,622	1,683	1,747	1,813	1,882	1,953	2,027	2,103	2,183	2,266	2,351	2,440	2,532
5.3	1,101	1,142	1,185	1,229	1,276	1,323	1,373	1,425	1,478	1,533	1,591	1,651	1,713	1,777	1,843	1,913	1,984	2,059	2,136	2,216	2,299	2,386	2,475	2,568
5.4	1,124	1,166	1,209	1,254	1,301	1,349	1,399	1,452	1,506	1,562	1,620	1,680	1,742	1,807	1,874	1,944	2,016	2,091	2,169	2,250	2,333	2,420	2,510	2,604
5.5	1,148	1,190	1,234	1,279	1,327	1,376	1,426	1,479	1,534	1,590	1,649	1,710	1,773	1,838	1,906	1,976	2,049	2,124	2,203	2,284	2,368	2,456	2,546	2,640
5.6	1,172	1,215	1,259	1,305	1,353	1,402	1,454	1,507	1,562	1,619	1,678	1,740	1,803	1,869	1,938	2,008	2,082	2,158	2,237	2,319	2,403	2,491	2,582	2,677
5.7	1,197	1,240	1,285	1,332	1,380	1,430	1,482	1,535	1,591	1,649	1,709	1,770	1,835	1,901	1,970	2,041	2,115	2,192	2,272	2,354	2,439	2,528	2,619	2,714
5.8	1,222	1,266	1,311	1,358	1,407	1,458	1,510	1,564	1,621	1,679	1,739	1,802	1,866	1,934	2,003	2,075	2,150	2,227	2,307	2,390	2,475	2,564	2,657	2,752
5.9	1,248	1,292	1,338	1,386	1,435	1,486	1,539	1,594	1,651	1,710	1,770	1,834	1,899	1,966	2,037	2,109	2,184	2,262	2,342	2,426	2,512	2,602	2,694	2,790
6.0	1,274	1,319	1,366	1,414	1,464	1,515	1,569	1,624	1,682	1,741	1,802	1,866	1,932	2,000	2,071	2,144	2,219	2,298	2,379	2,463	2,550	2,640	2,733	2,829
6.1	1,301	1,346	1,393	1,442	1,493	1,545	1,599	1,655	1,713	1,773	1,835	1,899	1,965	2,034	2,105	2,179	2,255	2,334	2,416	2,500	2,588	2,678	2,772	2,869
6.2	1,328	1,374	1,422	1,471	1,522	1,575	1,630	1,686	1,745	1,805	1,868	1,932	1,999	2,069	2,140	2,215	2,291	2,371	2,453	2,538	2,626	2,717	2,811	2,909
6.3	1,356	1,403	1,451	1,501	1,552	1,606	1,661	1,718	1,777	1,838	1,901	1,967	2,034	2,104	2,176	2,251	2,328	2,408	2,491	2,577	2,665	2,757	2,851	2,949
6.4	1,385	1,432	1,481	1,531	1,583	1,637	1,693	1,751	1,810	1,872	1,935	2,001	2,069	2,140	2,213	2,288	2,366	2,446	2,530	2,616	2,705	2,797	2,892	2,991
6.5	1,414	1,462	1,511	1,562	1,615	1,669	1,725	1,784	1,844	1,906	1,970	2,037	2,105	2,176	2,250	2,326	2,404	2,485	2,569	2,656	2,745	2,838	2,933	3,032

TABLE 14–1. (CONTINUED)

Abdominal Circumferences

Bi-parietal diameters	15.5	16.0	16.5	17.0	17.5	18.0	18.5	19.0	19.5	20.0	20.5	21.0	21.5	22.0	22.5	23.0	23.5	24.0	24.5	25.0	25.5	26.0	26.5	27.0	27.5	28.0
6.6	614	635	656	678	701	724	748	773	799	826	853	882	911	942	973	1,006	1,039	1,074	1,110	1,147	1,185	1,225	1,266	1,308	1,352	1,397
6.7	632	653	675	697	720	744	769	794	820	848	876	905	935	965	997	1,030	1,065	1,100	1,136	1,174	1,213	1,253	1,294	1,337	1,381	1,427
6.8	651	672	694	717	740	765	790	816	842	870	898	928	958	990	1,022	1,056	1,090	1,126	1,163	1,201	1,241	1,281	1,323	1,367	1,411	1,458
6.9	670	691	714	737	761	786	811	838	865	893	922	952	983	1,015	1,048	1,082	1,117	1,153	1,190	1,229	1,269	1,310	1,353	1,397	1,442	1,489
7.0	689	711	734	758	782	807	833	860	888	916	946	976	1,008	1,040	1,074	1,108	1,144	1,181	1,219	1,258	1,298	1,340	1,383	1,427	1,473	1,521
7.1	709	732	755	779	804	830	856	883	912	941	971	1,002	1,033	1,066	1,100	1,135	1,171	1,209	1,247	1,287	1,328	1,370	1,414	1,459	1,505	1,553
7.2	730	753	777	801	827	853	880	907	936	965	996	1,027	1,060	1,093	1,128	1,163	1,200	1,238	1,277	1,317	1,358	1,401	1,445	1,491	1,538	1,586
7.3	751	775	799	824	850	876	904	932	961	991	1,022	1,054	1,087	1,121	1,156	1,192	1,229	1,267	1,307	1,348	1,390	1,433	1,478	1,524	1,571	1,620
7.4	773	797	822	847	874	901	928	957	987	1,017	1,049	1,081	1,114	1,149	1,184	1,221	1,259	1,297	1,338	1,379	1,421	1,465	1,511	1,557	1,605	1,655
7.5	796	820	845	871	898	925	954	983	1,013	1,044	1,076	1,109	1,143	1,178	1,214	1,251	1,289	1,328	1,369	1,411	1,454	1,499	1,544	1,592	1,640	1,690
7.6	819	844	870	896	923	951	980	1,009	1,040	1,072	1,104	1,137	1,172	1,207	1,244	1,281	1,320	1,360	1,401	1,444	1,487	1,533	1,579	1,627	1,676	1,727
7.7	843	868	894	921	949	977	1,007	1,037	1,068	1,100	1,133	1,167	1,202	1,238	1,275	1,313	1,352	1,393	1,434	1,477	1,522	1,567	1,614	1,663	1,712	1,764
7.8	868	894	920	947	975	1,004	1,034	1,065	1,096	1,129	1,162	1,197	1,232	1,269	1,306	1,345	1,385	1,426	1,468	1,512	1,557	1,603	1,650	1,699	1,749	1,801
7.9	893	919	946	974	1,003	1,032	1,062	1,094	1,126	1,159	1,193	1,228	1,264	1,301	1,339	1,378	1,418	1,460	1,503	1,547	1,592	1,639	1,687	1,737	1,787	1,840
8.0	919	946	973	1,002	1,031	1,061	1,091	1,123	1,156	1,189	1,224	1,259	1,296	1,333	1,372	1,412	1,453	1,495	1,538	1,583	1,629	1,676	1,725	1,775	1,826	1,879
8.1	946	973	1,001	1,030	1,060	1,090	1,121	1,153	1,187	1,221	1,256	1,292	1,329	1,367	1,406	1,446	1,488	1,531	1,575	1,620	1,666	1,714	1,763	1,814	1,866	1,919
8.2	974	1,001	1,030	1,059	1,089	1,120	1,152	1,185	1,218	1,253	1,288	1,325	1,363	1,401	1,441	1,482	1,524	1,567	1,612	1,657	1,704	1,753	1,803	1,854	1,906	1,960
8.3	1,002	1,030	1,059	1,089	1,120	1,151	1,183	1,217	1,251	1,286	1,322	1,359	1,397	1,436	1,477	1,518	1,561	1,605	1,650	1,696	1,744	1,793	1,843	1,895	1,948	2,002
8.4	1,032	1,060	1,090	1,120	1,151	1,183	1,216	1,249	1,284	1,320	1,356	1,394	1,433	1,473	1,513	1,555	1,599	1,643	1,689	1,735	1,784	1,833	1,884	1,936	1,990	2,045
8.5	1,062	1,091	1,121	1,151	1,183	1,216	1,249	1,283	1,318	1,355	1,392	1,430	1,469	1,510	1,551	1,594	1,637	1,682	1,728	1,776	1,825	1,875	1,926	1,979	2,033	2,089
8.6	1,093	1,122	1,153	1,184	1,216	1,249	1,283	1,318	1,354	1,390	1,428	1,467	1,507	1,548	1,589	1,633	1,677	1,722	1,769	1,817	1,866	1,917	1,969	2,022	2,077	2,134
8.7	1,125	1,155	1,186	1,218	1,250	1,284	1,318	1,353	1,390	1,427	1,465	1,505	1,545	1,586	1,629	1,673	1,717	1,764	1,811	1,859	1,909	1,960	2,013	2,067	2,122	2,179
8.8	1,157	1,188	1,220	1,252	1,285	1,319	1,354	1,390	1,427	1,465	1,504	1,543	1,584	1,626	1,669	1,714	1,759	1,806	1,854	1,903	1,953	2,005	2,058	2,113	2,169	2,226
8.9	1,191	1,222	1,254	1,287	1,321	1,356	1,391	1,428	1,465	1,503	1,543	1,583	1,625	1,667	1,711	1,756	1,802	1,849	1,897	1,947	1,998	2,050	2,104	2,159	2,216	2,274
9.0	1,226	1,258	1,290	1,324	1,358	1,393	1,429	1,466	1,504	1,543	1,583	1,624	1,666	1,709	1,753	1,799	1,845	1,893	1,942	1,992	2,044	2,097	2,151	2,207	2,264	2,322
9.1	1,262	1,294	1,327	1,361	1,396	1,432	1,468	1,506	1,544	1,584	1,624	1,666	1,708	1,752	1,797	1,843	1,890	1,938	1,988	2,039	2,091	2,144	2,199	2,255	2,313	2,372
9.2	1,299	1,332	1,365	1,400	1,435	1,471	1,508	1,546	1,586	1,626	1,667	1,709	1,752	1,796	1,841	1,888	1,936	1,984	2,035	2,086	2,139	2,193	2,248	2,305	2,363	2,423
9.3	1,337	1,370	1,404	1,439	1,475	1,512	1,550	1,588	1,628	1,668	1,710	1,753	1,796	1,841	1,887	1,934	1,982	2,032	2,083	2,135	2,188	2,242	2,298	2,356	2,414	2,475
9.4	1,376	1,410	1,444	1,480	1,516	1,554	1,592	1,631	1,671	1,712	1,755	1,798	1,842	1,887	1,934	1,982	2,030	2,080	2,132	2,184	2,238	2,293	2,350	2,407	2,467	2,527
9.5	1,416	1,450	1,486	1,522	1,559	1,597	1,635	1,675	1,716	1,758	1,800	1,844	1,889	1,935	1,982	2,030	2,080	2,130	2,182	2,235	2,289	2,345	2,402	2,460	2,520	2,582
9.6	1,457	1,492	1,528	1,565	1,602	1,641	1,680	1,720	1,762	1,804	1,847	1,892	1,937	1,984	2,031	2,080	2,130	2,181	2,233	2,287	2,342	2,398	2,456	2,515	2,575	2,637
9.7	1,500	1,535	1,572	1,609	1,647	1,686	1,726	1,767	1,809	1,852	1,895	1,940	1,986	2,033	2,082	2,131	2,181	2,233	2,286	2,340	2,396	2,452	2,510	2,570	2,631	2,693
9.8	1,544	1,580	1,617	1,654	1,693	1,733	1,773	1,815	1,857	1,900	1,945	1,990	2,037	2,085	2,133	2,183	2,234	2,286	2,340	2,395	2,451	2,508	2,567	2,627	2,688	2,751
9.9	1,589	1,625	1,663	1,701	1,740	1,781	1,822	1,864	1,907	1,951	1,996	2,042	2,089	2,137	2,186	2,237	2,288	2,341	2,395	2,450	2,507	2,565	2,624	2,684	2,746	2,810
10.0	1,635	1,672	1,710	1,749	1,789	1,830	1,871	1,914	1,958	2,002	2,048	2,094	2,142	2,191	2,241	2,292	2,344	2,397	2,452	2,507	2,564	2,623	2,682	2,743	2,806	2,870

TABLE 14–1. (CONTINUED)

Bi-parietal diameters	Abdominal Circumferences																							
	28.5	29.0	29.5	30.0	30.5	31.0	31.5	32.0	32.5	33.0	33.5	34.0	34.5	35.0	35.5	36.0	36.5	37.0	37.5	38.0	38.5	39.0	39.5	40.0
6.6	1,444	1,492	1,542	1,594	1,647	1,702	1,759	1,817	1,878	1,941	2,006	2,073	2,142	2,213	2,287	2,364	2,443	2,524	2,609	2,696	2,786	2,879	2,975	3,075
6.7	1,474	1,523	1,574	1,626	1,679	1,735	1,792	1,852	1,913	1,976	2,042	2,109	2,179	2,251	2,326	2,403	2,482	2,564	2,649	2,737	2,827	2,921	3,018	3,117
6.8	1,505	1,555	1,606	1,658	1,713	1,769	1,827	1,887	1,949	2,012	2,078	2,147	2,217	2,290	2,365	2,442	2,522	2,605	2,690	2,778	2,869	2,964	3,061	3,161
6.9	1,537	1,587	1,639	1,692	1,747	1,803	1,862	1,922	1,985	2,049	2,116	2,184	2,255	2,329	2,404	2,482	2,563	2,646	2,732	2,821	2,912	3,007	3,104	3,205
7.0	1,570	1,620	1,672	1,726	1,781	1,839	1,898	1,959	2,022	2,087	2,154	2,223	2,295	2,368	2,444	2,523	2,604	2,688	2,774	2,863	2,955	3,050	3,149	3,250
7.1	1,603	1,654	1,706	1,761	1,817	1,875	1,934	1,996	2,059	2,125	2,193	2,262	2,334	2,409	2,485	2,564	2,646	2,730	2,817	2,907	2,999	3,095	3,193	3,295
7.2	1,636	1,688	1,741	1,796	1,853	1,911	1,971	2,034	2,098	2,164	2,232	2,302	2,375	2,450	2,527	2,607	2,689	2,773	2,861	2,951	3,044	3,140	3,239	3,341
7.3	1,671	1,723	1,777	1,832	1,890	1,948	2,009	2,072	2,137	2,203	2,272	2,343	2,416	2,491	2,569	2,649	2,732	2,817	2,905	2,996	3,089	3,186	3,285	3,388
7.4	1,706	1,759	1,813	1,869	1,927	1,987	2,048	2,111	2,176	2,244	2,313	2,384	2,458	2,534	2,612	2,693	2,776	2,862	2,950	3,041	3,135	3,232	3,332	3,435
7.5	1,742	1,795	1,850	1,907	1,965	2,025	2,087	2,151	2,217	2,285	2,354	2,426	2,501	2,577	2,656	2,737	2,821	2,907	2,996	3,088	3,182	3,279	3,380	3,483
7.6	1,779	1,833	1,888	1,945	2,004	2,065	2,127	2,192	2,258	2,326	2,397	2,469	2,544	2,621	2,700	2,782	2,866	2,953	3,042	3,134	3,229	3,327	3,428	3,531
7.7	1,816	1,871	1,927	1,985	2,044	2,105	2,168	2,233	2,300	2,369	2,440	2,513	2,588	2,666	2,746	2,828	2,912	3,000	3,090	3,182	3,277	3,376	3,477	3,581
7.8	1,855	1,910	1,966	2,025	2,085	2,146	2,210	2,275	2,343	2,412	2,484	2,557	2,633	2,711	2,792	2,874	2,959	3,047	3,137	3,230	3,326	3,425	3,526	3,631
7.9	1,894	1,949	2,006	2,065	2,126	2,188	2,252	2,318	2,386	2,456	2,528	2,603	2,679	2,757	2,838	2,921	3,007	3,095	3,186	3,279	3,376	3,475	3,576	3,681
8.0	1,934	1,990	2,048	2,107	2,168	2,231	2,296	2,362	2,431	2,501	2,574	2,649	2,725	2,804	2,886	2,969	3,056	3,144	3,235	3,329	3,426	3,525	3,627	3,733
8.1	1,975	2,031	2,089	2,149	2,211	2,275	2,340	2,407	2,476	2,547	2,620	2,695	2,773	2,852	2,934	3,018	3,105	3,194	3,286	3,380	3,477	3,577	3,679	3,785
8.2	2,016	2,073	2,132	2,193	2,255	2,319	2,385	2,462	2,522	2,594	2,667	2,743	2,821	2,901	2,983	3,068	3,155	3,244	3,336	3,431	3,529	3,629	3,732	3,838
8.3	2,059	2,116	2,176	2,237	2,300	2,364	2,431	2,499	2,569	2,641	2,715	2,791	2,870	2,950	3,033	3,118	3,206	3,296	3,388	3,483	3,581	3,682	3,785	3,891
8.4	2,102	2,160	2,220	2,282	2,345	2,410	2,477	2,546	2,617	2,689	2,764	2,841	2,920	3,001	3,084	3,169	3,257	3,348	3,441	3,536	3,634	3,735	3,839	3,945
8.5	2,146	2,205	2,266	2,328	2,392	2,457	2,525	2,594	2,665	2,739	2,814	2,891	2,970	3,052	3,135	3,221	3,310	3,401	3,494	3,590	3,688	3,790	3,894	4,000
8.6	2,192	2,251	2,312	2,375	2,439	2,505	2,573	2,643	2,715	2,789	2,864	2,942	3,022	3,104	3,188	3,274	3,363	3,454	3,548	3,644	3,743	3,845	3,949	4,056
8.7	2,238	2,298	2,359	2,423	2,488	2,554	2,623	2,693	2,765	2,840	2,916	2,994	3,074	3,157	3,241	3,328	3,417	3,509	3,603	3,700	3,799	3,901	4,005	4,113
8.8	2,285	2,346	2,408	2,472	2,537	2,604	2,673	2,744	2,817	2,892	2,968	3,047	3,128	3,210	3,295	3,383	3,472	3,565	3,659	3,756	3,855	3,958	4,063	4,170
8.9	2,333	2,394	2,457	2,521	2,587	2,655	2,725	2,796	2,869	2,944	3,021	3,101	3,182	3,265	3,351	3,438	3,528	3,621	3,716	3,813	3,913	4,015	4,120	4,228
9.0	2,382	2,444	2,507	2,572	2,639	2,707	2,777	2,849	2,923	2,998	3,076	3,155	3,237	3,321	3,407	3,495	3,585	3,678	3,773	3,871	3,971	4,074	4,179	4,287
9.1	2,433	2,495	2,559	2,624	2,691	2,760	2,830	2,903	2,977	3,053	3,131	3,211	3,293	3,377	3,464	3,552	3,643	3,736	3,832	3,930	4,030	4,133	4,239	4,347
9.2	2,484	2,547	2,611	2,677	2,744	2,814	2,885	2,958	3,032	3,109	3,187	3,268	3,350	3,435	3,522	3,611	3,702	3,795	3,891	3,989	4,090	4,193	4,299	4,408
9.3	2,536	2,599	2,664	2,731	2,799	2,869	2,940	3,014	3,089	3,166	3,245	3,326	3,409	3,494	3,581	3,670	3,761	3,855	3,951	4,050	4,151	4,254	4,361	4,469
9.4	2,590	2,653	2,719	2,786	2,854	2,925	2,997	3,070	3,146	3,224	3,303	3,384	3,468	3,553	3,641	3,730	3,822	3,916	4,013	4,111	4,213	4,316	4,423	4,532
9.5	2,644	2,709	2,774	2,842	2,911	2,982	3,054	3,129	3,205	3,283	3,362	3,444	3,528	3,614	3,701	3,791	3,884	3,978	4,075	4,174	4,275	4,379	4,486	4,595
9.6	2,700	2,765	2,831	2,899	2,969	3,040	3,113	3,188	3,264	3,343	3,423	3,505	3,589	3,675	3,763	3,854	3,946	4,041	4,138	4,237	4,339	4,443	4,550	4,659
9.7	2,757	2,822	2,889	2,958	3,028	3,099	3,173	3,248	3,325	3,404	3,484	3,567	3,651	3,738	3,826	3,917	4,010	4,105	4,202	4,302	4,404	4,508	4,615	4,724
9.8	2,815	2,881	2,948	3,017	3,088	3,160	3,234	3,309	3,387	3,466	3,547	3,630	3,715	3,802	3,890	3,981	4,074	4,170	4,267	4,367	4,469	4,573	4,680	4,790
9.9	2,874	2,941	3,009	3,078	3,149	3,222	3,296	3,372	3,450	3,529	3,611	3,694	3,779	3,866	3,956	4,047	4,140	4,236	4,333	4,433	4,536	4,640	4,747	4,857
10.0	2,935	3,002	3,070	3,140	3,211	3,285	3,359	3,436	3,514	3,594	3,676	3,759	3,845	3,932	4,022	4,113	4,207	4,303	4,400	4,501	4,603	4,708	4,815	4,924

Log (birth weight) = 1.7492 + 0.166(BPD) + 0.046(AC) −2.646 (AC + BPD)/1,000

SD = ±106.0 g/kg of birth weight.

From Shepard MJ, Richards VA, Berkowitz RL, et al. An evaluation of two equations for predicting fetal weight by ultrasound. Am J Obstet Gynecol. 1982;142:47–55, with permission.

TABLE 14–2. ESTIMATED WEIGHTS BASED ON FEMUR LENGTH AND ABDOMINAL CIRCUMFERENCE*

Abdominal circumference (cm)	Femur length (mm)																								
	32	34	36	38	40	42	44	46	48	50	52	54	56	58	60	62	64	66	68	70	72	74	76	78	80
18	350	395	431	484	543	609	683	766	859	954	1082	1213	1361	1527	1849	2082	2345	2641	2974	3349	3771	4247	4783	5386	6066
19	367	411	461	516	578	647	725	812	910	1019	1141	1278	1432	1604	1797	2012	2254	2525	2828	3167	3548	3973	4451	4985	5584
20	388	432	481	536	597	665	741	826	920	1025	1141	1272	1417	1578	1758	1959	2182	2431	2708	3017	3361	3744	4171	4647	5177
21	412	457	506	561	621	688	763	845	936	1038	1150	1274	1411	1564	1733	1920	2128	2358	2612	2895	3207	3554	3938	4363	4835
22	441	486	536	591	651	717	791	871	960	1058	1166	1285	1417	1561	1721	1896	2090	2303	2538	2797	3083	3398	3744	4127	4548
23	476	522	572	627	687	753	826	905	992	1087	1192	1306	1432	1570	1721	1886	2067	2266	2484	2723	2985	3271	3586	3931	4309
24	517	564	614	670	730	796	868	947	1032	1125	1227	1337	1458	1590	1733	1889	2060	2246	2448	2669	2910	3173	3459	3771	4112
25	566	613	665	721	782	848	920	997	1081	1173	1272	1379	1495	1621	1758	1906	2067	2242	2431	2636	2858	3100	3361	3645	3952
26	623	672	725	782	844	910	981	1058	1141	1231	1328	1432	1544	1666	1797	1938	2090	2254	2431	2622	2828	3050	3289	3548	3826
27	692	742	796	854	916	983	1054	1131	1213	1302	1396	1498	1607	1724	1849	1983	2128	2282	2448	2626	2817	3022	3242	3478	3731
28	774	826	881	940	1003	1070	1141	1218	1299	1386	1479	1578	1684	1797	1917	2045	2182	2328	2484	2650	2828	3017	3219	3434	3664
29	871	925	981	1041	1105	1173	1244	1321	1401	1487	1578	1675	1777	1886	2001	2124	2254	2392	2538	2694	2858	3033	3219	3416	3625
30	988	1043	1101	1162	1227	1295	1366	1442	1522	1607	1696	1790	1889	1994	2105	2222	2345	2475	2612	2757	2910	3072	3242	3422	3612
31	1129	1185	1244	1306	1371	1440	1511	1587	1666	1749	1836	1927	2023	2124	2230	2341	2457	2580	2708	2843	2985	3133	3289	3453	3625
32	1299	1357	1417	1479	1544	1613	1684	1758	1836	1917	2001	2090	2182	2278	2379	2484	2594	2708	2828	2952	3083	3219	3361	3509	3664
33	1506	1564	1624	1687	1752	1819	1889	1962	2038	2116	2198	2282	2370	2462	2557	2655	2757	2864	2974	3088	3207	3331	3459	3592	3731
34	1758	1816	1876	1938	2001	2067	2135	2206	2278	2353	2431	2511	2594	2679	2767	2858	2952	3050	3150	3254	3361	3472	3586	3704	3826
35	2067	2124	2182	2242	2303	2366	2431	2497	2566	2636	2708	2782	2858	2937	3017	3100	3184	3271	3361	3453	3548	3645	3744	3847	3952
36	2448	2502	2557	2612	2669	2728	2787	2848	2910	2974	3039	3105	3173	3242	3313	3385	3459	3535	3612	3691	3771	3854	3938	4024	4112
37	2921	2968	3017	3066	3116	3167	3219	3271	3325	3379	3434	3490	3548	3605	3664	3724	3785	3847	3910	3973	4038	4104	4171	4239	4309
38	3509	3548	3586	3625	3664	3704	3744	3785	3826	3868	3910	3952	3995	4038	4082	4127	4171	4217	4262	4309	4356	4403	4451	4499	4548
39	4247	4270	4293	4316	4340	4363	4387	4411	4435	4459	4483	4507	4531	4556	4581	4605	4630	4655	4681	4706	4732	4757	4783	4809	4835

* LnBW = (2.792 + .108 (FL) + .0036 (AC)^2 − .0027 (FL) (AC)), where BW = birth weight; FL = femur length; and AC = abdominal circumference.
From Warsof SL, Wolf P, Coulehan J, et al. Comparison of fetal weight estimation formulas with and without head measurements. Obstet Gynecol. 1986;67:569, with permission.

the BPD and the AC (error range 8.5% to 11%). In addition, when three parameters—the head, abdomen, and femur—were used, the random error was 15% to 25% less than with models of two parameters: BPD and AC. Regression models were based on measurements of AC, HC, BPD, and FL, both alone and in combinations. These researchers determined that the best results were obtained when 1 standard deviation was 7.5% of the actual weight.

Warsof et al,[15] in an effort to determine the best-fit formula with the lowest error for estimating fetal weight, used multiple stepwise regression analyses for AC and FL (Table 14–2), or FL alone. The mean error was 109 g per kilogram of fetal weight for AC and FL and 129 g per kilogram using FL alone.

Another interesting development was reported by Spinnato et al[19] in being able to predict birth weight at delivery from an ultrasound examination done remote from delivery. A regression equation uses interval to delivery as an adjunct to measurements of the head, abdomen, and femur for estimating fetal weight at delivery. With a mean time of approximately 16 days, their equation predicted birth weight to within ± 20%.

Since the development of the ultrasonic estimation of fetal weight in the mid-1970s, several studies attempted to improve the accuracy of fetal weight estimation. Major questions that must be addressed are: Just how accurate are in utero weight estimates, and what is the optimal combination of parameters for estimating fetal weight? The best way to answer these questions is to look at the studies in which all these parameters have been evaluated in the same population of fetuses. In this way, differences in population characteristics and imaging and measurement techniques can be eliminated as potential variables. It is important for such studies to evaluate fetuses throughout the entire weight spectrum, ideally extending from 500 g or less, to 5,000 g or more. The analysis of any changes in accuracy within various weight categories is also an important feature of such studies. The use of multiple parameters, particularly those including head, abdomen, and femur measurements, provides the most adequate measurements of fetal weight, with a 95% confidence interval in the range of 15% to 16%.[20]

Using the optimal modes for weight prediction will result in approximately 90% of fetal weight estimates being within ± 12% of the actual birth weight. It is important to understand, however, that these results assume a high level of image and measurement quality, and that this is the best one can expect to do in estimating fetal weight.

These models will not perform as well in the extreme low birth weight fetus. Townsend and coworkers[21] demonstrated that fetuses with birth weights less than 1,000 g had a 95% confidence interval of ± 24%. Moreover, factors that involve poor resolution, such as oligohydramnios or the thickness of the maternal abdominal wall, also decrease the accuracy of estimating fetal weight. With further improvement in the resolution of ultrasound, better estimation of birth weight may be feasible.

REFERENCES

1. Edouard L, Alberman E. National trends in the identified causes of perinatal mortality 1960–1978. *Br J Obstet Gynaecol.* 1980;87:833–838.
2. Frandsen V, Stakeman G. Urinary excretion of estriol during normal pregnancy. *Danish Med Bull.* 1960;7:95–99.
3. Van Leusden HA. Hormonal changes in pathological pregnancies. *Vitamins Hormones.* 1972;30:281–361.
4. Shearman RP. Some aspects of urinary excretion of pregnanediol in pregnancy. *Br J Obstet Gynaecol.* 1959;66:1.
5. Lubchenco LO, Hansman C, Dressler M, et al. Intrauterine growth as estimated from live born birth-weight data at 24 to 42 weeks of gestation. *Pediatrics.* 1963;32:793–800.
6. Lubchenco LO, Hansman C, Boyd E. Intrauterine growth in length and head circumference as estimated from live births at gestational ages from 26 to 42 weeks. *Pediatrics.* 1966;37:403–408.
7. Usher R, McLean F. Intrauterine growth of live-born caucasian infants at sea-level: standards obtained from measurements in 7 dimensions of infants born between 25 and 44 weeks of gestation. *Pediatrics.* 1969;74:901–910.
8. Shepard MJ, Richards VA, Berkowitz RL, et al. An evaluation of two equations for predicting fetal weight by ultrasound. *Am J Obstet Gynecol.* 1982;142:47–55.
9. Timor-Tritsch IE, Itskowitz J, Brandes JM. Estimation of fetal weight by real-time sonography. *Obstet Gynecol.* 1981;57:653–656.
10. Hadlock FP, Harrist RB, Carpenter M, et al. Sonographic estimation of fetal weight. *Radiology.* 1984;150:535–540.
11. Campbell S, Wilkin D. Ultrasonic measurement of fetal abdomen circumference in the estimation of fetal weight. *Br J Obstet Gynaecol.* 1975;82:689–697.
12. Hadlock FP, Harrist RB, Sharman RS, et al. Estimation of fetal weight with the use of head, body, and femur measurements: a prospective study. *Am J Obstet Gynecol.* 1985;151:333–337.
13. Hill LM, Breckle R, Gehrking WC, et al. Use of femur length in estimation of fetal weight. *Am J Obstet Gynecol.* 1985;152:847–852.
14. Woo JSK, Wan M. An evaluation of fetal weight prediction using a simple equation containing the fetal femur length. *J Ultrasound Med.* 1986;5:453–457.
15. Warsof SL, Wolf P, Coulehan J, et al. Comparison of fetal weight estimation formulas with and without head measurements. *Obstet Gynecol.* 1986;67:569–573.
16. Vintzileos AM, Campbell WA, Rodis JF, et al. Fetal weight estimation formulas with head, abdominal, femur, and thigh circumference measurements. *Am J Obstet Gynecol.* 1987;157:410–414.
17. Warsof SL, Gohari P, Berkowitz RL, et al. The estimation

of fetal weight by computer-assisted analysis. *Am J Obstet Gynecol.* 1977;128:881–891.

18. Ott WJ. Clinical application of fetal weight determination by real-time ultrasound measurements. *Obstet Gynecol.* 57:758–762,1981.

19. Spinnato JA, Allen RD, Mendenhall HW. Birth weight prediction from remote ultrasonographic examination. *Am J Obstet Gynecol.* 1989;161:743–747.

20. Hadlock FP. Sonographic estimation of fetal age and weight. *Radio Clin N Am.* 1990;28:39–50.

21. Townsend RR, Filly RA, Callen PW, et al. Factors affecting prenatal sonographic estimation of weight in extremely low birthweight infants. *J Ultrasound Med.* 1988;7:183–187.

15

Deviant Fetal Growth

The use of diagnostic ultrasound in obstetrics has made it possible to observe fetal growth in utero, and the recent development of normative biometric data for a number of fetal growth parameters allow objective evaluation of the growth process. Assessment of normal fetal growth and development is achieved by using the sonographic fetal growth profile; thus both the growth-retarded and the growth-accelerated fetus can be detected in utero.[1]

THE GROWTH-RETARDED FETUS

Intrauterine growth retardation has been well recognized in maternal fetal medicine. In 1961 the Committee on Maternal and Child Health of the World Health Organization recommended that infants weighing less than 2,500 g at birth be designated "low birth weight," rather than premature.[2] This recommendation was adopted for a short time because birth weight is a function of intrauterine growth and gestational age.

Today, premature and growth-retarded infants are differentiated by the various types of medical problems each experiences during the immediate postpartum period.[3,4] Fetal growth interests the clinician chiefly when it is disturbed. The intrauterine growth-retarded fetus and neonate carry a substantially increased risk of perinatal morbidity and mortality.[3,5–9] The incidences of long-term neurologic sequelae and intrauterine growth retardation appears to be related to growth inhibition, its duration, and severity.[6,7,9,10]

Ultrasonography has been used to detect growth retardation since the late 1960s; during the intervening years, attempts have been made to improve its diagnostic accuracy. A variety of sonographic parameters have been suggested for diagnosing altered fetal growth patterns. Serial cephalometry, head circumference (HC) to abdominal circumference (AC) ratio, femur length (FL) to AC ratio, qualitative estimation of amniotic fluid volume, estimation of fetal weight and, most recently, abnormal fetoplacental blood flow are all associated with fetal growth retardation.

Intrauterine growth retardation (IUGR) in a fetus is defined as weight at or below the tenth percentile for gestational age.[3,4] Because of the lack of uniformity in criteria used throughout the world in making this diagnosis the incidence of IUGR varies among institutions, reflecting differences in diagnostic criteria. For example, the tenth percentile in the Denver, Colorado growth curve[11] is analogous to the third percentile in the Montreal, Canada curve obtained at sea level.[12] In any event, the incidence of IUGR is estimated to be between 3% and 10% of all pregnancies.

Etiopathology

Normally, the fetus gains in length and weight as a function of time of the gestation; the rate of growth throughout pregnancy, however, is not constant. Researchers[11] have described different peak velocities for fetal intrauterine growth. Velocity in fetal growth peaks at 16 to 20 weeks and at 33 weeks for fetal weight. Fat represents less than 1% of total body weight of the fetus at 26 weeks but 12% at 38 weeks. Winick[13] described the three phases of cellular growth. The first consists of an increase in cell numbers (hyperplasia); the second phase is an increase in the number and size of the cells (hyperplasia and hypertrophy); and the third phase is further hypertrophy.

Fetal growth retardation is divided into two clinical types: type I (symmetric) and type II (asymmetric). These two types are likely to be the consequence of different times of onset of the disorder and different duration of the events that caused the retarded growth.

Type I, symmetric growth retardation, probably results from noxious injury very early in gestation, at a time when fetal growth is at the phase of cellular hyperplasia. Insult to the fetus at this time might be expected to produce profound effects. This type of growth-retarded fetus is thus intrinsic; approximately 20% of cases of growth retardation are symmetric.

Type II, asymmetric growth retardation, results mostly from adverse effects during the phase of cellular hypertrophy, that is, during later gestation. Thus, the majority of asymmetrically growth-retarded fetuses have an appropriate number of cells but those cells are smaller than normal. This type of asymmetric

191

growth retardation is usually caused by maternal diseases extrinsic to the fetus.

Growth inhibition will eventually be reflected in the fetal biometry that makes prenatal diagnosis feasible. Intrauterine growth retardation, or growth restriction, may result from maternal medical conditions, the presence of fetal diseases, and uterine and placental factors (Table 15–1).

Maternal Disease

A variety of medical conditions in the mother may be associated with intrauterine growth retardation in the fetus. Maternal hypertension, regardless of its cause, affects the placental vasculature and therefore interferes with the passage of nutrients by lowering the functional area of the placenta. Cardiac and pulmonary diseases are obvious sources of potential IUGR. The fetus shows the effects of chronically low oxygen levels when its metabolic demands increase in the third trimester. Maternal anemia, with its diminished oxygen content in the blood, will limit the amount of available oxygen for placental transfer. Maternal gastrointestinal diseases may cause IUGR when it is severe enough to limit the intake of nutrients. Renal disease complicated by protein-wasting nephropathies and by hypertension may be associated with fetal growth retardation. Smoking, drugs, and alcohol are causes of intrauterine growth retardation.[7] Other factors causing IUGR include maternal vasculopathy and autoimmune disease.[13]

TABLE 15–1. ETIOLOGY OF INTRAUTERINE GROWTH RETARDATION (IUGR)

Environmental
　Malnutrition
　Drugs and substance abuse
　　Aminopterin
　　Alcohol
　　Hydantoins
　　Narcotics
　　Prednisone
　　Trimethadione
　　Smoking
　　Antihypertensives
Uterine and placental anomalies and abnormalities
　Uterine
　　Bicornuate uterus
　　Septate uterus
　　Uterine myomas
　Placental
　　Circumvallation
　　Abruption and circulatory disturbances
　　Placental infection—villitis
　　Hemangiomatous placental tumors
　　Twin-to-twin transfusion syndrome
　　Abnormal cord insertion
　　Multiple gestations
Fetal infections
　Protozoan
　　Malaria
　　Toxoplasmosis
　Viral
　　Rubella
　　Cytomegalovirus
　　Varicella-zoster
　　Other viruses, including mumps, herpes simplex, vaccinia
　　　hepatitis A, and polio
Maternal conditions, diseases (genetic and nongenetic)
　Abnormal maternal nutrient metabolism
　Cyanotic heart disease
　Folate deficiency anemia
　Severe (iron-deficiency) anemia
　Sickle cell disease
　Gastrointestinal diseases (ulcerative colitis, Crohn's disease,
　　pancreatitis, and malabsorption states)

Maternal vascular disease
　Chronic hypertension
　Collagen vascular diseases
　Diabetes mellitus, classes D,F,R
　Renal disease
　Preeclampsia
　Reduced maternal plasma volume
　Neurofibromatosis (maternal) a.d. (IUGR, HTN)
　Phenylketonuria (maternal), a.r.
　Schmidt's syndrome
　High altitudes
Fetal genetic disorders
　Single gene disorders
　　Placental sulfatase deficiency x-linked
　　Dubowitz syndrome a.r.
　　Dwarfism
　　　Levi-Laron a.r.
　　　Snubnosed a.d.
　　Lissencephaly a.r.
　　Meckel's syndrome a.r.
　　Potter's syndrome a.d./multifactorial
　　Robert's syndrome a.r.
　　Russell–Silver syndrome a.d./sporadic
　Chromosomal disorders
　　XO (Turner's syndrome)
　　Trisomies
　　　21—Down syndrome
　　　18—Edwards' syndrome
　　　13—Patau's syndrome
　　Deletion syndromes
　　　4p—short arm
　　　5p—cri du chat
　　　18p—
　　　18q—
Congenital anomalies
　Gastroschisis
　Duodenal atresia
　Pancreatic agenesis
　Osteogenesis imperfecta (congenital)
　Omphalocele: noted, not seen
　Congenital heart disease

a.d. = autosomal dominant inheritance; a.r. = autosomal recessive inheritance.
From Lockwood CJ, Weiner S. Assessment of fetal growth. Clin Perinatol. 1986; 13:3, with permission.

Fetal Diseases

Congenital infections with rubella, cytomegalovirus, and toxoplasmosis are associated with symmetrically small infants.[14] A variety of genetically determined conditions result in IUGR and are associated with symmetrically impaired growth and development.[1,3]

Uterine and Placental Causes

Growth of many infants with IUGR secondary to uteroplacental insufficiency is asymmetric. Causes of decreased intrauterine space, for example fibromas, malformed uteri, and multiple gestations can also cause asymmetric growth retardation.[1,3,4] The etiologies of IUGR are described in Table 15–1.

Prenatal Diagnosis

Accurate prenatal diagnosis may prevent the fetal morbidity and even mortality associated with IUGR. Although the success of clinical diagnosis has been limited, the suspicion of growth delay may be based on the identification of maternal factors that suggest a high risk for IUGR. Careful evaluation of the growth of the uterine fundus offers a valuable index of fetal growth. Belizan et al[15] have demonstrated that fundal height measurement in centimeters from the symphysis pubis to the top of the fundus has a curvilinear relationship with gestational age and thus with fetal growth. The authors found an 86% positive predictive accuracy in the diagnosis IUGR when the fundal height fell below the tenth percentile. Fundal height, as a reflection of the total mass of the fetus, placenta, and amniotic fluid can provide an index of fetal growth, but imprecision and inconsistency in the application of this technique have prevented widespread confidence in this clinical tool. In addition, multiparous women with sagging abdominal muscles may worsen the predictive accuracy of this clinical tool. A diagnosis of IUGR should be suspected and confirmation sought when the fundal height lags more than 4 cm or 4 weeks below the gestational age.

Hormonal and biochemical assays were once popular in the assessment of fetal condition, but today these tests do not enjoy widespread popularity or use.[4]

One of the important components in any strategy for detecting IUGR in utero is the identification of women who are at high risk for delivering a growth-retarded fetus. The characteristic population at high risk are those with a history of growth-retarded fetuses, chronic hypertension, severe insulin-dependent diabetes mellitus, extremely poor weight gain during pregnancy, alcohol or drug abuse, and heavy smokers.[14]

Ultrasound technique is employed for determining intrauterine fetal biometry and is used to monitor fetal growth and diagnose fetal growth retardation. If the gestational age of the fetus is known, the diagnosis of IUGR is made relatively early by the observation of the biometric parameters markedly at variance with the predicted gestational age, weight, or both. A number of sonographic parameters have been used for the diagnosis of IUGR:

1. Biparietal diameter
2. Head circumference
3. Head to abdominal circumferences ratio
4. Femur length to abdominal circumference ratio
5. Amount of amniotic fluid
6. Transverse cerebellar diameter
7. Estimated fetal weight
8. Blood flow in the umbilical cord and uterine artery

The same parameters cannot be used to assess both age and growth. The establishment of the precise gestational age is the gold standard in detecting IUGR. It is for this reason that attempts at accurately establishing early gestational age are so important.

Biparietal Diameter (BPD)

Ultrasonic assessment of fetal growth revealed two types of growth retardation.[16] The first, called late BPD flattening, can be detected by serial measurements of the BPD, which shows normal growth until about 30 weeks, beyond which the rate of growth slows. A second type of growth retardation is called low profile. This growth pattern is characterized by a BPD that grows consistently slower than normal, at least after 20 weeks of gestation. Examination of small-for-gestational-age babies by Campbell[16] has shown that approximately 70% of these infants show a late flattening BPD growth pattern (asymmetric growth-retarded fetuses), and 30% show a low profile pattern (symmetric IUGR). Prenatal diagnosis of IUGR based on the BPD measurement alone is a poor and insensitive technique and detects between 43% and 75% of IUGR newborns.[17–22] The insensitivity observed may result from the inclusion of so-called brain sparing IUGR resulting from placental insufficiency. This phenomenon is probably related to the preferential preservation of blood flow to the brain at the expense of the blood flow to other organs. Because the brain is spared, the BPD may not be affected until late in the growth-retardation process.

The use of the BPD alone would result in low sensitivity, with a high number of false-negative results. Variation in the fetal head shape due to molding,[23] particularly dolichocephaly, which is observed in cases of ruptured membranes, multiple gestations, and breech presentation, will result in abnormally low values in normal fetuses, which leads to a high number of false-positive cases of IUGR. In one study, correction of the lack of sensitivity of the BPD in predicting growth-retarded fetuses was undertaken using serial BPD measurements for predicting IUGR. The results indicated a lack of accuracy in serial BPD measurements in the diagnosis of IUGR.[22]

Transverse Cerebellar Diameter (TCD)

The cerebellum can be easily visualized as early as the first trimester as a butterflylike figure in the posterior fossa of the fetal head, behind the thalami, and in front of the echolucent cisterna magna. The transverse cerebellar diameter (TCD) in millimeters correlates with the gestational age in weeks up to 24 weeks, after which growth curves turn upward and this uniform correlation no longer exists. Goldstein and Reece et al[24] constructed a nomogram of the TCD throughout pregnancy (Table 5–4 and Table 5–5).

Reece et al[25] subsequently evaluated the TCD measurement in IUGR fetuses. They reported that TCD measurements were not significantly affected by retarded fetal growth, and therefore the TCD could be used as a reliable predictor of gestational age even in cases of IUGR. This parameter was particularly helpful because it could be used as a standard against which other parameters could be compared. Duchatel et al[26] have corroborated these findings in their report of 12 cases of IUGR below the third percentile and in

which the TCD remained unaltered. Campbell and co-workers[27] have provided additional support for the utility of the TCD by constructing a nomogram of TCD to abdominal circumference (AC) ratio. In a small series they have shown that this ratio permits the identification of IUGR, demonstrating the fairly consistent growth of the TCD relative to the decrease in AC in cases of IUGR.

In another study Hill et al[28] reported that the TCD was within 2 SD in only 40% of IUGR cases and in 60% of cases was greater than 2 SD below the mean. At present these results are at variance with the three reports discussed earlier. The majority of available data suggest that the utility of the TCD is extremely valuable when the gestational age is unknown or IUGR is suspected. The accuracy of the TCD can be enhanced by the use of biometric ratios, especially FL to AC, as well as the amniotic fluid volume and the presence or absence of fetal ossification centers.

Head Circumference (HC)

The HC is a more shape-independent measurement of the fetal head size than the BPD; its use in the growth profile will eliminate the high number of false-positive diagnoses of IUGR when the BPD is used in cases of

TABLE 15–2. NOMOGRAM OF FETAL HEAD/ABDOMINAL CIRCUMFERENCE RATIO

Gestational Age (Wk)	Mean	2 SD	Percentile							N
			5th	10th	25th	50th	75th	90th	95th	
13										
14	1.24	0.04	1.22	1.22	1.2	1.26	1.26	1.26	1.26	3
15	1.18	0.04	1.17	1.17	1.17	1.18	1.20	1.20	1.20	2
16	1.20	0.08	1.14	1.14	1.16	1.20	1.22	1.28	1.31	16
17	1.23	0.1	1.15	1.15	1.16	1.23	1.27	1.30	1.30	7
18	1.20	0.1	1.14	1.14	1.16	1.20	1.20	1.20	1.20	7
19	1.20	0.1	1.13	1.13	1.13	1.19	1.27	1.38	1.38	6
20	1.14	0.06	1.10	1.10	1.11	1.16	1.17	1.18	1.18	6
21	1.15	0.1	1.00	1.00	1.09	1.14	1.22	1.25	1.25	8
22	1.18	0.06	1.12	1.12	1.14	1.20	1.22	1.22	1.22	10
23	1.15	0.12	1.08	1.08	1.08	1.13	1.22	1.22	1.22	3
24	1.16	0.1	1.07	1.07	1.14	1.15	1.20	1.24	1.24	9
25	1.13	0.1	1.03	1.03	1.09	1.13	1.19	1.21	1.21	10
26	1.12	0.1	1.03	1.05	1.09	1.11	1.16	1.21	1.26	17
27	1.09	0.1	0.94	0.98	1.08	1.10	1.12	1.17	1.17	16
28	1.09	0.1	1.01	1.01	1.03	1.09	1.14	1.20	1.20	19
29	1.08	0.08	1.01	1.02	1.05	1.09	1.10	1.13	1.17	22
30	1.08	0.1	0.98	1.00	1.03	1.07	1.13	1.17	1.21	28
31	1.08	0.1	0.99	0.99	1.01	1.09	1.13	1.18	1.21	20
32	1.04	0.1	0.93	0.96	1.00	1.04	1.10	1.14	1.16	19
33	1.04	0.06	0.97	1.00	1.02	1.04	1.07	1.09	1.12	29
34	1.05	0.14	0.94	0.97	1.00	1.04	1.10	1.17	1.20	28
35	1.02	0.1	0.92	0.94	0.99	1.02	1.05	1.10	1.13	30
36	1.02	0.1	0.92	0.94	0.97	1.02	1.06	1.11	1.12	34
37	1.00	0.14	0.87	0.91	0.97	1.00	1.05	1.10	1.12	34
38	0.98	0.12	0.86	0.89	0.92	0.97	1.02	1.07	1.11	35
39	0.94	0.14	0.71	0.88	0.91	0.96	0.98	1.02	1.05	23
40	0.96	0.14	0.84	0.85	0.91	0.95	1.00	1.09	1.10	14
41	0.95	0.12	0.76	0.86	0.91	0.95	0.99	1.04	1.07	22
42	0.91	0.12	0.83	0.83	0.86	0.88	0.96	1.04	1.04	9

dolichocephaly.[23] HC is also an integral part of the head to body ratio assessment. The HC is not typically the last fetal measurement adversely affected by the IUGR process (Table 13–1).

Abdominal Circumference (AC)

The fetal liver is the largest intra-abdominal organ; it is considered the first organ to be affected by the process of growth retardation. The AC is therefore an indirect measurement of the state of fetal nutrition. Animal and human studies have shown diminished hepatic glycogen stores and liver mass associated with IUGR.[29] The AC is the most sensitive single parameter for detecting IUGR, with a sensitivity of 83% and a false-positive rate of 10%. Warsof et al[30] prospectively studied the effectiveness of three ultrasonic growth parameters, BPD, HC, and AC, throughout gestation to determine the optimal gestational age to perform the scan. They found that an AC performed at 34 (± 1) weeks had a higher sensitivity and specificity than the other single parameters in detecting IUGR. The sensitivity and the specificity of the AC was 80% and 84%, respectively, and the predictive value of a positive test approached 50% (Fig. 13–4, Fig. 13–5, and Table 13–2).

The Head Circumference to Abdominal Circumference Ratio (HC/AC)

Since the liver comprises the bulk of the fetal abdomen, it is important to know the relationship in growth between HC and AC throughout gestation. Campbell and Thomas[31] studied the HC to AC ratio between 17 and 41 weeks' gestation. The normal mean ratio was 1.18 at 17 weeks' and 0.96 at 40 weeks' gestation. The HC to AC ratio was also evaluated in 31 growth-retarded fetuses and fell above the 95th percentile in 71% of the fetuses. This indicated that the HC to AC ratio could distinguish asymmetric (type II) (>95th percentile) from symmetric (type I) IUGR fetus as well as from growth within the normal range (Fig. 15–1A, Fig. 15–1B, and Table 15–2).

The Femur Length to Abdominal Circumference Ratio (FL/AC)

Hadlock et al[32] suggested that the FL to AC ratio is independent of gestational age. This ratio was found to be fairly constant, 22 ± 2, after 21 weeks' gestation. This ratio was suggested as an important adjunct in the diagnosis of IUGR. The theory behind the use of the FL to AC ratio was the apparent length-sparing effect frequently observed in growth-retarded neonates. The authors determined that the ratio in 30 cases using the 90th percentile was found to be 23.5, the upper limit of normal, and successfully identified 63% of the growth-retarded fetuses. Ott and coworkers[33] also studied the FL to AC ratio; they did not find a discriminatory value to permit the diagnosis of IUGR.

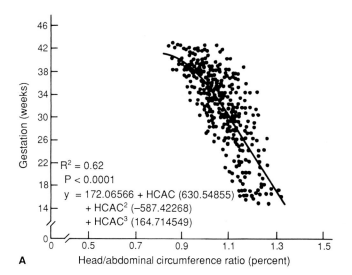

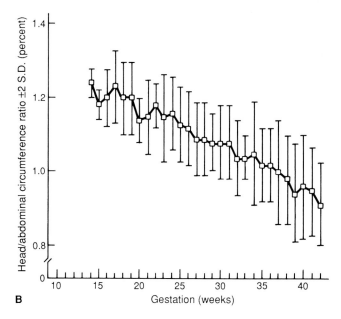

Figure 15–1. (A) Scattergram with a regression line depicting growth of the head to abdominal circumference ratio throughout gestation. **(B)** The mean ± 2 SD of the head to abdominal circumference ratio throughout gestation.

Ponderal Index (PI)

The ponderal index is a body mass measurement for diagnosis in the neonate. This procedure utilizes various morphometric measurements of the newborn. The ponderal index uses soft tissue and muscle mass measurements to describe the relationship between length and weight.

$$\text{Ponderal index} = \text{weight}/\text{length}^3 \times 100 = 2.2 \text{ to } 2.8.$$

The fetal ponderal index was introduced to predict intrauterine growth-retardation.[34] The estimated fetal length and weight were calculated using the fetal FL.[34] The fetal length, weight, and ponderal index were correlated with neonatal length, weight, and ponderal index. The fetal ponderal index was also evaluated as a predictor of IUGR and was found to have a sensitivity, specificity, and negative predictive value of 77%, 82%, and 96.4%, respectively; the positive predictive value, however, was 36%.

Estimated Fetal Weight (EFW)

While the pediatric evaluation of smallness for gestational age (SGA) is based on newborn weights, the estimation of fetal weight is based on the sonographic measurements and nomograms derived from mathematical models. Several investigators used multiple parameters to derive equations for *predicting* fetal weight. For example, the accuracy of the equation of Shepard et al[35] for predicting fetal weight was demonstrated to be within approximately 10% of the actual birth weight 85% of the time. (See Chapter 14 for further details.)

Amniotic Fluid Volume and Doppler Studies

The assessment of amniotic fluid and the Doppler waveform analysis in IUGR fetuses are described in Chapter 19 and Chapter 22.

In summary, the clinical diagnosis of impaired fetal growth can be based on clinical suspicion in cases with maternal high-risk factors, such as hypertension, or on the clinical observation of a uterus that is small for gestational age.

Evaluation of sonographic indices considered helpful in the diagnosis of IUGR relies on fetal weight and its deviation from normal. In addition, the indirect indices of fetal growth, such as systolic/diastolic (S/D) ratio, FL to AC ratio, HC to AC ratio, and qualitative amniotic fluid volume are useful adjuncts to improving diagnostic accuracy.[36]

MANAGEMENT AND OUTCOME

The prognosis for future growth and development for any neonate whose birth weight is below the 10th percentile for gestational age depends on the physiologic significance of the associated cause. Infants who are small for gestational age on a constitutional basis enjoy a good prognosis, although there appears to be an increase in perinatal mortality, even in this group.[14] An infant whose birth weight is below the 10th percentile for gestational age on a deprivational basis should also enjoy a good prognosis if delivery occurs without perinatal asphyxia.

THE GROWTH-ACCELERATED FETUS

Fetal macrosomia is multifactorial in its etiology. Although this condition is often associated with diabetes mellitus in pregnancy, especially in women without vasculopathy, macrosomia may also occur in nondiabetics. Fetal macrosomia is defined either as an estimated fetal weight (EFW) of more than 4,000 g at term or EFW above the 90th percentile for gestational age.

Macrosomic infants and their mothers are at increased risk for intrapartum injury, and perinatal mortality is more common among these fetuses. The principal causes of injury include shoulder dystocia, fractures, and neurologic damage.[37–40]

Prenatal Diagnosis

Accurate prenatal diagnosis of fetal macrosomia allows delivery by cesarean section, thus obviating the complications of macrosomia described above. On the other hand, widespread use of cesarean section may expose the mothers to unnecessary operative risks. Prenatal diagnosis of macrosomic fetuses is often difficult, since less than 40% of these infants are born with identifiable risk factors.[41]

A number of sonographic parameters have been used in an attempt to diagnose altered fetal growth such as the BPD, HC, HC to AC, thigh–calf circumference (Table 15–3), or HC to thoracic circumference ratio, the macrosomic index, and the EFW. Miller et al[42] conducted a study of 382 patients with singleton pregnancies whose infants were born within 1 week of the ultrasound examination. Of the 382 pregnancies, 58 delivered macrosomic infants (>4500 g). Ultrason-

TABLE 15–3. ULTRASOUND FETAL THIGH AND CALF CIRCUMFERENCES FROM 20 WEEKS' GESTATION TO TERM*

Gestational Age (Wk)	Fetal Thigh Circumference (cm)	Fetal Calf Circumference (cm)
20	6.5 ± 1.3	4.9 ± 1.5
21	6.3 ± 0.8	4.5 ± 1.0
22	7.8 ± 1.2	6.0 ± 1.3
23	7.9 ± 1.4	6.0 ± 1.3
24	8.3 ± 1.3	6.5 ± 0.9
25	8.6 ± 1.4	6.6 ± 1.4
26	9.2 ± 1.3	7.1 ± 1.1
27	9.6 ± 1.0	7.5 ± 1.2
28	10.3 ± 1.6	8.1 ± 0.6
29	10.5 ± 1.3	8.2 ± 1.7
30	10.5 ± 1.0	8.4 ± 0.7
31	11.3 ± 1.7	8.9 ± 1.7
32	12.0 ± 2.8	9.7 ± 1.0
33	12.4 ± 1.8	9.6 ± 1.1
34	13.5 ± 2.1	10.5 ± 1.1
35	13.9 ± 2.4	10.6 ± 1.0
36	14.1 ± 2.7	11.1 ± 1.5
37	14.2 ± 2.5	11.0 ± 0.9
38	14.8 ± 2.0	11.7 ± 0.6
39	15.3 ± 2.2	11.8 ± 0.6
40	15.7 ± 1.0	12.1 ± 0.8

* Values are expressed as means ± 2 SD.
From Vintzileos AM, Neckles S, Campbell WA, et al. Ultrasound fetal thigh–calf circumferences and gestational age-independent fetal ratios in normal pregnancy. J Ultrasound Med. 1985;4:287–292, with permission.

ically determined BPD, FL, AC, and EFW were analyzed as to their ability to predict the macrosomic newborn. EFW was superior to BPD or FL in the prenatal diagnosis of fetal macrosomia. Elliott et al[43] calculated a macrosomic index for 70 diabetic pregnancies by subtracting the BPD from the chest diameter. Thirty-three macrosomic infants (weight >4,500 g) were delivered. In this study 20 of 23 (87%) of the infants weighing more than 4,500 g had a chest diameter minus BPD equal to or greater than 1.4 cm. The authors reported four cases of shoulder dystocia among 15 infants with macrosomic indices of over 1.4. They recommended cesarean section for all fetuses with a chest diameter minus BPD equal to or greater than 1.4 cm, since such an approach would decrease the incidence of traumatic morbidity from 27% to 9%.

Tamura et al[44] showed that EFW by Shepard et al,[35] when greater than the 90th percentile, correctly predicted macrosomia at birth in 74% of cases. When both the AC and the EFW exceeded the 90th percentiles, macrosomia was correctly diagnosed in 88.8% of pregnant women with diabetes mellitus. The BPD and HC percentiles were significantly less predictive of macrosomia.

In summary, the prenatal diagnosis of macrosomia is best done by the use of the EFW. Caution ought to be exercised, however, in light of the fact that there is a margin of error with weight estimation via sonography. EFW is reported to be accurate within 10% of the birth weight 85% of the time. In the remaining 15%, EFW is less accurate, and the error can range from 15% to as high as 20% of the actual birth weight.

Management and Outcome

Following prenatal diagnosis of the macrosomic fetus, delivery should be made in the most atraumatic manner. When the estimated fetal weight is about 4,500 g or more, the fetus should be delivered by cesarean section. At an EFW between 4,000 and 4,500 g there is controversy. Some investigators recommend cesarean section, while others advocate a trial of labor. Clinical judgment based on historical facts, past obstetric performance, and the size of the pelvis should assist in the decision on the optimal route of delivery within this weight range. Based on the work of Elliott et al,[43] when the chest diameter minus BPD is more than 1.4 cm, strong consideration should be given to cesarean section delivery, especially when the EFW is greater than 4,000 g.

REFERENCES

1. Lockwood CJ, Weiner S. Assessment of fetal growth. *Clin Perinatol.* 1986;13:3–35.
2. World Health Organization. Public health aspects of low birth weight: third report of Expert Committee on Maternal and Child Health. *WHO Tech Rep Surv.* 1961; 217;3–16.
3. Cunningham FG, MacDoland PC, Gant NF. Preterm and postterm pregnancy and an appropriate fetal growth. In: *Williams Obstetrics Book.* 18th ed. Norwalk, Conn: Appleton & Lange; 1989:764–765.
4. Creasy RK, Resnik R. Intrauterine growth retardation. In: Creasy RK, Resnik R, eds. *Maternal Fetal Medicine.* Philadelphia, Pa: WB Saunders Co; 1984;491–494.
5. Koops BL, Morgan LJ, Battaglia FC. Neonatal mortality risk in relation to birth weight and gestational age: update. *Pediatrics.* 1982;101:969–977.
6. Low JA, Galbraith RS, Muir D, et al. Intrauterine growth retardation: a preliminary report of long term morbidity. *Am J Obstet Gynecol.* 1978;130:534–544.
7. Low JA, Gabraith RS, Muir D, et al. Intrauterine growth retardation: a study of long term morbidity. *Am J Obstet Gynecol.* 1982;142:670–677.
8. Winer EK, Tejani NA, Atluru VL, et al. Four-to-seven-year evaluation in two groups of small-for-gestational age infants. *Am J Obstet Gynecol.* 1982;143:425–429.
9. Starfield B, Shapiro S, McCormick M, et al. Mortality and morbidity in infants with intrauterine growth retardation. *Pediatrics.* 1982;101:978–983.
10. Lubchenco LO, Hansman C, Boyd E. Intrauterine growth in length and head circumference as estimated from live birth at gestational ages from 24 to 42 weeks. *Pediatrics.* 1966;37:403–408.
11. Battaglia FC. Lubchenco LO. A practical classification of newborn infants by weight and gestational age. *J Pediatr.* 1967;71:159.
12. Usher R, MacLean F: Intrauterine growth of liveborn caucasian infants at sea level: standards obtained from measuring 7 dimensions of infants born between 25 and 44 weeks of gestation. *J Pediatr.* 1969;74:901–910.
13. Winick M. Cellular changes during placental and fetal growth. *Am J Obstet Gynecol.* 1971;109:166–176.
14. Seeds JW. Impaired fetal growth: definition and clinical diagnosis. *Obstet Gynecol.* 1984;64:303–310.
15. Belizan JM, Villar J, Nardin JC, et al. Diagnosis of intrauterine growth retardation by a simple clinical method: measurement of uterine height. *Am J Obstet Gynecol.* 1978;131:643–646.
16. Campbell S. The assessment of fetal development of diagnostic ultrasound. *Clin Perinatol.* 1974;1:507–525.
17. Deter RL, Harrist RB, Hadlock FP, et al. The use of ultrasound in the detection of intrauterine growth retardation: a review. *J Clin Ultrasound.* 1982;10:9–16.
18. Wittmann BK, Robinson HP, Aitchison T, et al. The value of diagnostic ultrasound as a screening test for intrauterine growth retardation: comparison of 9 parameters. *Am J Obstet Gynecol.* 1979;134:30–35.
19. Queenan JT, Kubarych SF, Cook LN, et al. Diagnostic ultrasound for detection of intrauterine growth retardation. *Am J Obstet Gynecol.* 1976;124:865–873.
20. Sholl JS, Woo D, Rubin JM, et al. Intrauterine growth retardation risk detection for fetuses of unknown gestational age. *Am J Obstet Gynecol.* 1982;144:709–714.
21. Whethand JCG, Muggah H, Davis S. Assessment of in-

trauterine growth retardation by diagnostic ultrasound. *Am J Obstet Gynecol.* 1976;125:577–600.

22. Persson PH, Grennert L, Gennser G. Diagnosis of intrauterine growth retardation by serial ultrasonic cephalometry. *Acta Obstet Gynaecol Scand.* [suppl] 1978;78:40–48.

23. Hadlock FP, Deter RL, Carpenter RJ, et al. Estimating fetal age: effect of head shape on BPD. *AJR.* 1981;137:83–85.

24. Goldstein I, Reece EA, Pilu G, et al. Cerebellar measurements with ultrasonography in the evaluation of fetal growth and development. *Am J Obstet Gynecol.* 1987;156:1065–1069.

25. Reece EA, Goldstein I, Pilu G, et al. Fetal cerebellar growth unaffected by intrauterine growth retardation: a new parameter for prenatal diagnosis. *Am J Obstet Gynecol.* 1987;157:632–638.

26. Duchatel F, Mennesson B, Berseneff H, et al. Antenatal echographic measurement of the fetal cerebellum: significance in the evaluation of fetal development. *J Gynecol Obstet Biol Reprod.* 1989;18:879–883.

27. Campbell WA, Nardi D, Vintzileos AM, et al. Transverse cerebellar diameter/abdominal circumference ratio throughout pregnancy: a gestational age-independent method to assess fetal growth. *Obstet Gynecol.* 1991;77:893–896.

28. Hill LM, Guzick D, Fries J, et al. The transverse cerebellar diameter cannot be used to assess gestational age in the small for gestational age fetus. *Obstet Gynecol.* 1990;75:981–985.

29. Evans MI, Mukherjee AB, Schulman JD. Animal models of intrauterine growth retardation. *Obstet Gynecol Surv.* 1983;38:183–192.

30. Warsof SL, Cooper DJ, Little D. Routine ultrasound screening for antenatal detection of intrauterine growth retardation. *Obstet Gynecol.* 1986;67:33–39.

31. Campbell S, Thomas A. Ultrasound measurement of the fetal head to abdomen circumference ratio in the assessment of growth retardation. *Br J Obstet Gynaecol.* 1977;114:165–174.

32. Hadlock FP, Deter RL, Harrist RB, et al. A date-independent predictor of intrauterine growth retardation. *AJR.* 1983;141:979–983.

33. Ott WJ. Defining altered fetal growth by second trimester sonography. *Obstet Gynecol.* 1990;75:1053–1059.

34. Vintzileos AM, Loderio JG, Feinstein SJ, et al. Value of fetal ponderal index in predicting growth retardation *Obstet Gynecol.* 1986;67:584–588.

35. Shepard MJ, Richards VA, Berkowitz RL, et al. An evaluation of two equations for predicting fetal weight by ultrasound. *Am J Obstet Gynecol.* 1982;142:47–54.

36. Divon MY, Guidetti DA, Braverman JJ, et al. Intrauterine growth retardation: a prospective study of the diagnostic value of real-time sonography combined with umbilical artery flow velocity. *Obstet Gynecol.* 1988;72:611–614.

37. Sack RA. The large infant: a study of maternal, obstetric, fetal and newborn characteristics, including a long-term pediatric follow-up. *Am J Obstet Gynecol.* 1969;104:195–204.

38. Nelson JH, Rovner IW, Barter RH. The large baby. *South Med J.* 1958;51:23–25.

39. Posner AC, Friedman S, Posner LB. The large fetus: A study of 547 cases. *Obstet Gynecol.* 1955;5:268–278.

40. Parks DG, Ziel HK. Macrosomia: a proposed indication for primary cesarean section. *Obstet Gynecol.* 1978;52:407–409.

41. Boyd ME, Usher RH, McLean FH. Fetal macrosomia: prediction, risks, proposed management. *Obstet Gynecol.* 1983;61:715–722.

42. Miller JM, Brown HL, Khawli OF, et al. Ultrasonographic identification of the macrosomic fetus. *Am J Obstet Gynecol.* 1988; 159:1110–1114.

43. Elliott JP, Garite TJ, Freeman RK, et al. Ultrasonic prediction of fetal macrosomia in diabetic patients. *Obstet Gynecol.* 1982; 60:159–162.

44. Tamura RK, Sabbagha RE, Depp R, et al. Diabetic macrosomia: accuracy of third trimester ultrasound. *Obstet Gynecol.* 1986; 67:828–832.

16

Fetal Organ Maturity

INTRODUCTION

The use of ultrasonography in obstetrics has significantly improved the ability to estimate fetal age and weight. The accuracy of fetal biometry for predicting gestational age in the first trimester is within 3 to 5 days, and between 12 and 18 weeks' gestation, the error is approximately 7 days.[1] There is an inverse relationship between the accuracy of fetal age estimation and the advancement of the pregnancy, such that accurate sonographic estimation of age is precluded in the third trimester.

An alternative method for evaluating gestational age is via the maturity indices of fetal organs reflected by changes in their tissue characterization during pregnancy. Since these changes are a function of biologic growth and aging, they have become useful parameters to assess fetal age. These nonbiometric parameters include:

1. Heel ossification center
2. Distal femoral epiphyseal ossification center and proximal tibial epiphyseal ossification center
3. Proximal humeral ossification center
4. Echogenicity of fetal lung
5. Intestinal grading
6. Placental grading

EMBRYOLOGY

Epiphysis

Ossification begins in the long bones by the end of the embryonic period. It initially occurs in the diaphyses of the long bones, from the primary center of ossification. By 12 weeks' gestation primary centers have appeared in nearly all bones of the limbs. The secondary ossification centers of the bones at the heel and the knee are the first to appear. The part of bone ossified from the secondary center is called the epiphysis. The development of irregular bones is similar to that of the primary center of long bones, and only one, the calcaneus in the heel, develops a secondary center of ossification.[2]

Meconium

Meconium first accumulates in the small bowel at 13 to 14 weeks' gestation, after which the distal segment of the small intestine begins to fill with meconium.[3] The anal sphincter becomes patent at 22 weeks' gestation in the normal fetus, and thus meconium begins to accumulate and remain in the gastrointestinal tract; otherwise, there is fetal distress. By birth, the entire colon is filled with 69 to 200 mL of meconium.[4]

Small Intestine

Auerbach's plexus, found in the small intestine, develops at 9 weeks of gestation, and Meissner's plexus develops at 13 weeks.[3]

Haustra

The colonic haustral clefts have been documented histologically in 10-week abortuses.[5]

Placenta

It is not until the sixth to seventh week of pregnancy that the placenta and its margins can be clearly delineated. At the end of the first trimester, the chorionic plate, the substance of the placenta, and the basal areas can be identified.[1]

SONOANATOMY

Epiphysis

Calcaneus and talus. The fetal heel ossification centers have a characteristic pattern of growth and development throughout gestation. The calcaneus and the talus ossification centers can be identified sonographically by visualizing the tibia (or fibula) at its distal end, then locating the echogenic structures in the fetal heel (Fig. 16–1).[6]

Distal femoral and proximal tibial ossification centers. The distal femoral and proximal tibial epiphyseal ossification centers have a characteristic appear-

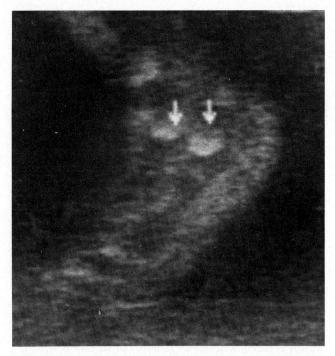

Figure 16–1. Echogenic structures in fetal heel representing ossification centers (arrows).

ance, growth, and development in the normal fetus throughout gestation.[7]

The distal femoral epiphysis is identified by visualizing the femur at its distal end and locating the echogenic epiphyseal structure near the distal end. Similarly, the proximal tibial epiphysis is identified by visualizing the proximal tibia and locating the echogenic epiphyseal structure adjacent to the head of the tibia. Measurements are obtained from the outer-to-outer margins in an axial (anteroposterior to the maternal abdomen) plane along the medio–lateral surfaces of the epiphyses (Fig. 16–2).

Lung and Liver Echogenicity

Studies have attempted the sonographic characterization of fetal lung development by assessing differences between lung and liver echogenicity.[8] The fetal lung will always appear more echogenic than the liver; it is depicted as a triangular-shaped structure (Fig. 16–3 and Fig. 16–4).[8]

Colon

Colonic echogenicity changes during gestation. The intraluminal changes in echogenicity appear to reflect the progressive increase in volume of meconium and decrease in water content in the fetal colon over the course of the pregnancy. The echogenicity of the colon was assessed and graded[9] in comparison with the echogenicity of the bladder, stomach, and liver. This grading system is shown below:

Grade 0: The abdomen is uniform in appearance, and the colon is not identified.
Grade 1: The colonic contents have an echo-free appearance. This is essentially identical to that of the bladder and the stomach; the colonic haustra can be identified.
Grade 2: Intermediate. The colon appears more echo-dense than the bladder but less than the liver.
Grade 3: The colonic contents have an echogenicity essentially equal to that of the liver (Fig. 9–5, Fig. 9–6, Fig. 9–7, and Fig. 9–8).

Small-Intestinal Peristalsis

Early peristalsis is characterized by a sporadic and fleeting movement, with a duration of less than 3 seconds. Later peristaltic waves are more vigorous, ubiquitous, and of longer duration. The nature of small-intestinal peristalsis was also graded[9] and shown below.

Grade 0: Small-intestinal peristalsis is absent.
Grade 1: Few sporadic waves of small-intestinal peristalsis in up to three discrete areas, present for short durations of less than 3 seconds.
Grade 2: Moderate waves of small-intestinal peristalsis in more than three discrete areas, present for a longer duration (more than 3 seconds).
Grade 3: Active waves of small-intestinal peristalsis are seen throughout the observation interval.

Semiquantitative evaluation of the small-intestinal peristalsis was compared with fetal gestational age.

Figure 16–2. Ultrasound of fetal femur bone with separate echogenic structure at distal end (arrows). This structure represents the distal femoral epiphysis (DFE).

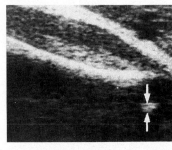
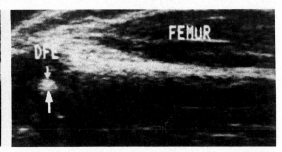

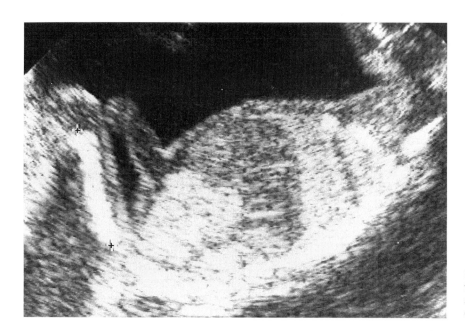

Figure 16–3. Sagittal view of ultrasound of fetus demonstrating echogenic triangular-shaped structure in the fetal chest representing the lung. Calipers(+'s) identify the femur.

Placenta

Many factors are thought to be associated with the maturation of the placenta. Since calcium has been noted in both the decidua and villi of normal-term placentas, it is reasonable to postulate that calcium and fibrous depositions are responsible for the characteristic appearance of the placenta. Grannum et al[10] developed a grading system based on this concept of placental maturation with the goal of predicting lung maturation. This system has not proven to be clinically useful, however.

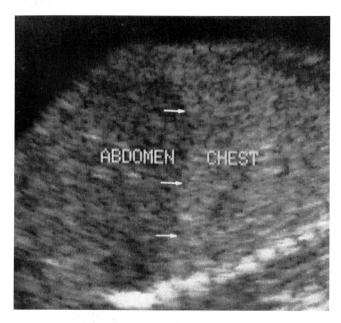

Figure 16–4. Sagittal view of ultrasound of fetus demonstrating the difference in echogenicity between abdomen (liver) and chest (lung). Arrows demarcate the diaphragm.

CLINICAL APPLICATION

Epiphysis

Heel Ossification Centers. The calcaneus ossification center can be sonographically visualized as early as 14 weeks' gestation in 25% of the cases, 18 weeks' in 80%, and 19 weeks' in 100% of the cases. The talus ossification center was identified as early as 17 weeks' gestation in 16% of the cases, and in 90% at 22 weeks' gestation.

The presence or absence of the calcaneus discriminates between gestations of less than 18 weeks and those of 18 weeks or more. Similarly, the presence or absence of the talus can distinguish between gestations of less than 22 weeks and those of 22 weeks' or more (Table 16–1).[6]

TABLE 16–1. PRESENCE AND ABSENCE OF CALCANEUS AND TALUS OSSIFICATION CENTERS OF THE FETAL HEEL

Gestational Age (wk)	Calcaneus		Talus	
	Absent (%)	*Present (%)*	*Absent (%)*	*Present (%)*
14	75	25	100	0
15	57	43	100	0
16	26	74	84	16
17	22	78	78	22
18	20	80	60	40
19	0	100	60	40
20	0	100	55	45
21	0	100	50	50
22	0	100	11	89

From Goldstein I, Reece EA, Hobbins JC. The sonographic appearance of the heel ossification centers and foot length measurements provide independent markers for gestational age estimation. Am J Obstet Gynecol. 1988; 159:923–926, with permission.

Knee Ossification Centers. The distal femoral epiphysis is not visualized before 28 weeks' gestation, but it is observed in 94% of fetuses at 34 weeks' gestation. If the distal femoral epiphysis measures 1 or 2 mm in an axial plane, the gestational age is usually greater than 33 weeks in 87% of fetuses. Moreover, a distal femoral epiphysis measuring 3 mm or more is associated with a gestational age of greater than 37 weeks in 84% of fetuses (Fig. 16–2). The absence or presence of the distal femoral epiphysis discriminates between gestations of less than or greater than 32 weeks with high sensitivity and specificity (Fig. 16–5 and Table 16–2).

The proximal tibial epiphysis is not visualized before 34 weeks' gestation, but it is observed in 35% of fetuses at 35 weeks, 80% at 37 weeks, and 100% of fetuses at 39 weeks of gestation. Figure 16–6 shows the distribution of proximal tibial epiphysis at each gestational age. If the proximal tibial epiphysis measures 1 to 2 mm, the gestational age is usually greater than 37 weeks in 77% of fetuses. A proximal tibial epiphysis equal to or greater than 3 mm is associated with a gestational age of more than 38 weeks in 94% of fetuses. The absence or presence of proximal tibial epiphysis discriminates between a gestational age of less than or greater than 34 weeks with good sensitivity and specificity (Table 16–3).

Characterization of the distal femoral and proximal tibial ossification centers in normal fetuses can improve the estimation of gestational age during the third trimester. The distal femoral epiphysis discriminates between gestational age of less than or greater than 32 weeks.

The distal femoral and proximal tibial ossification centers can also assist in predicting pulmonic maturity. In uncomplicated pregnancies the combination of a distal femoral epiphysis equal to or greater than 3 mm, and the presence of proximal tibial epiphyses was highly correlated with a lecithin to sphingomyelin (L/S) ratio equal to or greater than 2, with positive

TABLE 16–2. SPECIFICITY, SENSITIVITY, AND p VALUE FROM χ^2 TEST FOR DISTAL FEMORAL EPIPHYSIS

Gestational Age (wk) (Measurement of Distal Femoral Epiphysis)	SN (%)	SP (%)	PPV (%)	NPV (%)
< 32/>33 Absent/present	94	93	81	98
< 34/>35 Absent/1 or 2 mm	100	81	65	100
< 36/>37 1 or 2 mm/≥3 mm	70	85	81	75

SN = sensitivity; SP = specificity; PPV = positive predictive value; NPV = negative predictive value.
p < 0.0001.
From Goldstein I, Lockwood C, Balanger K, et al. Ultrasonographic assessment of gestational age with the distal femoral and proximal tibial ossification centers in the third trimester. Am J Obstet Gynecol. 1988; 158:127–130, with permission.

predictive value of close to 100% in the nondiabetic patient.[11]

Colon

The intracolonic echogenicity throughout pregnancy may predict gestational age.[9] Grade 0 is present in 82% of fetuses with a gestational age of less than 29 weeks; Grade 3 is present in 85% of fetuses greater than 39 weeks' gestation (Table 16–4).

Small-Intestinal Peristalsis

Intestinal peristalsis can be visualized sonographically at 18 weeks' gestation. Grade 1 is observed in 88% of fetuses before 29 weeks' gestation and grade 3 in 80% of fetuses between 37 and 38 weeks' gestation (Table 16–5).[9]

Haustra

The colonic haustra can be visualized sonographically at 30 weeks' gestation, providing an independent

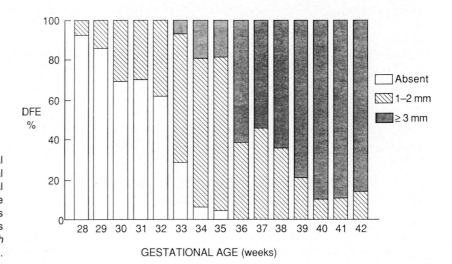

Figure 16–5. Bar graph demonstrating the normal distribution of the ossification centers during fetal development. The distribution of the distal femoral epiphysis (DFE) is shown. The blank areas of the bar graph represent absent DFE; the hatched areas represent DFE at 1 to 2 mm; and the black areas represent DFE at 3 mm or more. (*Reproduced with permission from* J Matern-Fet Med. *2;152:1993*).

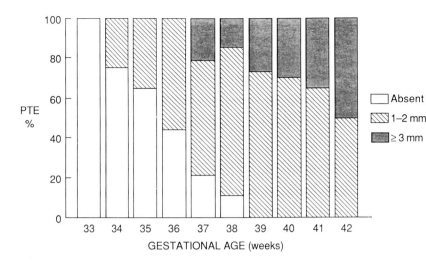

Figure 16–6. Bar graph demonstrating the normal distribution in the development of the proximal tibial epiphysis (PTE). The blank areas represent absence of PTE; the hatched areas represent PTE of 1 to 2 mm; and the black areas represent PTE of 3 mm or more. (*Reproduced with permission from* J Matern-Fet Med. *2;152:1993*).

marker for gestational age greater than or less than 30 weeks.

Lung versus Liver Echogenicity

The echogenicity of the fetal lung in relation to the echogenicity to the fetal liver throughout gestation was thought to be a promising technique for predicting gestational age.[8,12–15] This technique, however, is insensitive, and the interpretation of relative echogenicity of the lung compared with the liver is qualitative and not reproducible. Most institutions do not use this technique.

Placenta

The distribution of placental grades in normal pregnancies at term is: grade 1: 45%, grade 2: 55%, and grade 3: 5% to 10%.[16] There seems to be no meaningful correlation between placental grades and biparietal diameters (BPD). Examination of the placental maturation at or after 42 weeks' gestation shows: grade 2:

55%; grade 3: 45%. It is unusual, however, to find a grade 1 placenta at 42 weeks' gestation.

Correlation between placental grading and fetal pulmonic maturity is controversial. Grannum et al[10] reported that during the last 4 weeks of pregnancy in normal patients, 68% of those with grade 1 placenta have a positive L/S ratio, while 88% of those with grade 2, and 100% of those with grade 3 have positive L/S ratios. Harman et al[17] found an L/S ratio equal to or greater than 2 correlated with grade 3 placentas in 93% of cases; the false-positive rate was 7%. Quinlan and coworkers,[18] however, reported that grade 3 placenta occurred in only 7% of fetuses with pulmonic maturity, and that it falsely predicted fetal pulmonic maturity in 42% of pregnancies in which grade 3 placental changes were found. Kazzi et al[19] reported that placental grading may be affected by pregnancy complications; for example, chronic hypertension seems to accelerate maturation, while diabetes and isoimmunization seem to retard maturation.

POSTDATISM

Postdate pregnancy is defined as pregnancy that has exceeded 42 weeks or 294 days, documented from the

TABLE 16–3. SPECIFICITY, SENSITIVITY, AND p VALUE FROM χ^2 TEST FOR PROXIMAL TIBIAL EPIPHYSIS

Gestational Age (wk) (Measurement of Distal Femoral Epiphysis)	SN (%)	SP (%)	PPV (%)	NPV (%)
< 34/>35 Absent/present	95	82	96	79
< 36/>37 Absent/1 or 2 mm	85	92	77	95
< 37/>38 1 or 2 mm/≥ 3 mm	96	29	94	40

SN = sensitivity; SP = specificity; PPV = positive predictive value; NPV = negative predictive value.
p < 0.0001.
From Goldstein I, Lockwood C, Balanger K, et al. Ultrasonographic assessment of gestational age with the distal femoral and proximal tibial ossification centers in the third trimester. Am J Obstet Gynecol. 1988; 158:127–130, with permission.

TABLE 16–4. SEMIQUANTITATIVE EVALUATION OF COLONIC ECHOGENICITY: GRADES ACROSS GESTATIONAL AGE AND PERCENT OF CASES WITH A GIVEN GRADE

Gestational Age (wk)	Grade 0 (%)	Grade 1 (%)	Grade 2 (%)	Grade 3 (%)
<29	82.6	17.4	0	0
29–30	7.7	84.6	7.7	0
31–32	5.5	77.8	16.7	0
33–34	0	72.7	27.3	0
35–36	0	31.0	41.4	27.6
37–38	0	3.3	36.7	60.0
≥39	0	0	14.9	85.1

From Goldstein I, Lockwood C, Hobbins JC. Ultrasound assessment of fetal intestinal development in the evaluation of gestational age. Obstet Gynecol. 1987; 70:682, with permission.

TABLE 16–5. SEMIQUANTITATIVE EVALUATION OF THE SMALL-INTESTINAL PERISTALSIS: PERCENT OF CASES WITH A GIVEN GRADE ACROSS GESTATIONAL AGE

Gestational Age (wk)	Grade 0 (%)	Grade 1 (%)	Grade 2 (%)	Grade 3 (%)
<29	8.0	88.0	4.0	0
29–30	0	57.1	42.9	0
31–32	0	12.5	75.0	12.5
33–34	0	12.5	81.3	6.3
35–36	0	9.0	22.7	68.2
37–38	0	0	20.0	80.0
≥39	0	0	0	100.0

From Goldstein I, Lockwood C, Hobbins JC. Ultrasound assessment of fetal intestinal development in the evaluation of gestational age. Obstet Gynecol. 1987; 70:682, with permission.

onset of the last menstrual period. Postmaturity is a fetal condition due to uteroplacental insufficiency with consequent deprivation of nutrients.[20] Approximately 3.5% to 12% of pregnancies will complete 42 weeks of amenorrhea, and 1% to 4% of all pregnancies will complete 43 weeks.[21]

While fetal mortality in cases of postdate pregnancy has been significantly reduced, the associated morbidity continues to affect both neonates and mothers. Researchers[22] found that the incidence of cesarean section rose from 13.6% of term pregnancies to 25.6% of those in the postterm group. There were 10.2% of term infants compared with 25.2% of postterm infants weighing more than 4,000 g. Intrapartum fetal distress requiring cesarean section increased from 1% to 3.5% in postterm pregnancies.[23]

The infant with postmaturity syndrome is at increased risk of morbidity and mortality.[22] The undernourished neonate may show temperature instability and neurologic damage. These fetuses tolerate labor poorly in severe cases.

While 80% of postterm infants will not develop postmaturity syndrome, problems may still occur. The chance for long-term neurologic damage also rises with gestational age, and it is the most costly of all morbidity.[21] Meconium-stained amniotic fluid occurs twice as often in postdate pregnancies than in term pregnancies (25% vs 12%).[22]

Several investigators have evaluated the usefulness of ultrasound assessment of placental maturation and amniotic fluid volume in the management of postterm pregnancy.[24–26] When there is oligohydramnios, there is a greater risk for advanced signs of postmaturity compared to pregnancies with normal amounts of amniotic fluid. A significant decrease in the amount of amniotic fluid may thus suggest the presence of postmaturity in the fetus. Ultrasound findings of advanced placental maturation, grade 3 placenta, and decreased amniotic fluid may indicate a state of placental dysfunction associated with a decrease in the transfer of nutrients to the fetus.[24]

CLINICAL APPLICATION

Investigators[27] determined a sonographic model for evaluating the term fetus based on the above parameters. The presence of a proximal humeral epiphysis of 1 mm or greater, carries at least a 69% probability of a fetus being 40 to 42 weeks' gestation, independent of colonic grade (Fig. 16–7). Similarly, a colonic grade of 3 predicts a gestational age of 40 to 42 weeks with a probability of >0.67. If the above-mentioned parameters were present simultaneously, there would be a 95% probability of the gestation being 40 to 42 weeks.

It remains unsolved how to differentiate prospectively the term and postdate fetus presenting late with unknown or uncertain date of LMP.

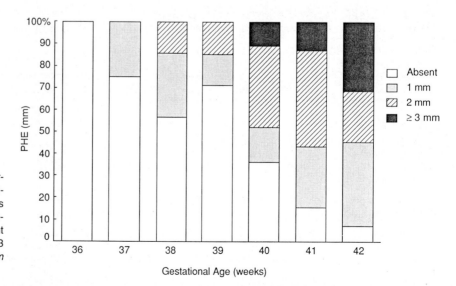

Figure 16–7. Bar graph demonstrating the normal distribution in the development of the proximal humeral epiphysis (PHE). The blank areas represent absence of PTE; the gray areas represent PTE of 1 mm; the hatched areas represent PTE of 2 mm; the black areas represent PTE of 3 mm or more. (*Reproduced with permission from J Matern-Fet Med. 2;152:1993*).

REFERENCES

1. Reece EA, Gabrielli S, Degennaro N, et al. Dating through pregnancy: a measure of growing up. *Obstet Gynecol Surv.* 1989;44:544–554.

2. Moore KL. The articular and skeletal system. In: *The Developing Human: Clinically Oriented Embryology.* 3rd ed. Philadelphia, Pa: WB Saunders Co; 1982:281–294.

3. Grand RJ, Watkins JB, Tori FA. Development of human gastrointestinal tract. *Gastroenterology.* 1976;70:790–810.

4. Arey LB. *Developmental Anatomy.* Philadelphia, Pa: WB Saunders Co; 1974:249–255.

5. Pace JL. The age of appearance of the haustra of the human colon. *J Anat.* 1971;109:75–85.

6. Goldstein I, Reece EA, Hobbins JC. The sonographic appearance of the heel ossification centers and foot length measurements provide independent markers for gestational age estimation. *Am J Obstet Gynecol.* 1988;159:923–926.

7. Goldstein I, Lockwood C, Balanger K, et al. Ultrasonographic assessment of gestational age with the distal femoral and proximal tibial ossification centers in the third trimester. *Am J Obstet Gynecol.* 1988;158:127–130.

8. Fried AM, Loh FK, Umer MA, et al. Echogenicity of fetal lung: relation to fetal age and maturity. *AJR.* 1985;145:591–594.

9. Goldstein I, Lockwood C, Hobbins JC. Ultrasound assessment of fetal intestinal development in the evaluation of gestational age. *Obstet Gynecol.* 1987;70:682–686.

10. Grannum PA, Berkowitz RL, Hobbins JC. The ultrasonic changes in the maturing placenta and their relation to fetal pulmonic maturity. *Am J Obstet Gynecol.* 1979;133:915–922.

11. Goldstein I, Lockwood CJ, Reece EA, et al. Sonographic assessment of the distal femoral and proximal tibial ossification centers in the prediction of pulmonic maturity in normal woman and woman with diabetes. *Am J Obstet Gynecol.* 1988;159:72–76.

12. Benson DM, Waldroup LD, Kurtz AB, et al. Ultrasonic tissue characterization of fetal lung, liver and placenta for purpose of assessing fetal maturity. *J Ultrasound Med.* 1983;2:489–494.

13. Carson PL, Meyer CR, Bowerman RA. Prediction of fetal lung maturity with ultrasound. *Radiology.* 1985;155:533.

14. Cayea PD, Grant DC, Doubilet PM, et al. Prediction of fetal lung maturity: inaccuracy of study using conventional ultrasound instrument. *Radiology.* 1985;155:473–475.

15. Birnholz C, Farrell EE. Fetal lung development: compressibility as a measure of maturity. *Radiology.* 1985;157:495–498.

16. Grannum PA, Hobbins JC. The placenta. *Radiol Clin North Am.* 1982;20:353–365.

17. Harman CR, Manning FA, Stearns E, et al. The correlation of ultrasonic placental grading and fetal pulmonary maturation in five hundred sixty-three pregnancies. *Am J Obstet Gynecol.* 1982;143:941–943.

18. Quinlan RW, Cruz A, Buhi W, et al. Changes in placental ultrasonic appearance, I: incidence of Grade III changes in placenta in correlation of fetal pulmonary maturity. *Am J Obstet Gynecol.* 1982;144:468–473.

19. Kazzi GM, Gross TL, Rosen, et al. The relationship of placental grade, fetal lung maturity, and neonatal outcome in normal and complicated pregnancies. *Am J Obstet Gynecol.* 1984;148:54–58.

20. Lagrew DC, Freeman RK. Management of postdate pregnancy. *Am J Obstet Gynecol.* 1986;154:8–13.

21. Vorherr H. Placental insufficiency in relation to postterm pregnancy and fetal postmaturity. *Am J Obstet Gynecol.* 1975;123:67–101.

22. Callenebach JC, Hall RT. Morbidity and mortality of advanced gestational age: post-term or post-mature. *Obstet Gynecol.* 1979;53:721–724.

23. Sachs BP, Friedman EA. Results of an epidemiologic study of postdate pregnancy. *J Reprod Med.* 1986;31:162–166.

24. Moya F, Grannum PA, Pinto K, et al. Ultrasound assessment of post-mature pregnancy. *Obstet Gynecol.* 1985;65:319–322.

25. Rayburn W, Motley M, Stempel L, et al. Antepartum prediction of the post-mature infants. *Obstet Gynecol.* 1982;60:148–151.

26. Crowley P. Nonquantitative estimation of amniotic fluid volume in suspected prolonged pregnancy. *J Perinatol.* 1980;8:249.

27. Goldstein I, Reece EA, O'Connor T, et al. Estimating gestational age in the term pregnancy with a model based on multiple indices of fetal maturity. *Am J Obstet Gynecol.* 1989;161:1235–1238.

17

The Umbilical Cord

EMBRYOLOGY

The umbilical vessels of the 2.9-mm embryo enter the body stalk and unite to form a plexus intimately associated with the allantois. The body stalk has a single umbilical vein that approaches the embryo. The right and left umbilical arteries of the 3.4-mm embryo also unite to form a single vessel on entering the body and do not divide until they reach the chorion. Then it travels with a single umbilical vein arising from vessels in the chorion. The latter pattern persists and is seen in the 4- and 5-month fetus.[1]

SONOANATOMY

The umbilical cord usually contains two arteries and one vein surrounded by mucoid connective tissue, often called Wharton's jelly (Fig. 17–1 and Fig. 17–2).

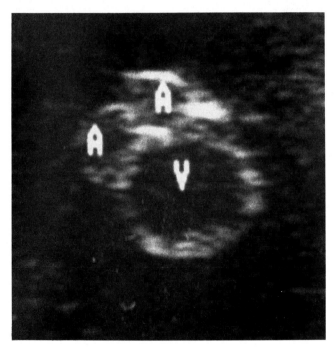

Figure 17–2. Cross-sectional scan of a normal umbilical cord showing the two arteries (A) and the single vein (V), which is larger and is thin walled.

Because the umbilical vessels are longer than the cord, twisting and bending of the vessels are common.

The umbilical cord is usually 1 to 2 cm in diameter and 30 to 60 cm in length. On one side it inserts into the fetal anterior abdominal wall, and on the other side it inserts into the placenta (Fig. 17–3 and Fig. 3–2).

SINGLE UMBILICAL ARTERY

The incidence of a single umbilical artery is 0.72% of single live births,[2] and 2.4% in twins. The ratio between female and male is 1.4 to 1.

Etiology

A single umbilical artery may result from aplasia, or atrophy of the missing vessel. It is also possible that it can be due to persistence of the normally transient

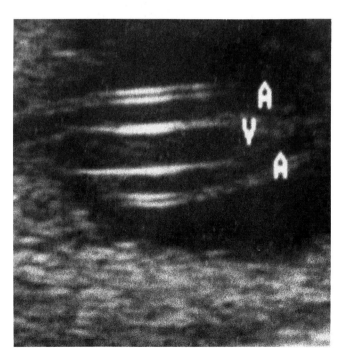

Figure 17–1. Longitudinal scan of a normal umbilical cord demonstrating the two arteries (A) on either side of the vein (V).

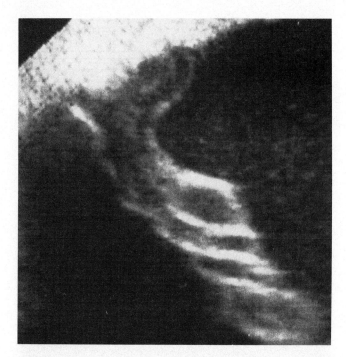

Figure 17–3. Ultrasound scan of the umbilical cord as it inserts into the placenta. Note the tortuous nature of the arteries wrapping around the vein.

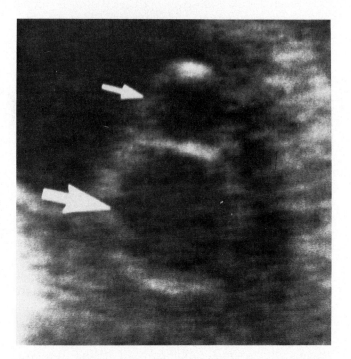

Figure 17–4. Ultrasound picture of a cross section of the umbilical cord demonstrating a single umbilical artery (small arrow). The large vessel (large arrow) represents the umbilical vein.

single umbilical artery of early development in association with degeneration of the truncal portion of either the right or the left umbilical artery.[1] This might explain why, when a single umbilical artery occurs, traces of the absent artery are seldom found in the cord. It has been suggested that a single umbilical artery results in hypoxia that leads to embryonic abnormality (Fig. 17–4).

Clinical Application

The occurrence of a single umbilical artery is associated with an 18% incidence of other malformations in infants, in the largest series, the figure ranges from 15% to 48%. These malformations may occur in all parts of the body, and at multiple sites. The organ systems most often involved are the gastrointes-

tinal, skeletal, cardiovascular, and central nervous system.[2–4]

REFERENCES

1. Moore KL. The circulatory system: The cardiovascular and lymphatic systems. In: Moore KL, ed. *The Developing Human: Clinically Oriented Embryology,* 3rd ed. Philadelphia, Pa: WB Saunders Co.; 1982:298–303.
2. Bryan EM, Kohler HG. The missing umbilical artery. I. Prospective study based on a maternity unit. *Arch Dis Child.* 1974;49:844–852.
3. Harris RJ, Van Leeuwen G. Single umbilical artery. *J Pediatr.* 1968;72:98–99.
4. Byrne J, Blanc WA. Malformations and chromosome anomalies in spontaneously aborted fetuses with single umbilical artery. *Am J Obstet Gynecol.* 1985;151:340–342.

18

The Placenta

Significant advances in our understanding of the placenta have occurred in the last decade. These advances result from our ability to visualize the placenta throughout pregnancy with ultrasound. Studies of placental sonography with clinical applications are summarized here.

EMBRYOLOGY

The decidua, or endometrium of the pregnancy, is divided into three regions according to their relationship to the implantation site.[1] The region underlying the conceptus and forming the maternal component of the placenta is the decidua basalis; the portion overlying the conceptus is the decidua capsularis; and the remaining decidua is called the decidua parietalis.[1]

By the fourth week of pregnancy, the arrangements necessary for physiologic exchanges between the mother and the embryo are established. The maternal component of the placenta is formed by the decidua basalis. This comprises all the endometrium beneath the fetal component of the placenta except the deepest part, which is often called the decidual plate. The fetal component of the placenta consists of the chorionic plate and the chorionic villi that arise from it and project into the intervillous spaces. The intervillous spaces form a large blood sinus, which is bounded by the chorionic plate and decidua basalis.[1]

SONOANATOMY

The earliest sonographic sign of pregnancy is thickening and increased echogenicity of the uterine endometrium (decidua), which occurs in the third to fourth weeks of gestation.[2] By the fourth[3] to fifth[4] weeks of gestation one can demonstrate sonographically the early gestational sac within the uterus, which is surrounded by a prominent echogenic decidual reaction. The placenta, which will form at the site of interaction of the decidua basalis of the uterus and the chorionic villi of the fetus, is not seen until 8 to 10 weeks' ges-

tation.[2] At this time, the site of placental development can usually be identified as an area of relatively increased thickness and echogenicity in the decidual change surrounding the gestational sac. The chorionic plate is formed by fusion of the amnionic and chorionic mesoderms at approximately 12 weeks of gestation. The chorionic plate usually produces a strong acoustic interface between the amniotic cavity and the fetal surface of the placenta.[2]

During the early second trimester the normal placenta maintains a fine granular echogenic pattern with a smooth well-defined chorionic plate after approximately 20 weeks' gestation; gradual changes in the sonographic appearance of a normal placenta may occur, however.[5,6] These changes may include undulation in the chorionic plate, calcification and separation within the placental substance, development of sonolucent areas beneath the chorionic plate and in the placental parenchyma, and development of large draining venous sinuses in the myometrium at the base of the placenta. Grannum et al[6] described a classification of the placenta according to the degree to which these changes occur. Grannum's classification is: (Fig. 18–1).

Grade 0: All placentas start with this morphologic configuration. The chorionic plate is smooth. The placental substance is completely homogeneous. The basal layer is devoid of echogenic densities.

Grade I: The chorionic plate assumes subtle undulations. The placental substance shows randomly dispersed echogenic densities, which are linear, measure 2 to 4 mm in length, and have their long axis parallel to the long axis of the placenta. The basal layer remains devoid of densities.

Grade II: The chorionic plate becomes more markedly indented. There may be extensions, commalike densities, from the chorionic plate into the placental substance, but not extending all the way to the basal layer. The placental substance maintains the randomly dispersed echogenic densities, although the latter may become more prominent. The basal layer shows basal echogenic densities that represent the hallmark of the grade II pla-

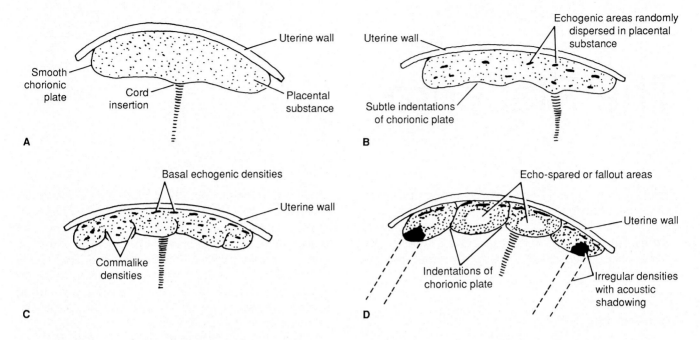

Figure 18–1. Diagrams showing the ultrasonic appearance of the placenta. **(A)** Grade 0, **(B)** grade I, **(C)** grade II, and **(D)** grade III.

centa. These are linear, and their long axis is parallel to the long axis of the placenta.

Grade III: The chorionic plate may be markedly indented. The extensions from the chorionic plate reach all the way to the basal layer, dividing the placenta into compartments, the fetal cotyledons. At least two complete extensions from the chorionic plate to the basal layer should be present to constitute a grade III placenta. The substance of the placenta can have sonolucent "fallout" areas, which probably represent the central portions of the cotyledons devoid of villi. The basal echogenic densities seen in a grade II placenta persist in a grade III placenta, but they may become more confluent and dense enough to cast their own shadows. Two different placental grades are commonly noted on a scan. The highest grade is assigned in these situations.

By the sixth to seventh week of pregnancy the placenta and its margins can be clearly delineated. The chorionic plate, the substance of the placenta, and the basal area can be identified at the end of the first trimester.

An echo-free area can be seen between the chorionic plate and the placental parenchyma. These areas are probably not of any pathologic significance. Blood flow can also be demonstrated in these echo-free areas.[2] Similar echo-free areas of different sizes can be identified within the placental parenchyma; at pathologic examination these spaces typically contain blood and are free of villi. Again, these "placental lakes" are

not thought to have any pathologic significance except for a reported association of elevated maternal serum alpha-fetoprotein, probably from enhanced protein transfer.

The retroplacental areas at the junction of the basal plate and the myometrium are frequently not echogenic, probably as a result of the presence of large mural veins. These echo-free areas can be mistaken for abruptio placenta. Furthermore, these vessels may produce significant bleeding if transversed during invasive procedures such as amniocentesis, percutaneous umbilical cord sampling, or cesarean section.[7]

CLINICAL APPLICATIONS

Placental Growth

Placental volume depends on the amount of placental tissue and the amount of fetal and maternal blood. The volumetric growth of the human placenta reaches a maximum volume by late gestation and decreases in volume and size toward the end of gestation.[8] Researchers have reported that the thickness of the placenta gradually decreases after 32 weeks' gestation.[6] The thickness of a grade I placenta was 3.8 cm, while that of a grade III placenta was 3.5 cm. Placental size increases in cases of diabetes mellitus, Rh isoimmunization, and nonimmune hydrops fetalis.[9] These sonographic images of the placental volume and size are not currently used to make any clinical decision.

Placental Location

The clinical significance of sonographic findings of placenta previa in the second trimester of pregnancy has been evaluated by several investigators.[9-12] The reported incidence of placenta previa in the second trimester detected by ultrasound in asymptomatic patients referred for genetic amniocentesis is approximately 5%, but the incidence of placenta previa at term in these patients is less than 1%.[13] This explains the hypothesis of placental migration,[12] in which early placenta previa was thought to migrate away from the internal cervical os as pregnancy advanced. Artis and coworkers[10] reported a high number of false-positive diagnoses of placenta previa made during this time in pregnancy. They suggested that high-resolution sector scanning with a near-empty bladder can help identify the cervix and placenta and thereby avoid a false-positive diagnosis (Fig. 18–2 and Fig. 18–3).

If a question of precise placental location with respect to the internal os exists after sonographic examination in the second trimester, a repeat scan at 36 weeks' gestation must confirm the diagnosis of placenta previa.

Placental Separation

The reported sensitivity of sonographic detection of placental abruption varies from 2 to 20%.[14,15] The

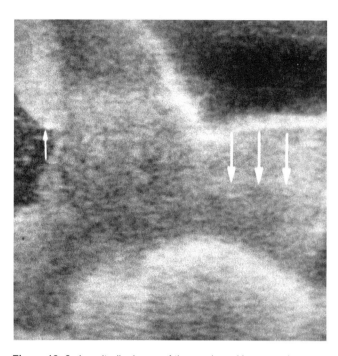

Figure 18–3. Longitudinal scan of the cervix and lower uterine segment using transabdominal ultrasound. The three larger arrows designate the midline of the cervical canal, and the single smaller arrow shows the lower border of the placenta. These findings are suggestive of a marginal placenta previa.

range of sonographic appearance contributes to the range of sensitivities for detection of placental abruption. Nyberg et al[7] concluded that a wide variety of sonographic findings in women who present with vaginal bleeding may be overlooked or misdiagnosed.

The diagnosis of abruptio placenta is best made clinically. Ultrasound can assist in the conservative management of this condition. The lack of ultrasound evidence for abruptio placenta, however, does not exclude the diagnosis. This diagnosis can be made by ultrasound following the demonstration of a retroplacental clot and a retromembranous clot. These clots appear as sonolucent areas between the uterine wall and the placenta, or the membranes and the placenta, respectively. A separation of the placenta from the underlying uterine wall appears as "tenting up" of the membranes by a retromembranous clot in close proximity to the placental margin.[16] Ultrasonography can be used to follow the progress of the abruptio placenta. The dimensions of the clots can be quantified, and serial scans will determine whether the clot is regressing or increasing in size. As the clot becomes more organized, it may appear more echogenic.[16]

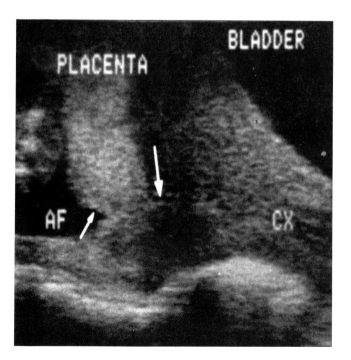

Figure 18–2. Longitudinal scan of the cervix and lower uterine segment using transabdominal ultrasound. The bladder can be seen in this view. The cervix (CX) and the central cervical canal can also be seen. The placenta (large arrow) is seen coursing down to the level of the midcervical area. The small arrow demarcates the edge of the placenta, findings consistent with a partial placenta previa. The amniotic fluic (AF) is also seen within the amniotic cavity.

REFERENCES

1. Moore KL. The fetal membranes and placenta. In: *The Developing Human: Clinically Oriented Embryology.* 3rd ed. Philadelphia, Pa: WB Saunders Co, 1982:111–118.

2. Hadlock FP, Athey PA. Sonography of the placenta. In: Larvey JP, ed. *The Human Placenta: Clinical Prospectives.* Rockville, Md: Aspen Publishers Inc.; 1987:101–106.

3. Warren WB, Timor-Tritsch I, Peisner DB, et al. Dating the early pregnancy by sequential appearance of the embryonic structures. *Am J Obstet Gynecol.* 1989;161:747–753.

4. Goldstein I, Zimmer EA, Tamir A, et al. Evaluation of normal gestational sac growth: appearance of embryonic heartbeat and embryo body movements using the transvaginal technique. *Obstet Gynecol.* 1991;77:885–888.

5. Winsberg F. Echogenic changes with placental aging. *J Clin Ultrasound.* 1973;1:52–55.

6. Grannum, PA, Berkowitz RL, Hobbins JC. The ultrasonic changes in the maturity placenta and their relation to fetal pulmonic maturity. *Am J Obstet Gynecol.* 1979;133:915–922.

7. Nyberg DA, Cyr DR, Mack LA, et al. Sonographic spectrum of placental abruption. *AJR.* 1987;148:161–164.

8. Bleker OP, Kloosterman GJ, Breur W, et al. The volumetric growth of the human placenta: a longitudinal ultrasonic study. *Am J Obstet Gynecol.* 1977;127:657–661.

9. Scheer K. Ultrasonic diagnosis of placenta previa. *Obstet Gynecol.* 1973;42:707–710.

10. Artis AA, Bowie JD, Rosenberg JD, et al. The fallacy of placental migration: effect of sonographic technique. *AJR.* 1985;144:79–81.

11. Bowie JD, Rochester D, Cadkin AV, et al. The accuracy of placental location by ultrasound. *Radiology.* 1978;128:177–180.

12. King DL. Placental migration demonstrated by ultrasonography. *Radiology.* 1973;167–170.

13. Wexler P, Gottesfeld KR. Early diagnosis of placenta previa. *Obstet Gynecol.* 1979;54:231–234.

14. Mantoni M. Ultrasound signs in threatened abortion and their prognosis significance. *Obstet Gynecol.* 1985;65:471–475.

15. Goldstein SR, Subramanyam BR, Raghavendra BN, et al. Subchorionic bleeding in threatened abortion: sonographic findings and significance. *AJR.* 1983;141:975–978.

16. Grannum PA, Hobbins JC. The placenta. *Radiol Clin N Am.* 1982;20:353–365.

19

The Amniotic Fluid

INTRODUCTION

The epithelial structures lining the amniotic cavity and fetal organs, having direct communication with the amniotic fluid, serve as possible sites of origin or routes of exchange of amniotic fluid. The placenta and the amniotic membranes, the umbilical cord, the fetal skin, and the gastrointestinal, respiratory, and urinary tracts all take part in the production and exchange of the amniotic fluid.[1]

Normal amniotic fluid volume is approximately 30 mL at 10 weeks, 350 mL at 20 weeks, 1,000 mL at 35 weeks, and 250 mL at 43 weeks of gestation. No single factor controls amniotic fluid volume; rather, several relatively efficient pathways and mechanisms contribute to the maintenance of amniotic fluid homeostasis.[1] Amniotic fluid volume is thought to play an important role in the temperature control and cushioning of the fetal environment, as well as in fetal pulmonary development and extremity growth.[2]

Both polyhydramnios and oligohydramnios during the second and the third trimesters have been associated with poor pregnancy outcome, an increased anomaly rate, and increased perinatal morbidity and mortality.[3–14] The detection of amniotic fluid volume abnormalities in the second trimester may suggest fetal abnormalities, occult diabetes, or placental insufficiency.

POLYHYDRAMNIOS

Polyhydramnios is defined as an excess of amniotic fluid, exceeding 2,000 mL at birth. This condition occurs in 0.4 to 1.5% of pregnancies.[2,11]

Etiopathology

The etiology of polyhydramnios is poorly understood. In cases of polyhydramnios associated with maternal diabetes mellitus, it has been postulated that increased osmolality of the amniotic fluid results from increased glucose in the fetus. This increases amniotic fluid volume, mainly from fetal polyuria secondary to fetal hyperglycemia.

It has been theorized that polyhydramnios in association with fetal central nervous sytem malformations results from impaired fetal swallowing; polyuria due to lack of antidiuretic hormone, and transudation of fluid across the meninges.[1] Similarly, in cases of fetal gastrointestinal tract abnormalities, polyhydramnios may be due to diminished fetal swallowing or obstruction of the gastrointestinal tract. Polyhydramnios may be associated with the following specific and nonspecific conditions[5,6,11]:

1. Idiopathic: 34% to 66.7%
2. Diabetes mellitus: 7.8% to 24.6%
3. Congenital anomalies: 12.7% to 26.9%
4. Erythroblastosis fetalis: 11.5%
5. Multiple births: 4.9% to 8.4%
6. Acute polyhydramnios: 1.5%
7. Abnormalities of the central nervous system: 45%—anencephaly (80% of total CNS), meningocele, encephalocele, cebocephaly, hydrocephaly, hydranencephaly
8. Gastrointestinal anomalies: 30%—duodenal atresia, esophageal atresia, diaphragmatic hernia
9. Cardiovascular system: 7%—coarctation of aorta, fetal hydrops
10. Other anomalies

Prenatal Diagnosis

The sonographic diagnosis is made by measuring a single vertical amniotic fluid pocket of 8 cm or more, or an amniotic fluid index greater than 24 cm when using the four-quadrant technique (Table 19–1).[14] As the severity of polyhydramnios increases, so does the likelihood of determining an etiology related to increased amniotic fluid production.[11]

Management and Outcome

Polyhydramnios is associated with malpresentation and maternal respiratory distress, especially when the hydramnios is acute. In cases of malpresentation at term, external version of the fetus under sonographic guidance along with careful rupture of the membranes, may be useful to stabilize the fetus in the pelvis.

TABLE 19–1. AMNIOTIC FLUID (MEAN VALUES) FOR EACH GESTATIONAL AGE USING THE FOUR-QUADRANT TECHNIQUE

Gestational Age (wk)	No. of Patients	Amniotic Fluid Volume (cm)
36	19	12.8 ± 4.8
37	63	13.1 ± 4.3
38	83	13.4 ± 4.7
39	55	12.4 ± 4.9
40	33	12.4 ± 4.6
41	68	8.8 ± 4.5
42	32	8.5 ± 4.7

From Phelan JP, Smith CV, Broussard P, et al. Amniotic fluid volume assessment with the four-quadrant technique at 36–42 weeks' gestation. J Reprod Med. *1987; 32:540–542, with permission.*

Amniotic fluid drainage and decompression of the amniotic cavity is desirable in cases of acute polyhydramnios with maternal respiratory distress. Once the diagnosis of hydramnios is made, careful fetal ultrasonography is necessary to exclude structural anomalies.

Women whose pregnancies are found to have an amniotic fluid index greater than 24 cm at 32 weeks' gestation should be offered a detailed ultrasound examination. Fetal cytogenetic analysis should be recommended when fetal anomalies are detected.[14] Management in these cases is dependent on the severity of the fetal anomaly. If no anomaly is detected by ultrasonography, repeat ultrasound examination within 3 weeks to confirm the diagnosis of polyhydramnios is recommended. Amniotic fluid drainage is suggested if there is acute maternal respiratory distress.[2]

Carlson and coworkers[14] assessed 49 pregnancies with severe polyhydramnios using an amniotic fluid index of greater than 24 cm at 32 weeks' gestation to define polyhydramnios. They found 22 cases (44%) with recognized fetal malformations, 6 of which had an abnormal karyotype. There was also a 20% perinatal death rate.

REFERENCES

1. Wallenburg HCS. The amniotic fluid, I. water and electrolyte homeostasis. *Perinatal Med.* 1977;5:193–210.
2. Cunningham FG, MacDonald PC, Gant NF, eds. The morphologic and functional development of the fetus. In: *Williams Obstetrics.* 18th ed. Norwalk, Conn: Appleton & Lange; 1989:105–106.
3. Chamberlain PF, Manning FA, Morrison R, et al. Ultrasound evaluation of amniotic fluid volume, I: the significance of marginal and decreased amniotic fluid volume to perinatal outcome. *Am J Obstet Gynecol.* 1984;150:245–249.
4. Chamberlain PF, Manning FA, Morrison R, et al. Ultrasound evaluation of amniotic fluid volume, II: the significance of increased amniotic fluid volume to perinatal outcome. *Am J Obstet Gynecol.* 1984;150:250–254.
5. Murry SR. Hydramnios: a study of 846 cases. *Am J Obstet Gynecol.* 1964;88:65–67.
6. Jacoby HE, Charles D. Clinical conditions associated with hydramnios. *Am J Obstet Gynecol.* 1966;94:910–918.
7. Buckingham JC, Mcelin TW, Bowers VM, et al. A clinical study of hydramnios. *Obstet Gynecol.* 1960;15:652–655.
8. Hobbins JC, Grannum PAT, Berkowitz RL, et al. Ultrasound in the diagnosis of congenital abnormalities. *Am J Obstet Gynecol.* 1979;134:331–345.
9. Alexander ES, Spitz HB, Clark RA. Sonography of polyhydramnios. *AJR.* 1982;138:343–346.
10. Sivit CJ, Hill MC, Larsen JW, et al. Second-trimester polyhydramnios: evaluation with US. *Radiology.* 1987; 165:467–469.
11. Hill LM, Breckle R, Thomas ML, et al. Polyhydramnios: ultrasonically detected prevalence and neonatal outcome. *Obstet Gynecol.* 1987;69:21–25.
12. Zamah NM, Gillieson MS, Waltes JH, et al. Sonographic detection of polyhydramnios: a five-years experience. *Am J Obstet Gynecol.* 1982;143:523–526.
13. Barkin SZ, Pretorius DH, Beckett MK, et al. Severe polyhydramnios: incidence of anomalies. *AJR.* 1987;148:155–159.
14. Carlson DE, Platt LD, Medearis AL, et al. Quantifiable polyhydramnios: diagnosis and management. *Obstet Gynecol.* 1990;75:989–992.

OLIGOHYDRAMNIOS

Oligohydramnios is a clinically significant decrease in amniotic fluid volume which occurs in approximately 4% of pregnancies. This condition is also associated with decreased fetal growth. Since amniotic fluid is easily detectable sonographically, reduction in fluid volume can be a useful marker to predict altered fetal growth.

Prenatal Diagnosis

There are four principal methods to determine decreased amniotic fluid volume:

1. Measurement of total amniotic fluid volume
2. Measurement of a 1-cm pocket
3. Four-quadrant amniotic fluid volume
4. Subjective evaluation of amniotic fluid volume

Total Amniotic Fluid Volume
Gohari et al[1] used sonography to study the total intrauterine volume measurements of the uterus and its contents in order to determine the amount of amniotic fluid associated with both normal and growth-retarded pregnancies. They assessed total intrauterine volume (TIUV) by using a static scanner and obtaining a measurement of the largest sagittal dimension

between the level of the cervix and the top of the fundus. The transducer was then rotated 90 degrees to the longitudinal diameter (A) to perform the transverse (B) and anteroposterior (C) measurements. Volume was computed using the formula for an ellipse:

$$\text{Volume} = 0.5233 \times A \times B \times C$$

and a nomogram was generated. Ninety-six patients with fetuses at risk for intrauterine growth retardation were then examined ultrasonically. Twenty-eight patients delivered growth-retarded fetuses; in 21 of these 28 cases, the total intrauterine volume was greater than 1.5 standard deviations (SD) below the mean for gestational age, while the remaining 7 growth-retarded fetuses had amniotic fluid volumes between 1 and 1.5 SD below the mean for gestational age. There was no abnormal case in the normal range in that study. Since that original publication it has become clear that mild-to-moderate degrees of intrauterine growth retardation can be missed by this method. Furthermore, with the advent of real-time sonography, TIUV has become less useful.

One-Centimeter Pocket Sign

Manning et al[2] studied the relationship between amniotic fluid volume and growth-retarded fetuses. They found that a 1-cm pocket of amniotic fluid measured in a cord-free area was a critical discriminator for normal versus deviant fetal growth; 93.4% of pregnant women in the study delivered normal infants (appropriate for gestational age) if any amniotic fluid pocket exceeded 1 cm in the broadest diameter, and 89.9% delivered growth-retarded fetuses when the largest amniotic fluid pocket measured less than 1 cm. Other investigators[3,4] found a high false-negative rate using the 1-cm pocket sign.

Four-Quadrant Amniotic Fluid Index

Phelan et al[5] addressed the four-quadrant technique for assessing the normal amniotic fluid index. The uterine cavity was arbitrarily divided into four quadrants, and the vertical diameter of the largest pocket in each quadrant was measured. The sum of these four measurements was used to provide the amniotic fluid index. The normal amniotic fluid index at term is 12.9 ± 4.6 cm. A nomogram was generated recently for the amniotic fluid index throughout gestation.[6] The amniotic fluid index continues to increase through 30 weeks' gestation, reaching a plateau until it declines at about 37 weeks' gestation.

Subjective Evaluation of Amniotic Fluid Volume

Goldstein and Filly[7] compared a sonographically subjective assessment of the amniotic fluid volume with measurements of amniotic fluid pockets. They found excellent intraobserver and interobserver agreement among estimates obtained using both subjective and objective criteria.

Phillipson et al[3] also studied the relationship between oligohydramnios diagnosed by ultrasound screening and the antenatal detection of IUGR. They demonstrated that of pregnancies complicated by oligohydramnios, 40% of offspring were small for gestational age, while only 8% of infants resulted from pregnancies without oligohydramnios.

Moore[8] compared the 1-cm pocket technique versus an amniotic fluid index of less than the fifth percentile for gestational age (70 to 88 mm) to diagnose oligohydramnios. The ability of the maximum 1-cm pocket technique to identify cases of oligohydramnios that were diagnosed by amniotic fluid index was poor; the sensitivity was 42%, and the positive predictive value was 51%. Fifty-eight percent of cases with oligohydramnios by amniotic fluid index had normal values according to the 1-cm pocket technique. Thus, the amniotic fluid index was found to be a better predictor of oligohydramnios than the 1-cm pocket technique.

In yet another study, Mercer et al[9] found an association between decreased amniotic fluid before 27 weeks' gestation and neonatal malformation rate although no chromosomal abnormalities were identified.

Management and Outcome

Once decreased amniotic fluid is determined sonographically, a detailed fetal ultrasound should be performed. If no abnormality is detected and the estimated fetal weight is less than the tenth percentile, fetal well-being should be assessed with nonstress testing, biophysical profile, and Doppler measurements of fetoplacental blood flow. In cases of oligohydramnios with fetal weight appropriate for gestational age a repeat ultrasound examination is suggested. If normal growth is confirmed, management can be expectant. Delivery should be considered when there is severe oligohydramnios and fetal growth retardation.

REFERENCES

1. Gohari P, Berkowitz RL, Hobbins JC. Prediction of intrauterine growth retardation by determination of total intrauterine volume. *Am J Obstet Gynecol.* 1977;127:255–260.
2. Manning FA, Hill LM, Platt LD. Qualitative amniotic fluid volume determination by ultrasound: antepartum detection of intrauterine growth retardation. *Am J Obstet Gynecol.* 1981;139:254–258.
3. Phillipson EH, Sokol RJ, Williams T. Oligohydramnios: clinical association and predictive value for intrauterine growth retardation. *Am J Obstet Gynecol.* 1983;146:271–276.

4. Gross TL, Sokol RJ, Wilson M, et al. Using ultrasound and amniotic fluid determinations to diagnose intrauterine growth retardation before birth: a clinical model. *Am J Obstet Gynecol.* 1982;143:265–269.

5. Phelan JP, Smith CV, Broussard R, et al. Amniotic fluid volume assessment with the four-quadrant technique at 36–42 weeks' gestation. *J Reprod Med.* 1987;32:540–542.

6. Hallak M, Kirson B. Amniotic fluid index: gestational age specific values for normal human pregnancy. Presented at the Society of Perinatal Obstetricians 11th Annual Meeting 1991. Abstract No 432.

7. Goldstein RB, Filly RA. Sonographic estimation of amniotic fluid volume: subjective assessment versus pocket measurements. *J Ultrasound Med.* 1988;7:363–369.

8. Moore TR. Superiority of four-quadrant sum over single-deepest-pocket technique in ultrasonographic identification of abnormal amniotic fluid volumes. *Am J Obstet Gynecol.* 1990;163:762–767.

9. Mercer LJ, Brown LG, Peters RE, et al. A survey of pregnancies complicated by decreased amniotic fluid. *Am J Obstet Gynecol.* 1984;149:355–360.

AMNIOTIC BAND SYNDROME

The amniotic band syndrome is a collection of fetal structural anomalies associated with fibrous bands that appear to entangle or entrap various fetal parts in utero, causing amputations or disruptions of normal morphogenesis.[1,2]

Incidence

The incidence of amniotic band syndrome varies from 1 in 1,200 to 1 in 15,000 live births; however, approximately 1 in 2,000 neonates have some problem related to early amnion rupture.[2,3]

Etiopathology

Amniotic band syndrome is a collection of sometimes severe structural defects that occurs randomly and in no other genetic or chromosomal context (Table 19–2). The etiology of this syndrome remains unclear, although there are two main hypotheses (Table 19–3).

Streeter's endogenous theory[1] of the amniotic band syndrome proposes that there is no evidence that intrauterine amputation is due to amniotic bands or adhesions, since the fibrous bands often appear to originate beneath the fetal epithelium. The classic amniotic band was thought to be the degenerative result of defective development and not the cause of it. Streeter's view of a single intrinsic defect, however, fails to explain the tremendous variation and asymmetry of lesions involving structures formed at different embryologic time periods and derived from different germ layers. Absence of any consistent association with trauma or toxic exposure, moreover, fails to support an endogenous etiology.[2,3]

TABLE 19–2. ABNORMALITIES ASSOCIATED WITH AMNIOTIC BAND SYNDROME

Limb defects, multiple, asymmetric
  Constriction rings of limbs or digits
  Amputation of limbs or digits
  Pseudosyndactyly
  Abnormal dermal ridge patterns
  Simian creases
  Clubfoot
Craniofacial defects
  Encephalocele, multiple, asymmetric
  Anencephaly
  Facial clefting: lip, palate
    Embryologically appropriate
    Embryologically inappropriate
  Severe nasal deformity
  Asymmetric microphthalmia
  Incomplete or absent cranial calcification
Visceral defects
  Gastroschisis
  Omphalocele

Adapted from Seeds JW, Cefalo R, Herbert WB. Amniotic band syndrome. Am J Obstet Gynecol. 1982; 144:243–248, with permission.

Torpin[4] suggested that the nature of the lesions seen in amniotic band syndrome was exogenous and the result of entanglement with mesodermic bands. Once ruptured, the amniotic sac ceases to grow appropriately and gradually separates from the chorion. The amniotic fluid and the fetus exit the amnion and come to lie within the chorion, where the fetus may adhere to and fuse with the chorion, with subsequent deformation or disruption of the subadjacent fetal tissue.[5] Transient oligohydramnios will follow. Multiple mesodermic strands emanate from the chorionic side of the amnion. These may entangle and constrict the limbs, digits, cranium, and, if vulnerable at the time of the insult, the bowels of the fetus.[4]

The nature and severity of the deformations and disruptions that result from amnion rupture depend on the timing of the event. Amnion rupture early in gestation can lead to more severe craniofacial and visceral manifestations, such as anencephaly and abdominal or thoracic wall defects. Transient oligohydramnios leads to compression, crowding, cord tethering, and deformation of the extremities, such as clubbing of the feet and angulation of the spine.[2]

TABLE 19–3. ETIOLOGIES OF AMNIOTIC BAND SYNDROME

1. "Impressions" on mother during pregnancy
2. Gangrene of lost part
3. Inflammatory exudates of amnion
4. Abnormal disposition of amnion
5. Maldevelopment of amnion
6. Defective germ plasm
7. Penetration of amnion
8. Premature rupture of amnion

Adapted from Baker CJ, Rudolph AJ. Congenital ring constrictions and intrauterine amputation. Am J Dis Child. 1971; 400:393, with permission.

Sonoanatomy

Defects vary from digital band constrictions to amputations of limbs or craniofacial and visceral defects (Fig. 19–1). Diagnosis is based on sonographic visualization of either amniotic sheets or bands associated with fetal deformations or structural anomalies.[5] In contrast, antenatal sonographic demonstration of a sheet of aberrant tissue in the amniotic fluid surrounding the fetus, without evidence of associated deformity, does not imply the presence of amniotic band syndrome.

Prenatal Diagnosis

Approximately 77% of the cases of amniotic band syndrome manifest multiple anomalies.[6] Constriction ring defects of the extremities are the most common associated anomalies. Clubbing of the feet is found in up to one third of the cases.[2,4] A diagnosis of amniotic band syndrome can be made when antenatal sonography visualizes an aberrant sheet or multiple bands attached to the fetus with characteristic deformities and restriction of motion. Once a band is seen sonograph-

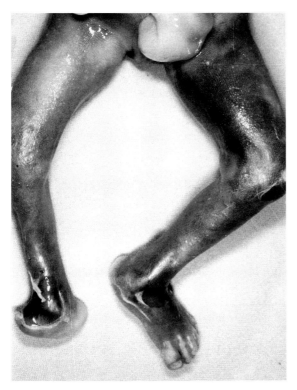

Figure 19–1. Fetal legs showing amputation of the right foot.

ically, careful evaluation of the fetus, with attention to the limbs and the fingers, should be performed. The multiple and asymmetric annular constrictions or amputations of limbs or digits are pathognomonic and can be visualized sonographically.[7]

Craniofacial deformities associated with amniotic bands occur in about one third of the cases.[6,8] Visceral manifestations of the syndrome are infrequent, but the most common is gastroschisis. Omphalocele and other defects have been reported, however.[2,3,9,10]

Management and Outcome

The defects are almost always external in location and nature and are irreversible. There is no known recurrence risk and no familial pattern of inheritance.[11] Genetic consultation is advised, however, for parental reassurance.

REFERENCES

1. Streeter GL. Focal deficiencies in fetal tissues and their relation to intrauterine amputation. *Contrib Embryol.* 1930;22:41–45.
2. Seeds JW, Cefalo R, Herbert WP. Amniotic band syndrome. *Am J Obstet Gynecol.* 1982;144:243–248.
3. Ossipoff V, Hall BD. Etiologic factors in amniotic band syndrome: a study of 24 patients. *Birth Defects.* 1977;13:117–132.
4. Torpin R. Amniochorionic mesoblastic fibrous strings and amniotic bands. *Am J Obstet Gynecol.* 1965;91:65–68.
5. Mahony BS, Filly RA, Callen PW, et al. The amniotic band syndrome: antenatal sonographic diagnosis and potential pitfalls. *Am J Obstet Gynecol.* 1985;152:63–68.
6. Beyth Y, Perlman M, Ornov A. Amniogenic bands associated with facial dysplasia. *J Reprod Med.* 1977;18:83–86.
7. Fiske CE, Filly RA, Golbus MS. Prenatal ultrasound diagnosis of amniotic band syndrome: a case report. *J Ultrasound Med.* 1982;1:45–47.
8. Jones KL, Smith DW, Hall BD, et al. A pattern of craniofacial and limb defects secondary to aberrant tissue bands. *Pediatrics.* 1974;84:90–95.
9. Stock RJ, Stock ME. Congenital annular constrictions and intrauterine amputations revised. *Obstet Gynecol.* 1979;53:592–598.
10. Baker CJ, Rudolph AJ. Congenital ring constrictions and intrauterine amputation. *Am J Dis Child.* 1971;121:393–400.
11. Higginbottom MC, Jones KL, Hall BD, et al. The amniotic band disruption complex: timing of amniotic rupture and variable spectra of consequent defects. *Pediatrics.* 1979;95:544–549.

20

Behavioral Status of the Fetus

INTRODUCTION

Antepartum assessment of fetal well-being can be obtained simply through direct observation of the fetus using ultrasound; the results are immediately available to the clinician. Fetal behavior is an indirect means of assessing fetal well-being and is somewhat independent of gestational age. Observation of the fetus permits recognition of different types of fetal movements, including gross body movements, fetal breathing motions, movements of upper and lower limbs, fetal heartbeats, lens movements, swallowing, and small-intestinal peristaltic movements. Sonographic visualization of most of these movements usually indicates fetal well-being.

The concept of rest and activity cycles in the human fetus has become well accepted. Fetal risk assessment based on fetal behavior in utero may be a method of antepartum fetal surveillance.[1-15]

PHYSIOLOGY

The First Movements

Using transvaginal ultrasound, the embryonic heartbeat can be imaged when the mean gestational sac diameter (the mean of the longitudinal, transverse, and anteroposterior diameters) measures 2 cm, or the gestational age is 6½ weeks by last menstrual period (LMP), or when the crown–rump length (CRL) measures 5 mm.[16] Fetal body movements can be observed at 8 weeks' gestational age by LMP, when the mean gestational sac reaches 3 cm, or when the CRL measures 15 mm.[16]

Fetal Swallowing

Fetal swallowing is considered a part of normal fetal activity that occurs intermittently.[17] Activities observed can be classified as follows: hand-to-mouth, chewing (mandibular), swallowing (pharyngeal), and tongue movements. Hand movements toward the face can be visualized at 16 weeks' gestation and may be associated with the sucking of fetal digits.[18]

Swallowing activity is part of the normal turnover of amniotic fluid and may represent a homeostatic mechanism. Horimoto et al[19] studied the relationship between mouth and eye movements. The authors demonstrated that regular mouth movement was correlated with nonrapid eye movement from 35 weeks' gestation to term, while random mouth movement, which occurred over a wide range of intervals, was observed during periods of rapid eye movement and was unrelated to advanced gestational age.

Fetal Eye Movements

Studies have been conducted on the patterns of eye movements in the developing fetus using real-time ultrasonography.[20,21] There are two types of eye movement patterns, a rapid eye motion of over 6 seconds and a nonrapid eye movement of less than 6 seconds. In the third trimester of pregnancy there was a proportionate increase in the amount of time the fetus spent in maintaining rapid eye movement; this movement increased throughout gestation.[21]

Fetal Activity

Natale et al[11] studied the body and breathing movements of normal fetuses between 24 and 32 weeks' gestation 2 and 3 hours following an 800 kilocalorie maternal meal. The percent of time the fetus spent in body movements during the 2-hour period decreased from about 11% at 24 to 26 weeks' gestation, to 9%, 7%, and 6.8% at 26 to 28, 28 to 30, and 30 to 32 weeks' gestation, respectively.

Fetal breathing movements increased progressively from 6% at 24 to 26 weeks' gestation to 11%, 19%, and 30% at 26 to 28, 28 to 30, and 30 to 32 weeks' gestation, respectively.

Investigators addressed the importance of daily fetal movement using the subjective maternal percep-

219

tion.[1] Movements of the normal fetus in utero are believed to be expressions of fetal well-being. Daily fetal movements increase from the 18th week of gestation, reaching a maximum between the 29th and 38th weeks. In cases of fetuses at risk due to placental insufficiency and fetal disease, however, there is a decrease in fetal movements. In severe cases, moreover, there is significant diminution or cessation of fetal movements before the occurrence of fetal death in utero.

Others[2] have reported that in normal pregnancies the number of fetal movements between 31 and 41 weeks' gestation did not vary significantly during a given period of time (12.8 ± 3.5 fetal movements in 20 minutes). Roberts et al[3] studied the incidence of fetal trunk and respiratory movements between 28 and 39 weeks' gestation and reported that the overall mean percentage of fetal trunk and respiratory movements during daylight was approximately the same: 16% and 18%, respectively. These authors demonstrated that the maximum frequency of fetal activity occurred between 7:00 and 10:00 PM for respiratory movements, and between 10:00 PM and 1:00 AM for trunk movements. Total fetal activity rarely fell below 10% during the observation time.

Patrick and Challis[13] demonstrated that the incidence of fetal breathing movements increased significantly during the second and the third hours following maternal meal ingestion, as well as overnight while the women slept. Their research also showed that during the last 10 weeks of gestation the fetuses did not manifest apnea for longer than 45 minutes during the second and third hours following meals. Patrick and Challis failed to show an effect of gestational age on fetal breathing movements during the last trimester of pregnancy. They did demonstrate that in the last 10

weeks' gestation, fetal breathing movements occurred about 30% of the time per day[13] (a higher percentage of breathing movements than was shown by Roberts et al[3]).

CLINICAL APPLICATION

Assessment of the overall behavioral activities (biophysical profile) offers indirect information about central nervous system (CNS) function and is analogous to extrauterine neurologic examination of the infant. Patrick and Challis[13] showed clear evidence that short-term periodicity (20 to 40 minutes) in biophysical activities such as fetal breathing movements were analogous to sleep states in the newborn infant, while long-term periodicity was similar to diurnal rhythms seen in extrauterine life.[14] Any factor resulting in fetal CNS depression will, in general, reduce or abolish fetal biophysical activities. Hypoxemia produces a dramatic decrease in fetal breathing movements, and when severe or associated with acidemia (asphyxia), can result in a reduction or cessation of gross body movements.[2] Drugs that depress the CNS activity, such as sedatives, analgesics, and anesthetics, usually abolish fetal biophysical activities.[22]

Interpretation of fetal biophysical activities as an index of fetal health is facilitated by an understanding of the regulation of the CNS activities. The presence of normal variability is, in general, a powerful indicator of an intact and well-functioning CNS. When variability is reduced or absent, the differential diagnosis must include hypoxemia. In practical terms, the differentiation of the normal fetus in quiet sleep from an asphyxiated, comatose fetus can be very difficult when based on the assessment of a single biophysical activ-

TABLE 20–1. TECHNIQUE OF BIOPHYSICAL PROFILE SCORING

Biophysical Variable	Normal (Score = 2)	Abnormal (Score = 0)
Fetal breathing movements	At least 1 episode of at least 30 seconds' duration in 30 minutes' observation	Absent or no episode of ≥ 30 seconds in 30 minutes
Gross body movement	At least 3 discrete body/limb movements in 30 minutes (episodes of active continuous movement considered as a single movement)	Two or fewer episodes of body/limb movements in 30 minutes
Fetal tone	At least 1 episode of active extension with return to flexion of fetal limb(s) or trunk; opening and closing of hand considered normal tone	Either slow extension with return to partial flexion or movement of limb in full extension or absent fetal movement
Reactive fetal heart rate	At least 2 episodes of acceleration of ≥15 bpm and at least 15 seconds' duration associated with fetal movement in 30 minutes	Less than 2 accelerations or acceleration <15 bpm in 30 minutes
Qualitative amniotic fluid volume	At least 1 pocket of amniotic fluid that measures at least 1 cm in two perpendicular planes	Either no amniotic fluid pockets or a pocket <1 cm in two perpendicular planes

From Manning FA, Platt LD, Sipos L. Antepartum fetal evaluation: development of fetal biophysical profile. Am J Obstet Gynecol. 1980; 136:787–795, with permission.

ity. Assessment of multiple activities is helpful in making this differentiation. Combinations of fetal biophysical variables (fetal breathing, movement, tone, amniotic fluid volume, and the nonstress test) are useful in lowering the false-positive rate.

There are, however, no significant differences in the accuracy of predicting outcomes for each single abnormal variable considered. The false-positive rate can be between 50% and 80%, depending on the fetal test used. Combination of these variables results in a progressive fall in false-positive results; the lowest false-positive rate (20%) occurs when all five variables are considered (Table 20–1).

The biophysical profile has been interpreted as follows for clinical use: a score of 8 to 10 is considered normal, 4 to 6 points equivocal, and 0 to 2 abnormal. A prospective study[5] of 1184 high risk patients, using the biophysical profile as the principal testing parameter resulted in a gross perinatal mortality rate of 5.06 per 1,000. This was significantly less than the predicted rate for a similar high-risk group (65 per 1,000) or the general population (14 per 1,000).

During the last two decades the biophysical profile score has become an acceptable means of managing high-risk patients. The biophysical profile is an adjunctive means of sonographic evaluation. It is easy and simple to use, and aids in identifying the fetus at risk of fetal jeopardy.

Biophysical profile scoring, however, remains an incomplete method for risk assessment. The exact relationship between the duration and the degree of insult and the sequence of loss of activities is unknown. Similarly, the rate and duration of change in the fetal condition are also frequently unknown. The optimum interval for fetal testing is thus not well documented (Table 20–1).

REFERENCES

1. Sadovsky E, Yaffe H. Daily fetal movement recording and fetal prognosis. *Obstet Gynecol.* 1972;41:845–850.
2. Manning FA, Platt LD, Sipos L. Fetal movements in human pregnancies in the third trimester. *Obstet Gynecol.* 1979;54:699–702.
3. Roberts AB, Little D, Cooper D, et al. Normal patterns of fetal activity in the third trimester. *Br J Obstet Gynaecol.* 1979;86:4–9.
4. Manning FA, Platt LD, Sipos L. Antepartum fetal evaluation: development of fetal biophysical profile. *Am J Obstet Gynecol.* 1980;136:787–795.
5. Manning FA, Baskett TF, Morrison I, et al. Fetal biophysical profile scoring: a prospective study in 1184 high-risk patients. *Am J Obstet Gynecol.* 1981;140:289–293.
6. Platt LD, Eglinton GS, Sipos L, et al. Further experience with the fetal biophysical profile. *Obstet Gynecol.* 1983; 61:480–485.
7. Vintzileos AM, Campbell WA, Ingardia CJ, et al. The fetal biophysical profile and its predictive value. *Obstet Gynecol.* 1983;62:271–278.
8. Baskett TF, Gray JH, Prewett SJ, et al. Antepartum fetal assessment using a fetal biophysical profile score. *Am J Obstet Gynecol.* 1984;148:630–633.
9. Natale RN, Nasello C, Turliuk R. The relationship between movements and accelerations in fetal heart rate in twenty-four to thirty-two weeks' gestation. *Am J Obstet Gynecol.* 1984;148:591–594.
10. Manning FA, Morrison I, Lange I, et al. Fetal assessment based on fetal biophysical profile scoring: experience in 12,620 referred high-risk pregnancies, I: perinatal mortality by frequency and etiology. *Am J Obstet Gynecol.* 1985;151:343–350.
11. Natale R, Paterson CN, Turliuk R. Longitudinal measurements of fetal breathing, body movements, heart rate, and heart rate accelerations and decelerations at 24 to 32 weeks of gestation. *Am J Obstet Gynecol.* 1985;151:256–263.
12. Boddy K, Dawes GS. Fetal breathing. *Br Med Bull.* 1975;31:3–7.
13. Patrick J, Challis J. Measurements of human fetal breathing movements in healthy pregnancies using a real-time scanner. *Semin Perinatol.* 1980;4:275–285.
14. Patrick J, Fetherston W, Vick H, et al. Human fetal breathing movements and gross fetal body movements at 34–35 weeks gestational age. *Am J Obstet Gynecol.* 1978;130:693–699.
15. Patrick J, Campbell K, Carmichael L, et al. A definition of human fetal apnea and the distribution of fetal apneic intervals during last ten weeks of pregnancy. *Am J Obstet Gynecol.* 1980;136:471–477.
16. Goldstein I, Zimmer EA, Tamir A, et al. Evaluation of normal gestational sac growth: appearance of embryonic heartbeat and embryo movements using the transvaginal technique *Obstet Gynecol.* 1991;77:885–888.
17. Pritchard JA. Fetal swallowing and amniotic fluid. *Obstet Gynecol.* 1966;28:606–610.
18. Bowie JD, Clair MR. Fetal swallowing and regurgitation: observation of normal and abnormal activity. *Radiology.* 1982;144:877–878.
19. Horimoto N, Koyanagi T, Nagata S, et al. Concurrence of mouthing movement and rapid eye movement/non-rapid eye movement phases with advance in gestation of the human fetus. *Am J Obstet Gynecol.* 1989;161:344–351.
20. Inoue M, Koyanagi T, Nakahara H, et al. Functional development of human eye movement in utero assessed quantitatively with real-time ultrasound. *Am J Obstet Gynecol.* 1986;155:170–174.
21. Horimoto N, Koyanagi T, Satoh S, et al. Fetal eye movement assessed with real-time ultrasonography: are there rapid and slow eye movements? *Am J Obstet Gynecol.* 1990;163:1480–1484.
22. Boddy K, Dawes GS. Fetal breathing. *Br Med Bull.* 1975;31:3–7.

21

Diagnostic Procedures in Obstetrics

Invasive procedures in obstetrics have been made possible with improvement and the adjunctive use of ultrasound. This adjunctive use of ultrasound provides the means for monitoring these procedures to ensure greater accuracy, safety, and success. This chapter discusses the following prenatal diagnostic procedures: 1) amniocentesis, 2) chorionic villus sampling, 3) fetal cord blood sampling and, 4) embryoscopy.

Amniocentesis

Genetic amniocentesis is most often performed between 16 and 18 weeks gestation. The amniotic fluid volume is approximately 150cc at this stage in pregnancy. Moreover, the ratio of viable to nonviable cells is greatest at this gestational age.[1] Some procedures are performed, however, as early as 10 weeks.

Prior to amniocentesis a thorough ultrasound examination should be performed to 1) document fetal viability, 2) determine the number of fetuses, 3) detect major fetal structural abnormalities, 4) locate the placenta, 5) confirm gestational age, 6) confirm adequate amniotic fluid volume, 7) select an optimal pocket of fluid for sampling, and 8) rule out significant uterine or adnexal pathology.

TECHNIQUE

The optimal site for needle placement is selected following a thorough ultrasound examination. This site should ideally be where there is adequate amniotic fluid volume in the absence of fetal parts. Inserting the needle through the placenta should not be considered a contraindication. This may occur without any adverse effects. The area where the umbilical cord inserts into the placenta should always be avoided because of the possibility of perforating one of the large chorionic plate vessels.

The sampling site and the surrounding abdominal wall should be thoroughly cleansed with iodine solution. The ultrasound transducer, either sector or linear-array is then enclosed in a sterile plastic bag or glove. A sector transducer should be placed several centimeters away from the needle, whereas a linear-array transducer should be placed immediately adjacent to the needle. Sterile gel is placed on the abdomen.

A 20- or 22-gauge needle is inserted under direct visualization into the amniotic cavity using the free-hand technique. Once satisfactory placement of the needle is obtained the stylet is removed and in most instances free flow of amniotic fluid will follow. A 10- to 30-cc syringe is then attached to the needle and 20 to 30 cc of fluid are removed. The first few drops often contain contaminated maternal cells or blood-tinged fluid and should be discarded. Occasionally, there is difficulty in obtaining the fluid, and reinsertion may be necessary if in situ manipulations fail to produce fluid. One common cause of failure to obtain fluid is tenting of the membranes. This can usually be seen on ultrasound. Withdrawing the needle a few centimeters and then thrusting it forward in a quick controlled motion will often overcome this problem. Cessation of flow of amniotic fluid may in some cases be due to a uterine contraction at the insertion site. Fetal cardiac activity should be monitored both before and after the procedure and should be shown to the woman for reassurance.[2]

No more than two needle insertions should be performed on any given occasion. If an initial attempt to obtain amniotic fluid is unsuccessful, a second needle can be inserted in another location. The procedure should be reattempted several days or a week later. The fetal loss rate has been shown to increase in proportion to the number of needle insertions, but not to the number of separate procedures performed. If the patient is Rh-negative, she should be given Rh immune globulin (300 mg). After the procedure she can resume normal activities.

RISKS

The United States and Canadian collaborative studies involved about 1,000 cases each with matched controls. The amniocentesis group had a total fetal loss rate (spontaneous abortions, stillbirths, and neonatal deaths) that was comparable with controls. Increasing numbers of needle insertions per procedure and the use of needles 18-gauge size, or larger, were correlated with a higher fetal loss rate. The number of separate procedures performed to obtain fluid, and whether or not the placenta was traversed, did not affect the loss rate. Immediate complications included vaginal bleeding and leakage of fluid. There was no significant difference in other outcome variables.

In contrast to previous studies, the British collaborative study of almost twice the number of cases concluded that there was a significant excess in fetal losses in the amniocentesis group of 1% to 1.5%. In addition, infants born to amniocentesis subjects had a higher incidence of unexplained respiratory difficulties lasting more than 24 hours and orthopedic postural abnormalities than the controls. The latter study has been criticized for a number of potential confounding variables, including a significant proportion of women who underwent amniocentesis because of elevated maternal serum alpha-fetoprotein, which, in itself, is associated with adverse pregnancy outcome, and an unusually low incidence of pregnancy complications in the control group.[2]

The Danish collaborative study[3] is the only randomized trial performed to date. The study population consisted of 4,606 low risk women ranging in age from 25 to 34 years, who were randomized to either have amniocentesis or no procedure. All amniocenteses were done under direct ultrasound guidance, and the majority (83.5%) of the controls underwent ultrasound examination at comparable gestational ages (16 to 17 weeks). The rate of spontaneous abortion was 1.7% in the study group compared with 0.7% in the control group. This difference was statistically significant. The observed difference of 1% corresponded to a relative risk of 2.3 for the amniocentesis group. There was no correlation between the rate of spontaneous abortion and the location of the placenta, the number of needle insertions, or the experience of the operator. There was no significant difference in the perinatal mortality rates. The frequency of malformations was the same in both groups, but in the study group, respiratory distress syndrome was diagnosed more often and more babies were treated for pneumonia.

It seems reasonable to conclude that amniocente-

sis carries a risk that may approach 1%; this risk may be enhanced by certain factors, such as needle gauges less than 20, more than two needle insertions at any given time, a raised maternal alpha-fetoprotein level before the procedure, and the presence of discolored amniotic fluid.[2]

As is true for singletons, the technique of amniocentesis in twins requires a careful ultrasound exam before the procedure. In addition to the usual parameters, the physician must identify the membrane separating the sacs and the position of each fetus within its sac. The needle should be introduced into the first sac under ultrasound guidance. After aspiration of the amniotic fluid sample, a small amount of dye is injected before removal of the needle. Indigo carmine is the dye most commonly used. The other sac is then entered with a different needle; aspiration of clear fluid indicates that the initial reservoir has not been resampled.

Blue amniotic fluid, on the other hand, indicates that the same sac has been sampled twice, although a slight blue tinge may result from transmembranous diffusion of the dye in monochorionic pregnancies. If the same sac has been sampled twice, the needle should be removed, a different area identified and another amniocentesis performed in an attempt to aspirate clear fluid. No more than four needle insertions should be attempted at any given time. The use of adjunctive ultrasonography enhances the success rates. The spontaneous abortion rates in twin pregnancies (less than 28 weeks) ranges from 2 to 17%, but the significance of these figures is uncertain due to the small size of the studies.[2]

EARLY AMNIOCENTESIS

Amniocentesis can be performed as early as 9 weeks gestation, although genetic amniocentesis is most successfully performed at approximately 16 weeks gestation. The safety and success rate in obtaining a diagnosis by early amniocentesis is still unknown, as is the volume of fluid that can be safely removed from the uterus.

In 1987 Hanson et al[4] reported 541 amniocenteses performed between 11 and 14 weeks' gestation, although follow-up was available in only 298 of these cases. Volumes of amniotic fluid removed ranged from 15 to 35 cc, with an average of 25 cc. The procedures were performed with 20-gauge needles under ultrasound guidance. There were no amniotic fluid cell culture failures in this series. The total fetal loss rate was 4.7%, with 2.7% of the losses occurring before 28 weeks. The vast majority of the patients were in their 14th week; therefore the results cannot be extrapolated to earlier gestational ages.

Although there are variations in the gestational age of study populations, early amniocenteses have been generally performed between 10 and 14 weeks of gestation. The initial results have suggested fetal loss rates comparable to those of patients who have undergone second-trimester amniocentesis.[4] There are problems with the studies, however, that make the results difficult to evaluate. For example, the total number of patients in these studies was small, and the study populations were heavily laden with 14-week pregnancies. It would of course be unfair to a patient about to have an 11-week amniocentesis to quote a loss rate derived from a study comprised mostly of 14-week pregnancies. Of theoretical concern is the fact that proportionally more amniotic fluid is taken from the amniotic cavity in early amniocentesis than at 16 weeks or later.

The intra-amniotic fluid volumes in pregnancies between 14 and 16 weeks of gestation were evaluated using a vaginal ultrasound probe.[5] This new technique allows the visualization of both the amnion and chorion. In many cases there is a marked discrepancy between the intracavitary and the intra-amniotic volumes; in some 12- and 13-week pregnancies the intra-amniotic fluid volume is as little as 30 mL. If 13 mL of fluid were aspirated from one of these patients, the embryo would be temporarily deprived of almost one half its aquatic environment. This may not represent a problem to the fetus, but given the results from second-trimester studies in which higher rates of respiratory distress syndrome and pneumonia were found among infants born after amniocenteses, more information must be accumulated to assess the long-term effects of early amniocentesis. Until then, the physician cannot confidently counsel patients who wish to have an early amniocentesis about the potential risk of the procedure.

Chorionic Villus Sampling (CVS)

The placental villi and the fetus are derived from the same tissue, thus making CVS an attractive source of data for genetic studies on the fetus (Fig. 21–1 and Fig. 21–2). Furthermore, one major advantage is the fact that CVS can be performed early in gestation. In addition, these cells are actively growing; they come from a single cell line; and tissue culture of these cells can be obtained more rapidly than amniotic fluid cells. The indications for CVS are the same as those for genetic amniocentesis. Specimens can be directly examined for karyotyping or cultured for biochemical studies, gene mapping, or karyotypic analysis.

TRANSCERVICAL CVS PROCEDURE

Although Hahnemann and Mohr[6] first described an endoscopic technique to obtain trophoblast, Brambati

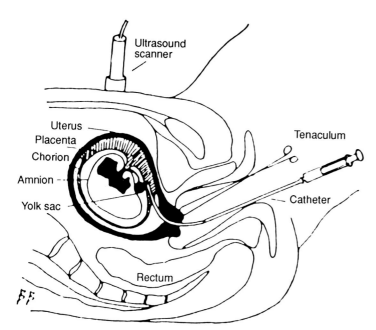

Figure 21–1. Schematic diagram of a chorionic villous sampling (CVS) done by the transvaginal route. Note the procedure is done under ultrasound guidance, and the catheter is passed transcervically along the chorion from which a biopsy is obtained. (*Hobbins JC and Reece EA. First-trimester prenatal diagnosis. In: Reece EA, Hobbins JC, Mahoney MJ, et al, eds.* Medicine of the Fetus and Mother. *Philadelphia, Pa.: JB Lippincott Co; 1992: 635, with permission.*)

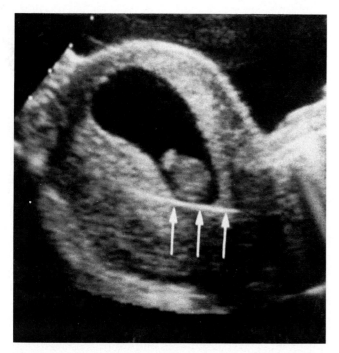

Figure 21–2. First-trimester ultrasound exam by transvaginal ultra-sonography. The view shows a sagittal scan of a uterus with a gestational sac and an embryo contained. An echolucent line is shown to pass inferior to the embryo and is outlined with arrows. This represents a catheter which is passed during a chorionic villous sampling (CVS) procedure. Note the catheter is passed on the outside of the gestation sac in the area of the chorion frondosum.

et al[7] was the first to describe the technique that is currently used. The procedure involves advancing a catheter, under ultrasound direction, into the thickest portion of the placenta. Trophoblastic material is aspirated through the catheter into a syringe, which is then attached to a catheter. In most cases, 5 mg or more is sufficient for direct chromosome analysis, although results can be obtained from smaller amounts after cell culture. More sophisticated DNA studies using restriction fragment-length polymorphisms or enzyme assays may require up to 40 mg of villus tissue.

TRANSABDOMINAL CVS PROCEDURE

Hahnemann and Mohr were also the first to introduce the transabdominal technique[6]. Its major advantage is the circumvention of the cervix which may increase the risk for infectious morbidity. The transabdominal CVS procedure is very similar to amniocentesis and can be performed with either a needle-aspiration transducer of a free-hand technique. The operator simply places a needle tangentially through the placental substance under ultrasound guidance. While aspirating through a syringe attached to the hub of the needle, the needle tip is moved up and down through the placenta until adequate tissue is obtained for analysis.

Some investigators prefer to use a double-needle technique, which requires a smaller needle to be advanced through an introducer needle.

ADVANTAGES AND DISADVANTAGES

The transcervical approach to CVS has been the most widely used. Despite the fact that more than 35,000 total procedures are estimated to have been performed worldwide before September 1987, the actual risks of the procedure have yet to be accurately measured. Patients undergoing CVS are at higher risk of pregnancy loss by virtue of their indications for the procedure (ie, chromosomally abnormal fetuses have a higher spontaneous abortion rate than do normal fetuses). Any comparison of pregnancy loss must be made with patients of similar maternal age. One source of information concerning CVS risks is a registry centered in Philadelphia presided over by Laird Jackson. The registry has accumulated data on more than 57,000 pregnancies.

There have been two prospective clinical trials, one from the United States[8] and one from Canada.[9] The results of the United States trial indicates a 0.7% greater risk for transcervical CVS as compared with second-trimester amniocentesis. A Canadian randomized clinical trial demonstrated similar findings. However, since some patients in the chromosomally normal CVS group chose to terminate their pregnancies, if one were to adjust the study subject denominator accordingly, the increased risk of CVS could attain 1.7%.[10,11] It appears from these data that CVS carries a slightly higher risk of pregnancy loss than does second-trimester amniocentesis.

Initial studies evaluating risks of transabdominal CVS indicate that this may well represent a safer procedure than transcervical CVS; the verdict on this must await completion of randomized clinical trials in progress.

Fetal Blood Sampling

Fetal cord blood sampling is performed as an outpatient procedure and obtained from a free-floating loop of cord or the placental insertion of the cord root, which is usually the preferred site. The type of transducer used varies from one operator to another, but linear array, sector scanner, or curvilinear transducers can all be used.

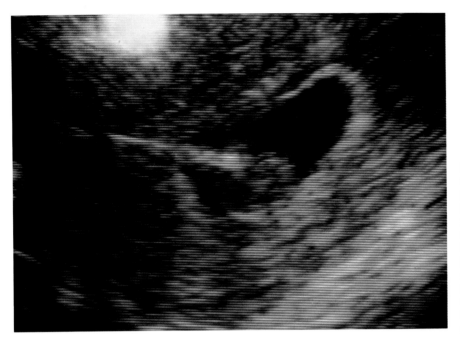

Figure 21–5. Ultrasound picture of a transcervical examination in progress in a pregnancy at approximately 9 weeks' gestation. Note the endoscope as it passes through the cervical canal into the amniotic cavity. Note the endoscope as it passes through the cervical canal into the exocoelomic space and comes in close proximity to the embryo. (*Hobbins JC and Reece EA. First-trimester prenatal diagnosis. In: Reece EA, Hobbins JC, Mahoney MJ, et al, eds.* Medicine of the Fetus and Mother. *Philadelphia, Pa.: JB Lippincott Co; 1992:638, with permission.*)

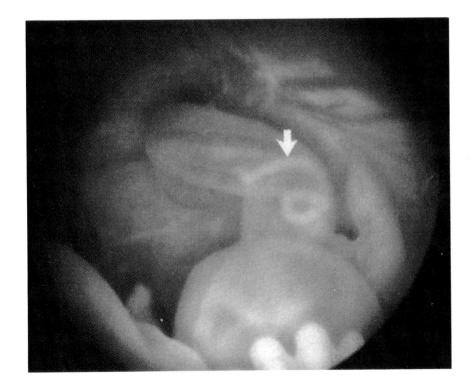

Figure 21–6. Embryoscopic examination of the fetal abdomen at 6 weeks' gestation. Note the umbilical cord inserting inferiorly into the fetal abdomen. The loops of bowel, indicated by the arrow, are seen within the umbilical stalk representing the physiologic hernia. (*Cullen MT, Reece EA, Whetham J, et al. Embryoscopy: description and utility of a new technique.* Am J Obstet Gynecol. *1990;162:85, with permission.*)

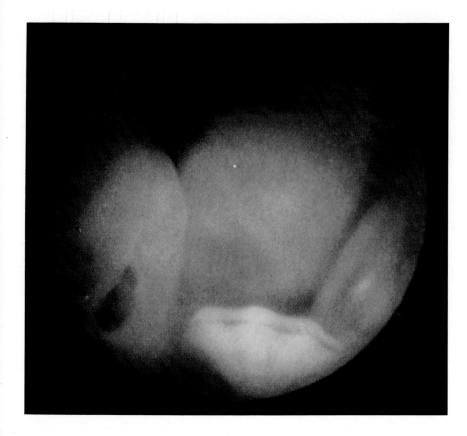

Figure 21–7. Direct visualization of fetus at 6 weeks (menstrual). The profile demonstrates a prominent forehead and widely spaced eyes. A hand paddle is seen at the bottom of the figure.

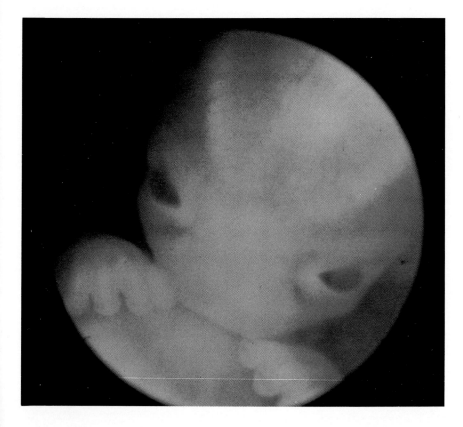

Figure 21–8. Direct visualization of fetus at 9 weeks (menstrual). Head is seen flexed on its chest with prominent forehead, normal separated eyes, and fused lips. Fingers at this age are only slightly webbed. (*Reece EA, Rotmensch S, Whetham J, et al. Embryoscopy: a closer look at first-trimester diagnosis and treatment. Am J Obstet Gynecol. 1992; 166:777, with permission.*)

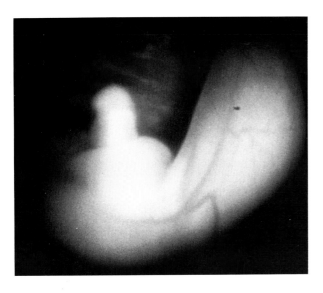

Figure 21–9. Note the male genitalia at 8 weeks' gestation. The scrotal sac and penis can be easily visualized.

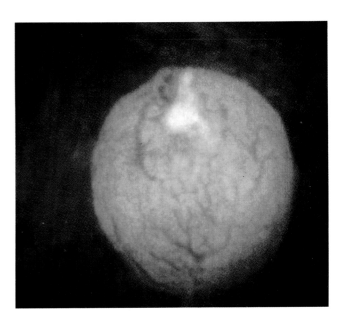

Figure 21–11. Photograph of the yolk sac at 6 weeks gestation.

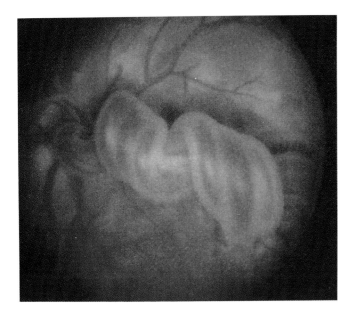

Figure 21–10. Embryoscopic examination of a 12-week fetus demonstrating the tortuous umbilical cord as it ramifies into the undersurface of the placenta. (*Cullen MT, Reece EA, Whetham J, et al. Embryoscopy: description and utility of a new technique. Am J Obstet Gynecol. 1990;162:85, with permission.*)

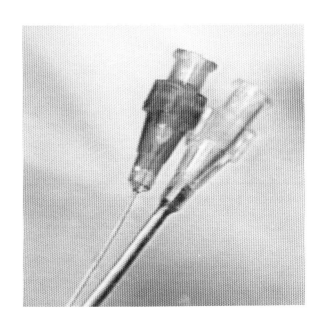

Figure 21–12. The specially designed 16-gauge double-barrel instrument sheath used to perform transabdominal embryoscopy. Two ports are seen; the one on the left is used for fetal blood sampling and the one on the right is used to pass the endoscope.

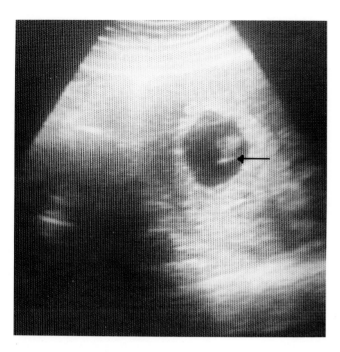

Figure 21–13. Ultrasound picture of an 8-week embryo. The end of the fiber-optic endoscope is seen as a bright white streak below the embryo as indicated by the arrow.

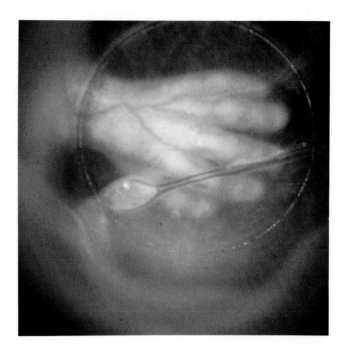

Figure 21–15. At 7 conceptual weeks a fully developed hand is observed without webbing. (*Reece EA. Embryoscopy: new developments in prenatal medicine. Current Opinion in Obstet Gynecol. 1992;4:452, with permission.*)

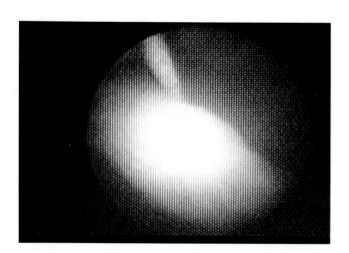

Figure 21–14. Photograph of 27-gauge needle entering the umbilical cord vessel for blood sampling.

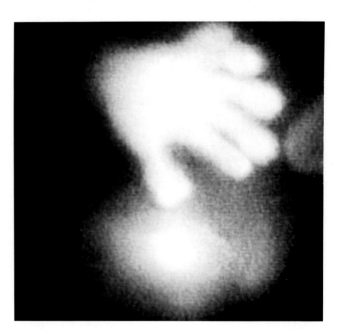

Figure 21–16. Embryoscopic examination of a fetus demonstrating polydactyly. (*Hobbins JC and Reece EA. First-trimester prenatal diagnosis. In: Reece EA, Hobbins JC, Mahoney MJ, et al, eds. Medicine of the Fetus and Mother. Philadelphia, Pa.: JB Lippincott Co; 1992:639, with permission.*)

TECHNIQUE

A 20- or 22-gauge needle is introduced under direct ultrasound guidance through the maternal abdominal wall into the targeted vessel (Fig. 21–3). Once the needle is in place, a 1-cc heparinized syringe is attached to the needle and gently aspirated. Once 2 to 4 cc of blood has been aspirated, its fetal origin should be confirmed. Upon confirmation, the needle is withdrawn, and the duration of bleeding from the puncture site is determined. Fetal cardiac activity should be assessed during and after the procedure

In the case of a posterior placenta, entry into the amniotic cavity becomes necessary. This poses a number of potential problems, most of which can be overcome by being cautious. In some cases paralyzing the fetus with a muscle blocker immediately after entry into the vessel is necessary to avoid complications such as fetal movements dislodging the needle. Fetal paralysis can also be achieved by administering the drug intramuscularly into the fetal thigh or buttock before the cord is punctured. Several neuromuscular blocking agents have been used including *d*-tubocurarine (1.5 to 3 mg/kg),[12] pancuronium (0.3 mg/kg),[13] and atracurium besylate (0.4 mg/kg).[14] Although paralyzing the fetus appears to be safe, it is usually unnecessary for fetal blood sampling because the sampling time is usually quite short. During long procedures such as intravascular transfusions, however, fetal paralysis is helpful.[2]

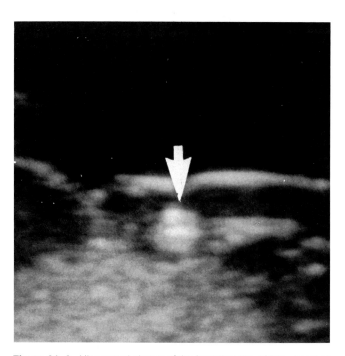

Figure 21–3. Ultrasound picture of the insertion site of the umbilical cord into a posterior placenta. The arrow indicates the point of a needle as it pierces the umbilical cord during a cordocentesis.

INDICATIONS

Fetal Karyotyping

Common indications for rapid fetal karyotyping are the detection of structural malformations or intrauterine growth retardation because management decisions may need to be made within days. If the need for karyotyping arises at a critical gestational age, ie, close to the time when legal termination of pregnancy is no longer possible, or if delivery is imminent, analysis of fetal blood is also indicated, and results can be available within 8 hours.

Fetal Infection

Toxoplasmosis, rubella, cytomegalovirus, varicella, and parvovirus have been diagnosed in utero by fetal blood analysis. Direct isolation of an organism in fetal blood or amniotic fluid is the most reliable evidence of fetal infection. This, however, is not always possible because culturing techniques may be either very difficult to perform or extremely lengthy. In these cases other evidence of infection may be helpful. As in the adult, fetal responses to infection may be either specific or nonspecific.

The former includes production of immunoglobulin M (IgM) antibodies that are specifically directed at the offending organism. The production of such antibodies, however, is dependent on the maturity of the fetal immune system and, consequently, on gestational age. In most cases detection of this marker of infection has proven to be reliable, when present, but its absence does not rule out fetal exposure to the organism.

Nonspecific evidence of infection has proven to be useful in these cases. Some of these signs include thrombocytopenia, erythroblastosis, leukocytosis, eosinophilia, elevated gamma-glutamyltransferase and lactose dehydrogenase, and elevated total IgM. These findings are not pathognomonic of fetal infection, and some of them can be seen in other fetal conditions such as intrauterine growth retardation. Nevertheless, when fetal infection is a possibility, positive nonspecific findings may be very helpful in either expediting a positive isolation of the organism or informing the patient that the chances of infection are high.[2]

Risks and Complications

The population of patients undergoing fetal blood sampling is unique because, in general, there is no alternative diagnostic procedure. Thus the risks of the procedure cannot be compared to those of any other, and controlled studies will never be done. In addition, some of these patients have very sick or anomalous fetuses already at a greater risk of death in utero so determining which poor outcomes are due to the procedure itself may be quite difficult.

Despite these drawbacks the fetal loss rate related to fetal blood sampling appears to be relatively low. Daffos et al[15] reported their experience with 606 procedures performed in 652 patients. In this series there was a total fetal loss rate of 1.9%, but only two of seven losses appeared to be related to the procedure. In 1989 the same group[16] reported 1,770 cases, with a total fetal loss rate of 2.3% and a procedure-related loss rate of 0.4%. The rate of premature delivery was 4.2%. As of October 1989, 3,002 procedures in 1,501 pregnancies had been reported from 16 centers in the United States and Canada. In this group 1.4% of the patients lost the pregnancy because of the sampling (1.2% loss rate per procedure).

The most common complication of fetal blood sampling is transient fetal bradycardia. Daffos et al reported that this occurred in 9% of their cases,[16] but the vast majority were of short duration. In some cases cord hematomas have been identified, but in the majority no obvious cause is found. Some postulate that when an umbilical artery is punctured instead of the vein, arterial vasospasm may occur. Since prolonged bradycardia is a potentially serious complication, cordocentesis should be performed in an area where immediate operative delivery is possible whenever the fetus is of a viable gestational age.[2]

Fetal bleeding from the puncture site can be observed in a number of cases when the needle is removed, but this also is usually very short lived. Many fetuses with severe coagulation defects have been sampled without complications. It appears that some hemostatic property of Wharton's jelly of amniotic fluid may have an important role in preventing significant fetal hemorrhage.

SKIN BIOPSY

Percutaneous insertion of the biopsy forceps under ultrasound guidance has replaced earlier methods. Because of the relatively large-bore instrument used, the placenta should never be punctured. In addition, the pocket selected should not contain loops of umbilical cord or fetal parts. The optimum site for fetal skin biopsy is the fetal back, buttocks, or thighs. However, for disorders of pigmentation, areas with abundant hair follicles (scalp) are preferred. A 3- to 4-mm incision is then made with a scalpel in the skin, down to the fascia, and under ultrasonic guidance a 14-gauge trocar with stylet is inserted into the amniotic cavity. The stylet is then removed, and a flexible fetal skin biopsy forceps with a diameter of 1 mm is introduced through the sleeve (Karl Storz Endoscopy-America, Inc, Culver City, California).

Several samples of fetal skin can be taken from the same general area or from different locales. Care

must be taken to always visualize the area being sampled with ultrasound because inadvertent biopsy of the amniotic sac may cause rupture of the membranes. Fetal heart activity should be monitored during and after the procedure.

The loss rate due to fetal skin biopsy is not known, but it is believed to be similar to that of fetoscopy, ie, 2% to 6%. Within the group of keratinizing disorders, the following disorders have been diagnosed: lamellar ichthyosis (nonbullous congenital ichthyosiform erythroderma),[17] epidermolytic hyperkeratosis (bullous ichthyosiform erythroderma),[18] and Harlequin syndrome.[19] Several forms of blistering disorders have also been diagnosed in utero, such as epidermolysis bullosa lethalis[20] and some of the recessive and dominant types of epidermolysis bullosa dystrophica.[21] Prenatal diagnosis of disorders of pigmentation such as oculocutaneous albinism has been possible by observing a lack of melanin synthesis in hair-bulb melanocytes.[22] This diagnosis can be made as early as 16 weeks' gestation because in the normal fetuses at least 50% of the melanosomes are fully pigmented at this age.[2]

Embryoscopy

The first direct transuterine visualization of the fetus was successfully performed by Westin[23] in 1954 using a 10-mm hysteroscope. In spite of the image quality being rather limited by the insufficient optical system, fetal parts and movements could be identified.[23,24]

Endoscopic visualization of the embryo (embryoscopy) is a new and evolving technology. The concept of direct visualization of the embryo reflects not only our ongoing quest for improved diagnostic techniques, but also the potential for direct, targeted embryonic therapy. Among the latest of such technologies is embryoscopy, which utilizes high-resolution fiber-optic equipment for direct visualization of the embryo or fetus.[23-29]

The widespread diagnostic and therapeutic use of fetoscopy in ongoing pregnancies became feasible when Hobbins and Mahoney[30] developed the Dyonics needlescope, which employed an ultrasonically guided percutaneous transabdominal technique under local anesthesia. Direct fetal visualization allows for the diagnosis of external structural anomalies; aspiration of fetal blood; skin, liver; fetal tumor biopsies; and intravascular infusion of blood and blood products.[28,31,32]

Major drawbacks of fetoscopy, however, are related to a fetal loss rate of 4% to 8%, as well as inconsistent success in obtaining fetal blood samples devoid of amniotic fluid contamination; risk-versus-benefit considerations limit the use of fetoscopy somewhat. Additionally, fetoscopy cannot be used when the amniotic fluid is discolored and is less efficacious in advanced pregnancies.

Embryoscopy is a technique that consists of either transcervical or transabdominal fiber-optic endoscopy of the first-trimester embryo or fetus. Currently, only a few centers in the world are involved in these procedures. These procedures allow direct visualization of the human embryo in vivo and access to its circulation. Multiple diagnoses of embryonic malformations have been made by embryoscopy; the diagnostic and therapeutic potential of this technique is just beginning to unfold.[25–28]

Originally, embryoscopy was performed using a transcervical approach. However, this approach requires passage through the vagina, cervical canal, and chorion. All of which increases the risks of the procedure. Recently, Reece et al[33] modified the transcervical technique to use a transabdominal approach. Both techniques will be described in the following sections.

TECHNIQUE FOR TRANSCERVICAL EMBRYOSCOPY

The technical aspects of the procedure have been described elsewhere.[25–29] In brief, transcervical embryoscopy uses a rigid fiber-optic endoscope, 30 cm in length, with diameters from 2.0 to 3.5 mm and a 0- or 30-degree-angle lens (Fig. 21–4). Under ultrasound guidance, the endoscope is passed transcervically into the extracoelomic cavity (chorionic cavity) without disturbing the amnion (Fig. 21–5). A complete examination of the embryo or fetus includes visualization of the head, face, dorsal and ventral walls, limbs, umbilical cord, and yolk sac (Fig. 21–6, Fig. 21–7, Fig. 21–8, Fig. 21–9, Fig 21–10, and Fig. 21–11). The average length of time for this procedure is 5 minutes. We have reported 95% success rates for visualization of the fetus.

A similar success rate has been reported by Dumez[34–35]. He performed embryoscopy, in over 50 continuing pregnancies to rule out head and limb anomalies. In his early attempts two pregnancies were lost, but no adverse outcome was noted in subsequent work. It should be emphasized that to date only a few ongoing pregnancies have been investigated, but this is expected to change with improvements in the technique and its applications to a variety of conditions and circumstances.

TECHNIQUE FOR TRANSABDOMINAL EMBRYOSCOPY

Recently, Reece et al[33] introduced a new endoscopic approach that utilizes a special 16-gauge, double-barrel instrument sheath, equipped with an 0.8-mm fiber-optic endoscope and a customized 27-gauge heparinized needle. This instrument is passed transabdominally under ultrasound guidance (Fig. 21–12) through the uterine wall and into the amniotic cavity in a manner very similar to performing amniocentesis (Fig. 21–13). As with the transcervical technique, a complete examination of the embryo/fetus is possible. In addition, a small aliquot of blood can be removed

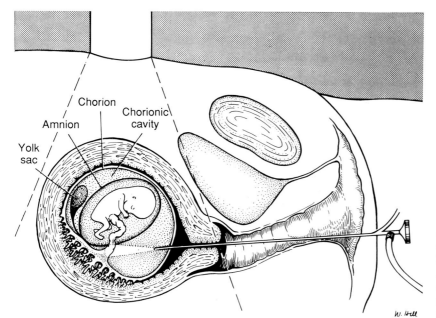

Figure 21–4. Schematic diagram of embryoscope inserted transcervically and passed through the chorion into the exocoelomic space. The entire conceptus can be easily visualized through the amnion. Note the anatomic landmarks as indicated. (*Reece EA, Rotmensch S, Whetham J. Embryoscopy: a closer look at first-trimester diagnosis and treatment. AM J Obstet Gynecol. 1992;166:776, with permission.*)

from the umbilical vessel through the heparinized needle (Fig. 21–14).[33] It is anticipated that this new transabdominal approach will be primarily used since it reduces the potential risk of infection and cervical trauma. That is theoretically associated, to a greater degree, with the transcervical approach.

CURRENT APPLICATIONS OF EMBRYOSCOPY

Morphologic Evaluation

Embryoscopy can be performed as early as 3 conceptional weeks' gestation as well as throughout the first and second trimesters. This procedure can be used to document developmental events and anomalies that are potentially diagnosable through the embryoscope.

The embryonic period extends from weeks 4 through 8 following conception, during which time all major external and internal structures develop. This is the period when the embryo is most vulnerable to the effects of teratogens. By the end of this period, there are recognizable features of human development.[25,35–37]

The Head and Neck

Growth of the fetal body tends to occur at a disproportionate rate, with the cephalic end developing before the remainder of the body. This disproportion begins very early, with the highest number of somites clustering in the future base of the head nurtured by a well-established blood supply. The brain and associated sense organs also develop early and remain disproportionately larger than other extracranial regions throughout embryonic life.[35]

The endoscopic view of the fetal face at 6 conceptional weeks demonstrates a prominent forehead, widely spaced eyes, as well as confluent oral and nasal cavities (Fig. 21–7). At 8 conceptional weeks, greater facial details are seen; by 10 conceptional weeks, normal human facial features are recognized (Fig. 21–8).

Head malformations that will have external manifestations include anencephaly, acrania, hydrocephaly, microcephaly. Anencephaly and acrania are the most probable disorders diagnosable in the first trimester • by embryoscopy. Potentially diagnosable anomalies of the face include micrognathia and cleft lip. The latter is usually unilateral (left more often than right) but can be bilateral. The lip is often the only affected area, but the bony upper jaw may also be involved.[25,36]

The eyes are initially located laterally and far from each other. This disproportion gradually decreases as broadening of the head occurs. Hypotelorism or hypertelorism and the absence of one or both eyes are potentially diagnosable anomalies via embryoscopy.

The ears develop around the first branchial groove and deepen to form the external meatus by 5 conceptional weeks; they shift to a higher and more lateral position by 10 conceptional weeks. Anomalies are often related to failure of upward shifting and also seem potentially diagnosable using embryoscopy during early gestation.[25,35]

The nose develops from a complex merging of frontonasal bones with maxillary processes; anomalies are not frequently seen.

The Trunk

The early embryo begins as a layered plate that undergoes infolding and results in a hollow cylinder, the trunk. In the dorsal region, the neural ridges undergo infolding and form a neural tube. The cephalic part of the neural tube rapidly grows to form the forebrain, midbrain, and hindbrain vesicles. The ventricles are formed by the lumina of the neural tube. The future axial skeleton and muscles are represented by somites located in this dorsal region. Development of the internal organs enhances the form and shape of this cylinder.[36]

Development of the gut occurs at a time when the abdominal cavity is still small; hence, herniation occurs in the body stalk at about 5 weeks. The gut remains extruded until about week 10 when reinsertion occurs followed by complete closure of the ventral wall.

These normal milestones of embryonic development can be visualized during embryoscopy. The neural tube is seen with the cephalic end open at about 5 conceptional weeks of gestation; by 7 conceptional weeks there is complete closure of the neural tube. The ventral hernia is seen as early as 4 conceptional weeks (Fig. 21–6); by 8 conceptional weeks, the hernia is almost completely resolved.[29] Occasionally the gut remains extruded after the eighth conceptional week.[25]

Both dorsal and ventral wall defects can be diagnosed by embryoscopy. Omphalocele results when the abdominal wall fails to close after the 10th conceptional week, and the bowels and even the liver persist in the body stalk. Gastroschisis occurs when the bowel protrudes from a defect that is located below and generally to the right of the umbilicus. The liver is rarely involved. Defects in dorsal wall closure are associated with spina bifida or rachischisis with or without saccular protrusions and herniation of neural elements.[25,26]

The Limbs

The limb buds are manifested first as lateral swellings or paddle-shaped structures in the late fourth conceptional week. Initially, arm buds are located lower on the trunk in the region of the lumbosacral somites.

Flattening constrictions will demarcate foot and hand, leg and thigh, and forearm and arm regions. Hand–radial ridges, suggested by grooves, predict the location of digits. Development of the lower limbs is slower. The thumbs and great toes separate earlier than the other digits in both upper and lower extremities.[35-37] The upper limb buds appear, attain normal appearance, and develop earlier. This disproportionate growth is maintained until the second year of postnatal life, when legs and arms become of equal length.

We have been able to document with embryoscopy many normal developmental events during the first trimester. The hand paddles are seen at 4 conceptional weeks with subtle demarcation of finger rays; by 6 conceptional weeks, webbed fingers are observed. At 7 conceptional weeks, a fully developed hand is seen (Fig. 21–15). The developmental progression of the upper limbs can be as much as 2 weeks ahead of the lower extremities.[29]

Since normal limb development can be documented with embryoscopy, it is likely that abnormalities of hands and feet could be easily identified. For example, polydactyly can be diagnosed at 9 conceptional weeks of gestation (Fig. 21–16). The potential exists to diagnose hemimelia, phocomelia, sirenomelia, missing digits, lobster claw, syndactyly, brachydactyly, or even clubhand or foot.[31]

EMBRYOSCOPIC CONFIRMATION OF EARLY SONOGRAPHIC PRENATAL DIAGNOSIS

With the continued improvement in high-resolution ultrasound equipment, prenatal diagnostic programs have been expanded to examine fetuses even in the early second trimester. When congenital anomalies are diagnosed and patients choose to undergo pregnancy termination, pathologic confirmation and careful anatomic studies can be performed via embryoscopy prior to a dilatation and extraction procedure.[27] Verification of prenatally diagnosed anomalies is vital to accurate patient counseling. Using embryoscopy, a direct view of the embryo can be obtained prior to evacuation and to document abnormalities by videotaping the examination. This procedure is invaluable in identifying additional anomalies not recognized by ultrasound and confirming others already detected sonographically.[25]

From a conceptual point of view, embryoscopy will be of increasing importance to general human embryology. Much of our knowledge of early human development is based on the investigation of human aborti or analogies drawn from animal research. The very same pathology that causes a miscarriage could affect fetal growth and development as well, thereby somewhat limiting the validity of the former approach. On the other hand, stages of embryonic development in animals are not necessarily representative of human development, thus limiting the validity of the latter approach. Embryoscopy visualizes the human embryo in vivo, unaffected by any pathology of the uterine or hormonal environment and representative of the intrinsic capability of a given fetus for early development.

A major question awaiting elucidation is the unclear role of the yolk sac in early human development. The yolk sac provides blood cell precursors, gonadocytes, and epithelia of the digestive and respiratory tracts, and has been demonstrated to be structurally altered when exposed to high glucose concentrations in embryo-culture experiments. It has been suggested that the yolk sac might play an essential role in the pathogenesis of congenital anomalies among fetuses of diabetic mothers.[38-40] Direct observation of the yolk sac by embryoscopy as well as aspiration of its contents for laboratory analysis might enhance our understanding of human malformations considerably.

THE FUTURE AND EMBRYOSCOPY

Embryoscopic examination, with the potential for embryonic therapy, is an extension of existing diverse prenatal diagnostic techniques, as well as the beginning of a new era of first-trimester intervention. Fetal tissue sampling, cell and/or gene therapy are goals to which embryoscopy can be applied (Table 21–1).

Tissue Sampling

First-trimester diagnoses of genetic diseases by organ tissue retrieval, embryonic blood sampling, or both also appear within reach. The evolution of sophisticated molecular techniques using gene probes for DNA analyses makes embryoscopy seem more attractive for the early prenatal diagnosis of many diseases.

Diagnosis can be done on the trophoblast via chorionic villous sampling between 9 and 12 menstrual weeks' gestation. However, in approximately

TABLE 21–1. POTENTIAL APPLICATIONS OF EMBRYOSCOPY

Prenatal diagnosis of structural anomalies

Confirmation of early sonographic diagnosis prior to pregnancy termination

Early blood or tissue sampling

Embryo access for cell and gene therapy

The biology of embryonic development

From Reece EA, Hobbins JC. Embryoscopy: an evolving technology for early prenatal diagnosis. In: Chapman M, Grudzinskas G, Chard T, eds. The Embryo: Normal and Abnormal Development and Growth. New York: Springer-Verlag; 1991:123–140.

1% of cases, an additional fetal source, such as the fetal blood, is needed to clarify initial aberrant chromosomal findings. With current technology such evaluation needs to wait until the second trimester. Embryoscopic blood sampling in the first trimester may soon be feasible and would reduce the anxiety-laden waiting period. Fetal blood sampling would also be indicated in patients presenting after the first trimester and desiring rapid prenatal diagnosis or early fetal blood typing in a mother with isoimmunization.[25]

Gene and Cell Therapy

Rapid progress has been made toward the concept of human gene and cell therapy.[41–42] If this concept becomes a reality, embryoscopy will permit accessibility to the human embryo at a time when embryos are immunologically naive and may therefore be receptive to these grafts.

Embryoscopy opens a new era in fetal medicine. Future prenatal diagnosis will change considerably, with more emphasis on the first trimester and performed directly on the embryo or on the placenta, as in chorionic villous sampling, rather than conducted in the second and third trimesters on the amniotic fluid and fetus. Perfection of embryoscopy should provide access to the entire conceptus, permitting both early diagnosis, as well as the potential for early treatment.

Gene or cell therapy has not yet been approved for clinical trials; in the coming era this new therapeutic approach will probably be used in the treatment of currently incurable diseases. The in utero application of this technology would be limited to serious genetic diseases that produce irreversible damage by the time of birth. At present, the only human tissue that can be used effectively for gene or cell transfer is bone marrow. More will be learned in the future about packaging the DNA, purifying stem cells, and making the DNA tissue-specific. It would then be feasible to use the intravenous route for injection of genetic material and for access to the embryo and its circulatory system.

The feasibility of this approach has been tested by Kantoff et al.[43] They demonstrated expression of the human adenosine deaminase (ADA) gene in the blood cells of irradiated monkeys that were reinfused with their own bone marrow cells. The cells had been treated in vitro with an ADA retroviral vector. The first attempts at postnatal human therapy of ADA deficiency are at advanced stages. Other genetic diseases, particularly those affecting the brain (eg, Lesch–Nyhan syndrome) will require in utero intervention in order to be effective. Since in utero transplantation of donor tissue might become necessary to achieve this goal, embryoscopy could be an invaluable access tool to the early embryo or fetus, which would allow for graft acceptance by a naive immune system.

Embryoscopy, therefore, is expected to have a major impact on fetal medicine in the years to come; prenatal diagnosis and therapy will undoubtedly change, with greater emphasis placed on intervention in the first trimester.

REFERENCES

1. Emery AE. Antenatal diagnosis of genetic disease. *Mod Trends Hum Genet.* 1970;1:267–273.
2. Lynch L, Berkowitz RL. Amniocentesis, skin biopsy and umbilical cord blood sampling in the prenatal diagnosis of genetic diseases. In: Reece EA, Hobbins JC, Petrie RH, et al., eds. *Medicine of the Fetus and Mother.* Philadelphia, Pa: JB Lippincott. 1992.
3. Tabov A, Philip J, Madsen M, et al. Randomized controlled trial of genetic amniocentesis in 4606 low-risk women. *Lancet.* 1986;1:1287–1293.
4. Hanson FW, Zorn EM, Tennany FR, et al. Amniocentesis before 15 weeks' gestation: outcome, risks and technical problems. *Am J Obstet Gynecol.* 1987;156:1524–1531.
5. Hobbins J, Green J. *Early Amniocentesis.* (Manuscript submitted for publication.)
6. Hahnemann N, Mohr J. Antenatal fetal diagnosis in the embryo by means of biopsy from the extra-embryonic membranes. *Bull Eur Soc Hum Genet.* 1968;2:33.
7. Brambati B, Oldrini A, Ferrazzi E, et al. Chorionic villus sampling: an analysis of the obstetric experience of 100 cases. *Prenatal Diagn.* 1987;7:157–169.
8. Rhoads GG, Jackson LG, Schlesselman SE, et al. The safety and efficacy of chorionic villus sampling for early prenatal diagnosis of cytogenetic abnormalities. *N Engl J Med.* 1989;320:609–617.
9. Canadian Collaborative CBS Amniocentesis Clinical Trial Group. Multicentre randomized clinical trial of chorion villus sampling and amniocentesis: first report. *Lancet.* 1989;1:1–6.
10. Ward RH, Lucas M. Chorionic villus sampling versus amniocentesis. *Lancet.* 1989;1:678.
11. Chorionic villus sampling or amniocentesis. *Lancet.* 1989;1:334–335.
12. Moise KJ, Carpenter RJ, Deter RL, et al. The use of fetal neuromuscular blockade during intrauterine procedures. *Am J Obstet Gynecol.* 1987;157:874–879.
13. Copel JA, Grannum PA, Harrison D, et al. The use of intravenous pancuronium bromide to produce fetal paralysis during intravascular transfusion. *Am J Obstet Gynecol.* 1988;158:170–171.
14. Bernstein HH, Chitkara U, Plosker H, et al. Use of atacurium besylate to arrest fetal activity during intravascular transfusions. *Obstet Gynecol.* 1988; 72:813–816.
15. Daffos F, Capella-Pavlovsky M, Forestier F. Fetal blood sampling during pregnancy with use of a needle guided by ultrasound: a study of 606 consecutive cases. *Am J Obstet Gynecol.* 1985;153:655–660.
16. Daffos F. Fetal blood sampling. Presented at the 27th annual meeting of the American College of Obstetrics & Gynecology. Atlanta, Georgia, May 1989.
17. Perry TB, Holbrook KA, Hoff MS, et al. Prenatal diag-

nosis of congenital nonbullous icthyosiform erythro-derma (lamellar icthyosis) *Prenat Diag.* 1987;7:145–155.

18. Golbus MS, Sagebiel RW, Filly RA, et al. Prenatal diagnosis of congenital bullous icthyosiform erythroderma (epidermolytic hyperkeratosis) by fetal skin biopsy. *N Engl J Med.* 1980;302:93–95.

19. Elias S, Mazur M, Sabbagha R, et al. Prenatal diagnosis of Harlequin ichthyosis. *Clin Genet.* 1980;17:275–280.

20. Rodeck CH, Eady RAJ, Gosden CM. Prenatal diagnosis of epidermolysis bullosa lethalis. *Lancet.* 1980;i:949–952.

21. Bauer EA, Ludmen MD, Goldberg JB, et al. Antenatal diagnosis of recessive dystrophic epidermolysis bullosa: collagenase expression in cultured fibroblasts as a biochemical marker. *J Invest Dermatol.* 1986;87:597–601.

22. Eady RA, Gunner DB, Garner A, et al. Prenatal diagnosis of oculocutaneous albinism by electron microscopy of fetal skin. *J Invest Dermatol.* 1983;80:210–212.

23. Westin B. Hysteroscopy in early pregnancy. *Lancet.* 1954; 267:872–876.

24. Galliant A, Leuken RP, Lindermann HJ. New instruments and new methods: a preliminary report about transcervical embryoscopy. *Endoscopy.* 1978;10:47–52.

25. Reece EA, Hobbins JC. Embryoscopy: an evolving technology for early prenatal diagnosis. In: Chapman M, Grudzinskas G, Chard T, eds. *The Embryo: Normal and Abnormal Development and Growth.* New York: Springer-Verlag; 1991:123–140.

26. Cullen MT, Reece EA, Whetham J, et al. Embryoscopy: description and utility of a new technique. *Am J Obstet Gynecol.* 1989;162:82–86.

27. Cullen MT, Reece EA, Viscarello RR, et al. Transcervical endoscopic visualization of prenatally diagnosed anomalies prior to second trimester termination. Proceedings of the Annual Meeting of the Society for Gynecologic Investigation, March 1989. San Diego.

28. Reece EA, Rothmensch S, Whetham J, et al. Embryoscopy: a closer look at first-trimester diagnosis and treatment. *Am J Obstet Gynecol.* 1992;166:775–780.

29. Reece EA. Embryoscopy: new developments in prenatal medicine. *Cur Opin Obstet Gynecol.* 1992;4:447–455.

30. Hobbins JC, Mahoney MJ. In utero diagnosis of hemo-globinopathies: technique for obtaining fetal blood. *N Engl J Med.* 1974;290:1065–1067.

31. Rodeck CH, Nicolaides KH. Fetoscopy. *Br Med Bull.* 1986;42:296–300.

32. Elias S. Fetoscopy in prenatal diagnosis. *Clin Perinatol.* 1983;10:357–367.

33. Reece EA, Goldstein I. New needle endoscopy permits first trimester transabdominal embryonic visualization and blood sampling. Society of Perinatal Obstetricians. 13th Annual Meeting. February 8–13, 1993. San Francisco. Abstract #51.

34. Dumez Y. *Embryoscopy and Congenital Malformations.* Proceedings of International Conference on Chorionic Villus Sampling and Early Prenatal Diagnosis. May 28–29, 1988, Athens, Greece.

35. Hobbins JC, Grannum P, Romero R, et al. Percutaneous umbilical blood sampling. *Am J Obstet Gynecol.* 1985; 152:1–6.

36. Moore KL. *The Developing Human. Clinically Oriented Embryology.* 4th ed. Philadelphia, Pa: WB Saunders Co; 1988.

37. Arey LB. *Development Anatomy.* 7th ed. (revised). Philadelphia, Pa: WB Saunders Co; 1974.

38. Hamilton WJ, Boyd JD, Mossman HW. *Human Embryology.* 3rd ed. Cambridge, UK: W. Heffner & Sons Ltd; 1964.

39. Reece EA, Pinter E, Leranth CZ, et al. Yolk sac failure in embryopathy due to hyperglycemia: horseradish peroxidase uptake in the assessment of yolk sac dysfunction. *Obstet Gynecol.* 1989;74:755–62.

40. Reece EA, Pinter E, Leranth CZ, et al. Ultrastructural analysis of malformations of the embryonic neural axis induced by hyperglycemic conceptus culture. *Teratology.* 1985;32:363–74.

41. Anderson WF. Human gene therapy: scientific and ethical considerations. *J Med Philos.* 1985;10:275–291.

42. Anderson WF. Prospects for human gene therapy. *Science;* 1984;226:401–409.

43. Kantoff PW, Gillis AP, McLachlin OR, et al. Expression of human adenosine deaminase in nonhuman primates after retrovirus-mediated gene transfer. *J Exp Med.* 1987; 166:219–234.

22

Doppler Ultrasound

Recent advances in Doppler ultrasound technology offer a unique opportunity to investigate the fetal hemodynamic state. The technique has been applied to the investigation of the fetal, fetoplacental, and uteroplacental circulations in normal and abnormal states. Application of Doppler ultrasound is not new in obstetrical practice. It has been used for many years to detect fetal heart activity and to determine fetal heart rate; this level of technology generates only audible Doppler signals.

PRINCIPLES OF DOPPLER IN OBSTETRICS

Sound

Sound is a form of mechanical kinetic energy that propagates in waves through a medium. The propagation is associated with pressure changes and causes alternating compression of particles in the medium. The wavelength of sound is composed of a single cycle of compression and refraction. The frequency of sound is the number of such cycles propagating in a second. One cycle is known as a hertz (Hz). Audible sound has a frequency ranging between 15 and 20 Hz. Ultrasound has a frequency greater than 20 Hz and is inaudible to the human ear. For obstetric diagnostic purposes, the frequency range of ultrasound is usually between 2 and 5 megahertz (MHz).

The Doppler Effect
When motion occurs between the source of ultrasound and the observer, there is a change in the observed frequency of the wave transmitted. When the source and the observer move closer, the frequency increases. When they move apart, the frequency decreases. This phenomenon was first described by Johann Christian Doppler[1] and is known as the Doppler effect. The change in frequency is known as the Doppler frequency shift, or Doppler shift. For example, when a train with a blaring whistle moves toward a stationary listener, the number of waves reaching the listener will be greater than when the train is stationary. Consequently, the frequency or pitch of sound reaching

the listener will be higher. Conversely, the pitch of sound will be less when the train moves away from the listener and will sound lower. Doppler shift will occur whether the source or observer moves.[2]

Backscattering
When an incident beam of ultrasound encounters the millions of moving cells in a circulation, it undergoes a reflection phenomenon. The red cells do not behave as point targets, but as volumes of distributed scatterers. The scattering power of blood becomes maximum at a hematocrit range of 25% to 30%.[3]

The Doppler Equation
The magnitude of the Doppler frequency shift (*Fd*) is expressed in the Doppler formula:

$$Fd = \frac{2F_0 \, v \cos \theta}{C}$$

In this equation, F_0 is the original frequency of the ultrasound beam (usually 3 to 5 MHz), v is the velocity of blood cells in the vessels studied, and θ is the incident angle between the ultrasound beam and the vessel and C, the velocity of sound in tissue. The cosine remains close to 1 as long as the angle is kept low, but at higher angles, especially more than 60 degrees, this factor has a significant impact.

Disadvantages
Flow is simply velocity times the cross-sectional area. It attempts to combine this derived value with two-dimensional diameters of the vessel, to calculate volume flow. Some factors must be considered before undertaking such measurements. Blood flow in vessels is not uniform. Close to the heart, however, there is relatively uniform blood flow, but as blood travels distally, in the umbilical circuit, for example, the gradual buildup of friction causes blood nearest the vessel wall to flow more slowly.[4]

Vessels are of different shapes. The aorta and pulmonary arteries are curved, and this may introduce errors into the measurements. Another factor of error in measurement is the cross-sectional area of a vessel that can be measured using the diameter of the vessel.

Any error in the measurement of the diameter is squared in the result.[4]

Doppler frequency shift signals that are returning from the circulation provide information on the speed or the velocity of the moving erythrocytes and, consequently, on the velocity of blood flow. The frequency shift is not the velocity. To determine the velocity, it is necessary to know the angle of the incident beam and to assume that the velocity of the ultrasound in the tissue and the transducer emission frequency are consistent during the examination.

In the velocity measurement technique it is necessary to measure the beam vessel angle to convert the frequency data into velocity data. The overall height of the velocity waveform depends on the angle between the ultrasound transducer and the blood vessel. Therefore, any measurements of the waveform should be angle-independent. The more acute the angle the greater the accuracy in determining velocity. Unfortunately, in order to measure vessel width most precisely (in attempting to make volume measurements), one must approach the vessel at right angles, which makes velocity measurements highly inaccurate. Conversely, approaching the vessel at an ideal angle for Doppler assessment requires that lateral resolution of the ultrasound equipment be put into play to measure vessel width. In many machines the lateral resolution is only accurate to 1 to 2 mm, which means that a vessel with a true diameter of 10 mm could give a reading of as much as 13 mm (1.5 mm on each side). Since this is squared in the volume formula, one could see the shortcomings of this technique. One such measurement is the percentage of time during which the waveform is in systole, calculated after the peaks and troughs are defined. This measurement is not commonly employed because of technologic limitations.

Modes of Doppler Ultrasonography

There are three modes of Doppler ultrasonography: continuous-wave (CW) Doppler, pulsed-wave (PW) Doppler, and two-dimensional Doppler color flow mapping (DCFM).

Continuous-Wave Doppler Ultrasound

Continuous-wave Doppler is so named because two transducers are used; one transmits and the other receives the reflected signals, with both operating continuously. The transducers are positioned so that the transmitted beam and the region most sensitive for receiving the backscattered echoes overlap. Any movement within this overlapped region will cause Doppler shift of the backscattered incident beam. Within this sensitive region a CW Doppler receives all Doppler shift signals; it cannot discriminate between different locations from which the Doppler signals are

originating. These instruments possess low acoustic energy output.

Pulsed-Wave Doppler Ultrasound

In the PW Doppler a single transducer element transmits pulses of the ultrasound beam. The machine transmits the signal 0.1% of the time; for the remaining 99.9% it receives returning echoes. The PW Doppler offers a major advantage because it has the ability to obtain flow velocity information from specific target vessels. The importance of the range resolution can be appreciated from the fact that it allows the collection of velocity information from fetal cardiac chambers, the aorta, and other deep vessels. The Doppler sample volume (DSV) is the three-dimensional region in the path of the transmitted ultrasound beam from which the Doppler shift signals are received.

Doppler Color Flow Mapping

In the DCFM mode two-dimensional flow patterns are superimposed on anatomic images in real time. Flow toward the transducer is usually red, and flow away from the transducer is blue.

HEMODYNAMIC EVALUATION BY DOPPLER ULTRASOUND

Doppler ultrasound has been used for several years to study the pattern of blood flow in fetal and maternal vessels. Vessels on both sides of the placenta have been studied, including the umbilical artery and vein, the fetal aorta, internal carotid, and branches of the maternal uterine artery. Both the uteroplacental and fetoplacental circulations are usually low-resistance systems in which downstream flow continues throughout the cardiac cycle. When vascular resistance increases, diastolic flow may decrease, stop, or even become reversed; this is reflected in the blood velocity waveform. The clinical value of Doppler is in identifying or predicting fetal growth retardation.

Doppler Indices

Gosling and King[5] first developed the pulsatility index (PI).

$$PI = \frac{systolic - diastolic}{mean}$$

It is the peak-to-peak height of the maximum-frequency envelope of the Doppler spectrum divided by the mean height over one cardiac cycle, both of which allow for reverse flow (Fig. 22–1).

Pourcelot[6] reported the resistance index (RI)

$$RI = \frac{systolic - diastolic}{systolic}$$

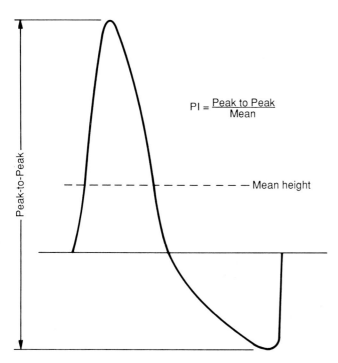

Figure 22–1. Pulsatility index (PI) is the peak-to-peak height of the waveform divided by the mean height over one cardiac cycle, with reverse flow allowed for in both.

while Stuart et al[7] described a simpler index of pulsatility called the A/B ratio, S/D ratio (Fig. 22–2).

$$S/D = \frac{\text{systolic}}{\text{diastolic}}$$

where S represents the peak systolic and D represents the end-diastolic maximum frequency shift. More equations were developed by others. The S/D ratio has been used most extensively, however, especially in the evaluation of the umbilical arterial hemodynamics.

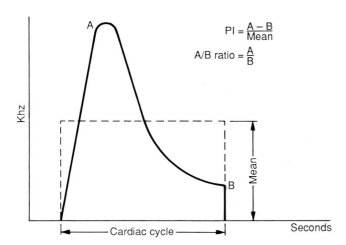

Figure 22–2. Schematic representation of a flow velocity waveform showing methods of calculation of pulsatility index (PI) and A/B ratio.

Sonoanatomy

Umbilical artery scanning is relatively simple. The fetal umbilical cord is identified within the amniotic fluid by the appearance of four parallel lines, using real-time ultrasound. The echo transducer is replaced with a CW Doppler instrument held in the same direction when the vessel has been identified. Doppler signals are then obtained from the vessel lying along the beam. The CW Doppler device is replaced with a range-gated, PW instrument to obtain signals from the individual blood vessel.

When the sample volume is set within the vein, a continuous low-frequency Doppler signal is heard. When the range gate is within the artery, a pulsatile high-frequency Doppler signal is heard. Doppler signals can also be obtained from vessels without real-time imaging. A CW Doppler device can be used to scan the maternal abdomen and locate the vessel by the pattern of an artery or a vein. The color Doppler makes it easier to recognize vessels by using the color as an indicator of blood steam in the vessels.

The spectral analysis computer program contains a section that automatically computes these waveform parameters. The program first computes the time, varying the waveform spectrum. It then outlines the waveform, and finally it identifies the individual cardiac cycles and computes the pulsatility index, percent systole, and heart rate. The maximum velocity envelope is represented by a solid line, and the peaks and troughs are identified by crosses. The extracted parameters are printed below their corresponding cardiac cycles.[8]

CHARACTERIZATION OF BLOOD FLOW IN THE VESSELS

Blood flow has traditionally been considered in terms of pressure and resistance. The velocity of blood flow is determined by a pressure gradient. If the resistance is high, the incident pressure pulse is highly reflected and returns to cancel the latter part of the pressure pulse. The result is zero or even negative pressures, which results in low or even reversed flow in diastole. If the vessels have low resistance, the pressure pulse wave is almost unaltered when high diastolic flow is present. The velocity waveform provides important physiologic indicators about the pumping heart, vessel wall condition, and peripheral resistance.[9]

The PI is the degree of pulse waveform damping, and it is indicative of downstream impedance to flow. For example, the internal carotid artery, which has a low termination impedance, has a PI of 1 to 2. In the femoral, popliteal, and tibial arteries, under resting conditions the PI ranges from 5 to 15 and falls to 1 to

2 after leg exercise, presumably as a result of arteriolar vasodilatation. Arterial waveforms can be recorded from various arteries; however, there are differences in the waveform position relative to zero flow line. The PI of the umbilical artery in the normal fetus declines from a value of 1.2 at 26 weeks to 0.8 at term. The PI in a fetus associated with pregnancy complications is elevated, indicating a greater placental impedance.

Umbilical Artery

Recording the umbilical artery's velocity waveform provides a direct measure of placental flow resistance. The systolic cardiac impulse propels blood down the arterial tree, and flow is maintained by pulsatile energy stored and then released from elastic vessel walls. Flow results from pressure acting against peripheral resistance. The extent of downstream impedance determines the degree of reflection of the incident pressure wave. The later diastolic part of the waveform is affected by the reflected wave. High impedance is associated with greater pressure-pulse-wave reflection and reduced or even reversed blood flow velocities in diastole (high A/B ratio). If reflection is low, high forward flow velocities continue (low A/B ratio). The A/B ratio provides a measure of impedance or resistance to blood flow downstream from the point of recording. A/B ratio, the angle of the ultrasound beam to the artery is unknown. Absolute velocity is thus not measured. What is measured is the ratio of systolic-to-diastolic, since the incident angle remains constant. By altering the transducer direction it is possible to estimate the maximum systolic velocity if the incident angle is within the range ±26 degrees of the direction to the flow.[9]

The fetal placental vascular tree is normally a low-resistance bed; resistance decreases with increasing gestational age, indicating a decrease in placental flow resistance relative to the proportion of cardiac output directed to the umbilical arteries (Fig. 22–3).

Uterine Arteries

When the Doppler probe is moved to the lower quadrants and to the parauterine area, the pelvic vessels can be identified. The nonpregnant uterine artery is similar to other vessels of the lower extremity in that it demonstrates high resistance (eg, zero, or reverse diastolic velocity and a prominent diastolic notch). In most women who are not pregnant there is persistent end-diastolic velocity at the end of the secretory phase. If the woman becomes pregnant, no further changes are seen in the first trimester and the systolic to diastolic ratio remains around 8.0.[9] Dramatic changes begin around the 14th week of pregnancy and culminate in the creation of the vessel that has a large persistent

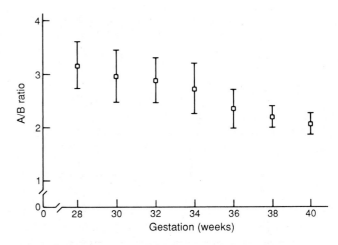

Figure 22–3. The mean (±SD) *A/B* ratio at each 2-week period in 15 normal pregnancies studied serially. *From Trudinger BJ, Warwick BG, Cook CM, et al. Fetal umbilical artery flow velocity waveforms and placental resistance: clinical significance. Br J Obstet Gynaecol. 1985;92:23–30, with permission.*

end-diastolic velocity and no diastolic notch. The rate of change may vary among women and also between the two uterine arteries.[9] One artery may be the primary provider to the placenta and will undergo these changes much earlier than the antiplacental vessel. This phenomenon may be of interest in women who develop preeclampsia. The evolutionary process of the uterine artery should be completed at week 26 of pregnancy.

Schulman[9] calculated a systolic to diastolic ratio of less then 2.7, which is an average of left and right uterine arcuate vessels, and also the complete disappearance of the diastolic notch. The physiologic basis of these changes is the development of the intervillous space and the trophoblastic invasion of the myometrial portion of the spiral arteries. The end-diastolic portion of the waveform is primarily influenced by the intervillous space perfusion; the diastolic notch is a marker of vascular tone at the myometrial level or higher.

DOPPLER FLOW AND INTRAUTERINE-GROWTH-RETARDED FETUSES

Umbilical Artery

Trudinger et al[10] studied umbilical artery flow velocity waveforms in intrauterine growth-retarded (IUGR) fetuses. The newborn weight of 43 infants was less than the 10th percentile and the birth weight of 22 infants was less than the 5th percentile. They demonstrated that the A/B ratio in 85% of the cases was above the 95th percentile. The authors, however, also found that 17.6% of the fetuses with A/B ratio above the 95th percentile did not become growth-retarded. The increase in A/B ratio was due to decreasing diastolic flow rather than to increasing systolic flow, resulting from high placental blood resistance.

Schulman and coworkers[11] reported the umbilical velocity wave S/D ratio in normal pregnancies declined from 2.8 at 25 weeks' gestation to 2.2 at 41 weeks' gestation. In pregnancies that resulted in a small-for-gestational age fetus the ratio is significantly higher, showing an average S/D ratio of 3.8 at 29 weeks' gestation with a decline to 3.0 at 40 weeks' gestation. Fleischer and others[12] determined that the peak S/D ratio of equal to or greater than 3 was defined as abnormal, as a reflection of vascular resistance distal to the point of measurement. The sensitivity and the specificity were 78% and 83%, respectively. The positive predictive value, however, was only 49%.

Umbilical Venous Flow

Gill and Kossof[13] studied the umbilical venous flow in normal and IUGR fetuses using pulsed Doppler techniques. The rate of umbilical venous flow increases steadily with gestational age and in parallel with fetal growth until a maximum is reached at 37 to 38 weeks, after which there is a reduction. The flow per kilogram of fetal weight (the umbilical venous flow measured in mL/min/kg) varies much less with gestational age. It remains constant until week 35, with an average of 120 mL/min/kg. Beyond 35 weeks a gradual decrease is seen, with an average value at 40 weeks of 90 mL/min/kg.

In growth-retarded fetuses the venous flow decreases. Low flow values in intrauterine growth retardation ranges from 69 to 85 mL/min/kg.[9] A formula of flow deficit was also generated.

$$\text{Flow deficit} = \frac{\text{median flow} - \text{actual flow}}{\text{median flow}}$$

The relationship between total flow deficit and perinatal complication showed that with increasing deficit IUGR increased, with an accuracy of 88%. The sensitivity, specificity, and negative predictive values were 70%, 90%, and 95%, respectively. The positive predictive value for flow deficit, however, was 50% in IUGR.

The flow is expressed in relation to the fetal weight; in normal pregnancies the results are relatively consistent and range from 110 to 125 mL/min/kg. The IUGR fetuses, however, have diminished umbilical vein blood flow.

Uterine Arteries

Brosens et al[14] studied the physiologic response of the vessels of the placental bed in normal and IUGR fetuses. The spiral artery opens into the intervillous space in the placenta. In every case there is complete absence of muscular and elastic tissue throughout the arterial wall. The lumen is widely dilated and tortuous. In IUGR fetuses, however, acute atherosclerosis affects the arteries.[15]

Most pregnant women who develop preeclampsia will demonstrate an abnormal uterine artery (UA) velocity wave pattern. There will be an elevated uterine artery S/D ratio, and a prominent diastolic notch will be present. This will be associated with an abnormal umbilical artery waveform in at least 60% of the cases. Earlier studies suggested that in women destined to develop preeclampsia the diastolic notch and S/D ratio are present since early pregnancy.

Campbell and colleagues[16] reported that an abnormal uterine waveform had a sensitivity and specificity of 68% and 69%, respectively, with a positive predictive value of 87%. Thus, while most complications were detected, a normal examination did not exclude pathology.

Fetal Aorta

The fetal aorta seemed to offer the potential to estimate body flow. Normal values have ranged from 191 to 276 mL/min/kg. The probable reason for this wide range is that there is a very low level of diastolic velocity, which creates the potential for significant calculation deviations. Jouppila and Kirkinen[17] studied blood velocity waveforms in the thoracic aorta. The mean velocity was 26.5 cm/sec (24.1 to 27.9 cm/sec); in cases of IUGR fetuses with distress the mean velocity decreased to 15.7 cm/sec (12.9 to 16.7 cm/sec). The mean end-diastolic velocity was 10.9 cm/sec and decreased to 1.9 in growth-retarded fetuses with distress. When there is absent or reversed diastolic flow, the aortic velocity waveform may be helpful as a predictor of fetal jeopardy. Griffin et al[18] studied the Doppler flow waveform in the descending thoracic aorta. In IUGR fetuses there was a significant reduction in the end-diastolic velocities and an increase in the pulsatility index. The normal fetal aorta pulsatility index

$$(\text{PI} = A - B/\text{mean})$$

was: mean 1.83 with a standard deviation of ± 0.22; and of the growth-retarded fetuses the PI was 2.78, ± 0.60. The authors determined also that the normal A/B ratio of the fetal aorta was 6.2, ± 1.9; the normal resistance index (RI = $A - B/A$) was 0.82, ± 0.05.

Fetal Carotid Vessels

Studies[19] have suggested that in some cases of fetal growth retardation there may be an increase in carotid velocity flow. This appears to complement the basic physiologic studies carried out in pregnant ewes that demonstrated a relative increase in brain blood flow in the fetus subjected to maternal–placental embolization. Evaluation of the fetal blood flow has been attempted in an effort to confirm the theory of head-sparing in growth retardation. If there is preferential blood flow to the brain, there would be maintenance, or perhaps even augmentation, of cerebral blood flow. Thus far, the carotid arteries are the cerebral vessels that can be identified reliably and that are straight enough for true volume flow measurements.[4]

These vessels, however, are too narrow to measure accurately, and if there is compensation for the compromised blood flow from the anastomotic circle of Willis, there will be reduced sensitivity in measurements.[4] Tonge and coworkers[4] compared the PI of the internal carotid artery with the umbilical artery. In IUGR fetuses, an increase in umbilical artery PI was identified concomitantly with a reduced carotid artery index.

Investigators are flooding the literature and various perinatal meetings with reports of Doppler's clinical utility in IUGR, Rh disease, twin to twin size discrepancies, diabetes, lupus (and when lupuslike antibodies are present), and in various fetal anomalies. Studies have included sampling sites in the fetus, in addition to the commonly sampled umbilical area, such as the middle cerebral artery, the internal carotid artery, the pulmonary artery, ascending aorta, ductus arteriosus, the descending aorta, across the A-V valves, the renal artery, the femoral artery and very recently, various fetal veins. Although initial reports tended to be very positive regarding the clinical efficacy of these evaluations, more recent investigations have begun to compare the usefulness of Doppler studies with other established indicators of fetal conditions, such as nonstress testing (NST) and the biophysical profile (BPP).

Thus far it appears that in IUGR fetuses initially there is a decrease in resistance in the cerebral vessels resulting in an increase in the diastolic component of the middle cerebral artery waveform. This causes a decrease in the pulsatility index, *S/D* ratio, and resistance index. As the deprivation worsens the indices begin to reverse to what would normally be present in appropriately grown fetuses. This, of course, can be misleading. In severe compromise the indices rise above normal, while the vessels supplying the lower part of the fetal body display increased resistance. Descending aorta, renal arteries, and forward arteries all show abnormally high indices. The umbilical artery, which reflects resistance in the placenta and indirectly the status of the overall fetal circulation, will display first an increased PI, *S/D* ratio, and resistance index in the face of fetal compromise, then later an absent end-diastolic flow. Very occasionally, in severely growth-retarded fetuses, there is the reversed end-diastolic

flow. Rarely does a fetus survive once the condition has progressed to this point.

Some physicians are beginning to use umbilical artery waveform indices clinically. It appears that in a sequence of progressive hypoxia in growth-retarded fetuses, the umbilical artery waveform indices rise about 95 confidence levels before fetal heart rate monitoring and fetal movement and breathing are affected. By the time there is absent diastolic flow other clinical parameters become abnormal. Therefore, although there have been exceptions to this scenario, a normal UA waveform should be reassuring in the presence of a nonreactive NST, which has an inherently high false-positive rate. On the other hand, an increased *S/D* ratio, for example, should not cause the clinician to deliver a fetus prematurely if the other clinical parameters are reassuring. It should, however, act as a signal to the clinician to increase fetal surveillance.

In conditions, other than IUGR the merit of Doppler waveform analysis of the umbilical artery is less clear. For example, in Rh disease waveform analysis anywhere in the fetal arterial circulation has been a poor predictor of fetal anemia. There is recent evidence, however, that measurement of Doppler flow in the inferior vena cava has some promise in this condition.

In diabetes, Doppler waveform has had mixed reviews. For example, in diabetics with end organ disease umbilical artery waveform is sometimes abnormal, but generally when the fetus is under grown. In twin size discrepancy sometimes there is a difference in waveform between the twins, while in other cases where twin to twin transfusion syndrome is documented at birth, there is no difference in umbilical artery waveform.

In some fetal structural anomalies UA *S/D* ratios were elevated and in others it is completely normal. Trisomy 21 fetuses tend to have normal waveforms, while trisomy 13 and 18 do not.

REFERENCES

1. White DN. Johann Christian Doppler and his effect: a brief history. *Ultrasound Med Biol.* 1982;8:583–591.
2. Maulik D. Biologic effects of ultrasound. *Clin Obstet Gynecol.* 1989;32:645–659.
3. Atkinson P. An ultrasonic fluctuation velocimeter. *Ultrasonics.* 1975;13:275–278.
4. Tonge HM, Wladimiroff JW, Noordam MJ, et al. Blood flow velocity waveform in the descending aorta: comparison between normal and growth-retarded pregnancies. *Obstet Gynecol.* 1986;67:851–855.
5. Gosling RG, King DH. Ultrasound angiology. In: Macus AW, Anderson J, eds. *Arteries and Veins.* Edinburgh: Churchill-Livingstone, 1975.
6. Pourcelot L. Application clinique de l'examen Doppler

transcutance. In: Pourcelot L, ed. *Velocimetric Ultrasonote Doppler*. IN-SERM; 1974:213.

7. Stuart B, Drumm J, FitzGerald DE, et al. Fetal blood velocity waveforms in normal pregnancy. *Br J Obstet Gynaecol.* 1980;87:780–785.

8. McCallum WD, Williams CS, Napeal S, et al. Fetal blood velocity waveforms. *Am J Obstet Gynecol.* 1978;132:425–429.

9. Schulman H. The clinical implications of Doppler ultrasound analysis of the uterine and umbilical arteries. *Am J Obstet Gynecol.* 1987;156:889–893.

10. Trudinger BJ, Giles WB, Cook CM. Ureteroplacental blood flow velocity-time waveforms in normal and complicated pregnancy. *Br J Obstet Gynaecol.* 1985;92:39–45.

11. Schulman H, Fleischer A, Stern W, et al. Umbilical velocity wave ratios in human pregnancy. *Am J Obstet Gynecol.* 1984;148:985–989.

12. Fleischer A, Schulman H, Farmakides G, et al. Umbilical artery velocity waveforms and intrauterine growth retardation. *Am J Obstet Gynecol.* 1985;151:502–505.

13. Gill RW, Kossof G. Umbilical venous flow in normal and complicated pregnancy. *Ultrasound Med Biol.* 1984; 10:349–363.

14. Brosens I, Robertson WB, Dixon HG. The physiological response of the vessels of the placental bed to normal pregnancy. *J Pathol Bacteriol.* 1967;93:569–578.

15. Brosens I, Dixon HG, Robertson WB. Fetal growth retardation and the arteries of the placental bed. *Br J Obstet Gynaecol.* 1977;84:656–663.

16. Campbell S, Pearce JM, Hackett G, et al. Qualitative assessment of uteroplacental blood flow: early screening test for high risk pregnancies. *Obstet Gynecol.* 1986; 68:649–652.

17. Jouppila P, Kirkinen P. Blood velocity waveforms of fetal aorta in normal and hypertensive pregnancies. *Obstet Gynecol.* 1986;67:856–860.

18. Griffin D, Bilardo K, Masini, et al. Doppler blood flow waveforms in the descending thoracic aorta of the human fetus. *Br J Obstet Gynaecol.* 1984;91:997–1006.

19. Wladimiroff JW, Wijngaard JA, Begali S, et al. Cerebral and umbilical arterial blood flow velocity waveform in normal and growth-retarded pregnancies. *Obstet Gynecol.* 1987;69:705–709.

23

Gynesonography

INTRODUCTION

Diagnostic images of the female pelvic organs can be obtained by using either transvaginal or transabdominal ultrasound. Transvaginal ultrasound has gained popularity with its technical advances in imaging and instrumentation and will be the focus of this chapter. Transvaginal ultrasound was first used in cases of infertility[1] for follicle surveillance in ovulation induction and oocyte retrieval for in vitro fertilization.[2] Subsequent applications of this technology included early pregnancy detection and evaluation.[3,4] Transvaginal ultrasound is used for diagnostic gynecology, since it is now possible to obtain a panoramic view of the pelvic area.[5–7] Furthermore, this approach avoids the thick abdominal wall and urine-filled bladder, which both increase sound attenuation and displace the region of interest. Transvaginal probes, generally of higher frequency, have better resolution as the probe moves closer to the objects of interest, unobstructed by layers of fat and muscles.[8–12]

Disadvantages of the transvaginal technique include patient uneasiness, which minimizes when the procedure is adequately explained to the patient and her questions answered prior to the examination.[2] Large masses greater than 7 to 10 cm or a mass relatively far from the vaginal fornix may be difficult to visualize. In addition, it is sometimes difficult for the transvaginal probe to penetrate the vagina in elderly women or young girls.[13,14]

PREPARATION OF PATIENTS

A detailed explanation of the procedure to the patient is important. The patient should know that transvaginal ultrasonography is similar to the bimanual pelvic examination but that there is probably less discomfort. Furthermore, there is no need to consume large amounts of liquid and wait for the bladder to fill. The use of a sterile rubber glove or condom on the transvaginal probe can virtually eliminate the risk of contamination and infection.[3,12]

THE TRANSVAGINAL PLANES

With transvaginal scanning, the uterus can be imaged in several different planes:[4,11] 1) sagittal, longitudinal, or long-axis planes (Fig. 23–1); 2) axial or cross-sectional planes (Fig. 23–2); and 3) coronal plane.

The uterine or endometrial line, which is echodense in appearance, should be imaged in its long-axis or sagittal plane (Fig. 23–3). The transvaginal probe enters the vaginal route at an angle of 45 degrees to the posterior fornix (or vs the cul-de-sac); then the probe is angled gently anteriorly or posteri-

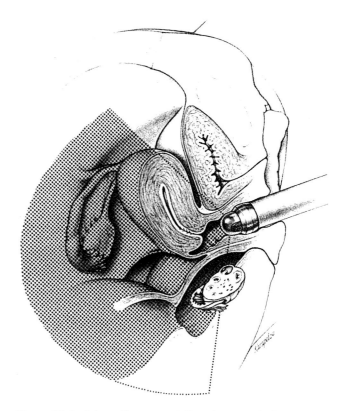

Figure 23–1. Schematic representation of transvaginal ultrasound showing the relationship between the ultrasound transducer and the uterus and bladder. The shaded area illustrates a sagittal view. (*From Zimmer EZ, Timor-Tritsch IE, and Rottem S. The technique of transvaginal sonography. In: Timor-Tritsch IE and Rottem S, eds.* Transvaginal Sonography. *New York: Elsevier; 1991:69, with permission*).

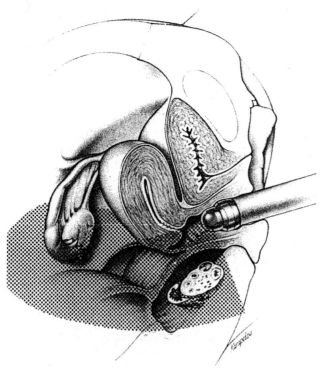

Figure 23–2. The shaded area illustrates an axial view of the same schematic representation presented in Figure 23–1. (*From Zimmer EZ, Timor-Tritsch IE, and Rottem S. The technique of transvaginal sonography. In: Timor-Tritsch IE and Rottem S, eds.* Transvaginal Sonography. *New York: Elsevier; 1991: 68, with permission*).

orly, depending on the position of the uterus (anteflexed or retroflexed).

The uterus and the endometrial line can be visualized in the axial plane once the entire endometrial line is identified, by turning the probe 90 degrees. Serial sections of the uterus from the fundus toward the cervix are obtained. In the normal uterus the endometrium should be seen in the midline, either in the longitudinal or in the axial planes.[4,11] Imaging of the

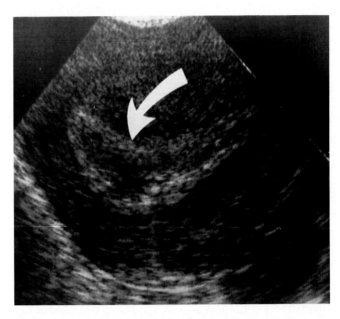

Figure 23–4. Semisagittal scan of the uterus. The curved arrow outlines the endometrium in a normal woman during the reproductive years.

uterus and the endometrium can be useful when the probe is either inserted or withdrawn from the vaginal fornices.[3,8,12] The uterus should also be visualized in semisaggital (Fig. 23–4), semiaxial, and semicoronal planes. Views of these planes are obtained when the long-axis plane is seen, and the probe can be turned 90 degrees and directed to both sides of the uterus.

Images of the cervix can be obtained after the probe is withdrawn into the midvagina once the

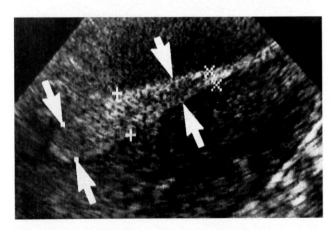

Figure 23–3. Sagittal scan of the uterus. Note the large thick arrows that outline the endometrium and the calipers(×'s) measuring the endometrial thickness near the internal cervical os.

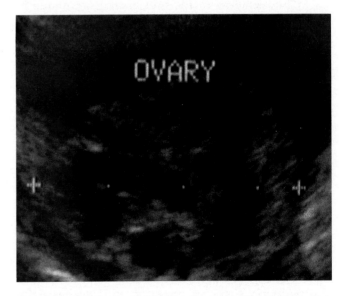

Figure 23–5. Cross-sectional view of an ovary demonstrating multiple follicles as evidenced by areas of echolucency throughout the substance of the ovary. The calipers(+'s) are placed at the borders of the ovary.

uterus and the endometrium are adequately visualized along the short- and long-axis planes. Now the entire view of the cervix can be seen in a long-axis view. When the probe is turned 90 degrees, the axial, or cross-sectional, view of the cervix can be visualized.[12]

During a woman's childbearing years, normal ovaries can be identified by directing the probe toward either side of the uterus. The ovaries can be located medially by using the iliac vessels as a marker. The ovaries are echodense in appearance and spherical in shape, with small sonolucent areas called *follicles* distributed throughout (Fig. 23–5).

REFERENCES

1. Schwimer SR, Lebovic J. Transvaginal pelvic ultrasonography. *J Ultrasound Med.* 1984;3:381–383.
2. Schwimer SR, Lebovic J. Transvaginal pelvic ultrasonography: accuracy in follicle and cyst size determination. *J Ultrasound Med.* 1985;4:61–63.
3. Timor-Tritsch IE, Rottem S, Thaler I. Review of transvaginal ultrasonography: a description with clinical application. *Ultrasound Q.* 1988;6:1–34.
4. Goldstein RB. Endovaginal sonography in very early pregnancy: new observation. *Radiology.* 1990;176:7–8.
5. O'Brien WF, Buck DR, Nash JD. Evaluation of sonography in the initial assessment of gynecologic patient. *Am J Obstet Gynecol.* 1984;149:598–602.
6. Goldstein SR. Incorporating endovaginal ultrasonography into the overall gynecologic examination. *Am J Obstet Gynecol.* 1990;162:625–632.
7. Timor-Tritsch IE. Is office use of vaginal ultrasonography feasible? *Am J Obstet Gynecol.* 1990;162:983–985.
8. Pennell RG, Baltarowitch OH, Kurtz AB, et al. Complicated first-trimester pregnancies: evaluation with endovaginal ultrasound versus transabdominal technique. *Radiology.* 1987;165:79–83.
9. Mendelson EB, Bohm-Velez M, Joseph N, et al. Endometrial abnormalities: evaluation with transvaginal sonography. *AJR.* 1988;150:139–142.
10. Rottem S, Thaler I, Goldstein SR, et al. Transvaginal sonographic technique: targeted organ scanning without resorting to "planes." *J Clin Ultrasound.* 1990;18:243–247.
11. Dodson MG, Deter RL. Definition of anatomical planes for use in transvaginal sonography. *J Clin Ultrasound.* 1990;18:239–242.
12. Timor-Tritsch IE, Rottem S, Elgali S. How transvaginal sonography is done. In: Timor-Tritsch IE, Rottem S, eds. *Transvaginal Sonography.* New York: Elsevier; 1988:15–25.
13. Mendelson EB, Bohm-Velez M, Joseph N, et al. Gynecologic imaging: comparison of transabdominal and transvaginal sonography. *Radiology.* 1988;166:321–324.
14. Coleman BG, Anger PH, Grumbach K, et al. Transvaginal and transabdominal sonography: prospective comparison. *Radiology.* 1988;168:639–643.

The Cervix

SONOANATOMY

The cervix appears more echodense in comparison to the body of the uterus.[1] During pregnancy, the internal os and the cervical canal are easily identified if the position of the uterus is known. The longitudinal plane of the cervical canal can be visualized as a thin echo-free line between the internal and the external cervical os, especially in cases of a dilated cervical canal. The entire cylindrical cervix in the longitudinal plane is approximately 4 cm. The entire dilated cervical canal, or specifically the internal os, can be assessed and measured in multiple cross-sectional planes of the cervix. The shape of the cervical canal should be assessed in high-risk patients. The internal os may also be dilated; it appears as a ballooning, *U* shape, or funneling, *V* shape.[1] In pregnancy the transvaginal probe should always be placed outside and around the cervix, and never inside the cervical canal.

SONOPATHOLOGY

Ultrasonographic examination of the cervix via transvaginal sonography has become popular in the second and third trimesters of pregnancy. It is used in the second trimester primarily to rule out cervical incompetence,[1] and for diagnosing placenta previa and malpresentations in the third trimester.

Sonographic examination of the cervix became part of the routine gynecologic evaluation of the female genitalia, to rule out cervical pathology, such as cysts, cervical pregnancy, or tumors.[2] Monitoring cervical dynamics may identify early changes in cervical dilation, necessitating cerclage procedures; it may even prevent unnecessary intervention.[2]

The Uterine Body

SONOANATOMY

The first step in using transvaginal pelvic scanning is identification of the uterus. The uterus is the most dominant structure in the normal female pelvis, usually in the midline, and relatively easy to visualize in the lower abdomen. The uterus appears prominent

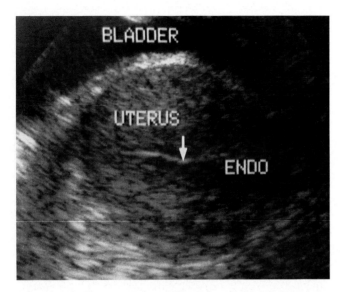

Figure 23–6. Cross-sectional scan of the female pelvis that reveals the bladder anteriorly, the globular uterus inferior to the bladder, and the midline echo representing the endometrium in a postmenopausal patient.

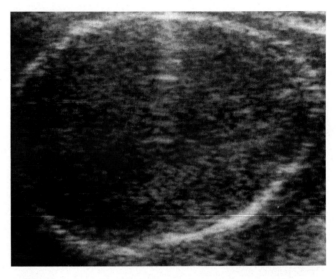

Figure 23–7. Transvaginal examination of a uterus demonstrating a large fibromyoma. Note the relatively homogeneous nature of the structure but, more important, the bright echodense borders of the fibromyoma representing calcifications within this structure.

during the reproductive period of the woman. It is more difficult to visualize the endometrial line in the prepubertal and menopausal period because it is very thin and barely echogenic in appearance (Fig. 23–6).

The normal corpus uteri in the patient of child-bearing age appears in longitudinal scans as a pear-shaped structure, 5 to 7 cm long. The entire uterine body appears in low echogenicity, and the central midline of the endometrium is identified with higher-intensity echoes.

The postmenopausal uterus is significantly smaller than it is during the reproductive years.[3] It has a uniform echogenicity, with the endometrial line barely distinguishable from the endometrial structure. The prepubertal uterus, similar to the postmenopausal uterus, is small and homogenous, with the endometrial line barely seen.

SONOPATHOLOGY

The sonographic assessment of the uterine body is necessary to identify intramural fibromas, the most common lesion of the corpus uteri. Fibromyomas, including any complicating degenerative changes, are readily detected by transvaginal sonography. Fibroids as small as 1 cm in diameter can be recognized.[4] Larger fibroids of the uterus are typically irregular and can contain either echo-free areas or echogenic areas, some with acoustic shadowing, which give the overall fibroid a nonhomogenous appearance (Fig. 23–7). Sonolucent cavities are sometimes present in the center.[4] Changes in uterine size, particularly when accompa-

nied by profuse intracavitary fluid, should alert the examiner of a malignant process.[5-9]

The postmenopausal uterus is small (Fig. 23–6), with absence of the endometrial line. This finding provides important information to the clinician about the possibility of malignancy.[4]

The Endometrium

SONOANATOMY

Endometrial thickening, as visualized by transvaginal ultrasonography, reflects the hormonal status of the patient. During the proliferative phase, the endometrium thickens between 4 to 8 mm and is iso-echogenic or slightly hyperechogenic in appearance relative to the outer myometrium.[8]

The ultrasound signs of proliferative endometrium include a triple-line sign, echo-free appearance, and minimal or absent posterior acoustic enhancement[9] (Fig. 23–8). The endometrium achieves a width of between 8 mm and 16 mm in the secretory phase.[8] The signs of secretory endometrium include absent triple-line sign, echo-dense functional layer, and strong posterior acoustic enhancement[10] (Fig. 23–9). The echogenicity of the secretory phase probably relates to increased mucus and glycogen within the glands, as well as to the increased number of inter-

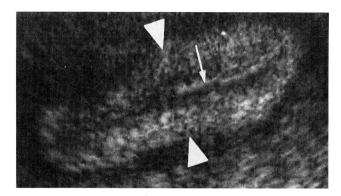

Figure 23–8. Sagittal scan of the uterus during the proliferative phase of the menstrual cycle. The large arrowheads indicate the walls of the endometrium undergoing proliferation; the small arrow indicates the midline echo of the uterus. This pattern is in contrast with the homogeneous echo pattern seen in the secretory phase of the menstrual cycle.

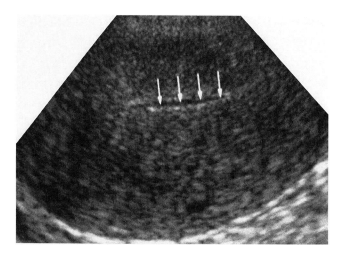

Figure 23–10. Sagittal scan of a uterus following menstruation. The walls of the endometrial cavity are almost in complete apposition to each other, except for a thin echolucent space (arrows).

faces created by tortuous glands presented in the secretory phase.[8]

The endometrium typically achieves its greatest thickness in the midsecretory phase of normal regular cycle, measuring approximately 14 mm in width. In the longitudinal plane of the uterus the single-line endometrium represents the postmenstrual phase (Fig. 23–10). Later on, in the early proliferative stage, corresponding to day 8 of the normal cycle, the sonographic endometrium appears as a thin echo-free functional layer, separated by the endometrial canal. There are well-defined triple lines and a thick echo-free functional layer separated by the endometrial canal in the late proliferative stage, which corresponds to day 14 of the normal cycle.[10]

The sonographic images demonstrate loss of triple line in the secretory endometrium, which corre-

sponds to day 25 of the cycle. The functional endometrium is echodense in appearance, with strong posterior acoustic enhancement.[10] The largest increase in endometrial thickness occurs between the early and the late proliferative stages; there is less of an increase between the proliferative and the secretory phases.

The endometrium appears as an echogenic interrupted layer of 1 to 4 mm in total anterior–posterior width during the menstrual phase[8] (Fig. 23–11).

The normal endometrium in the postmenopausal woman should be thin and histologically atrophic. Postmenopausal women taking estrogen or estrogen–progesterone replacement, however, may have a thick endometrium. The actual range of normal thickness

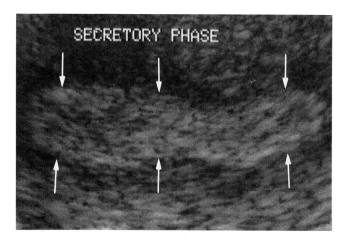

Figure 23–9. Transverse scan of a uterus by transvaginal ultrasound, which reveals the thickened endometrium (arrows) indicating the secretory phase of the cycle. Note the uniform echogenicity within the endometrium.

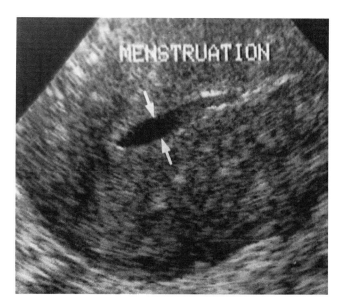

Figure 23–11. Sagittal scan of the uterus during menstruation. The arrows indicate the uterine walls. The echolucent area in the center of the uterus represents menstrual blood.

and texture has not been reported to date for this group of patients.

CLINICAL APPLICATION

It is impossible to definitely differentiate between benign and malignant endometrial lesions, based on transvaginal ultrasound findings, since only histology will provide a definite result. There are cases suggestive of abnormality, however, for which diagnostic curettage may be necessary. Transvaginal ultrasound can be useful to monitor high-risk patients. Endometrium greater than 12-mm thick in the perimenopausal period should be an indication for further evaluation, whereas in postmenopausal patients, endometrium over 8 mm should be considered abnormal.[6,8] An abnormally thick endometrium indicates the need in postmenopausal women for a diagnostic curettage, since this may represent a precancerous or cancerous lesion.[11] Transvaginal ultrasonography offers a potential tool for early detection of endometrial changes, especially in an at-risk population.[2]

Occasionally, incomplete curettage, unclotted blood, or fluid within the lumen can be easily visualized by transvaginal sonography. Problems related to an intrauterine contraceptive device (Fig. 23–12), such as a missing string, malposition, or incomplete removal, are diagnosed using transvaginal ultrasonography.

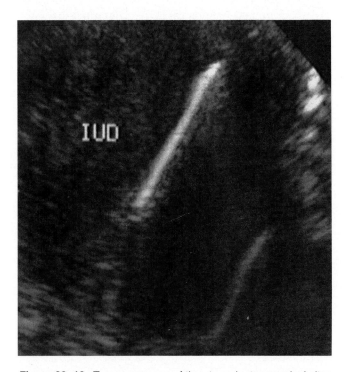

Figure 23–12. Transverse scan of the uterus by transvaginal ultrasound, which reveals an echodense foreign object, consistent with an intrauterine contraceptive device.

Malpai et al[12] studied the relationship between endometrial hyperplasia proven histologically, and thickening of the endometrium measured sonographically. They concluded that patients with endometrial hyperplasia had a mean endometrial thickness of 18.8 mm (range 8 to 45 mm) versus 5.4 mm (range 2 to 10 mm) in the normal group. New data support the value of ultrasonography in monitoring endometrial changes.

Polypoid tumors may cause an apparent distension of the endometrial lumen. Tumors extending into the myometrium can appear either echodense or echofree relative to the normal myometrial echogenicity.

The Ovary

SONOANATOMY

Scanning of the ovaries with the transvaginal probe has been valuable in: 1) infertility: measuring and assessing follicle growth and development, assessing the fluid collected in the cul-de-sac, and identification of the corpus luteum; 2) gynecology: early detection of simple, or multilocular cysts, or semisolid or solid masses (Fig. 23–13 and Fig. 23–14).

The normal ovary appears as an oval-shaped echogenic mass in the lateral fornices close to the iliac vessels. The ovaries contain a few spherical spaces, or follicles, that are small in diameter and scattered peripherally. Several follicles of different sizes normally

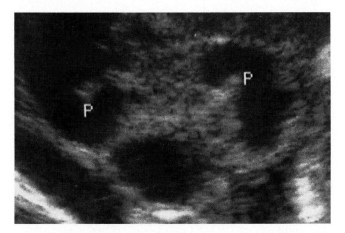

Figure 23–13. An ovary with semisolid and semicystic areas. Note the projections within the cystic cavities representing papillae (P). Below the semicystic ovary, note the iliac vessel that courses inferiorly and in its usual proximity. These ovarian findings suggest a neoplastic lesion.

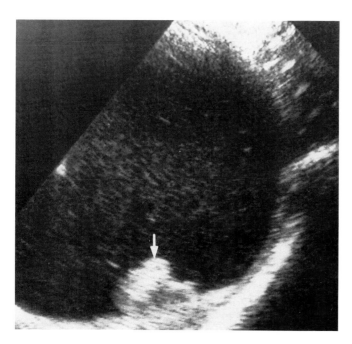

Figure 23–14. Cross section of an ovary, demonstrating the finger-like projection arising from the capsule of the ovary. This projection probably represents a papilla; overall findings suggest a neoplasm.

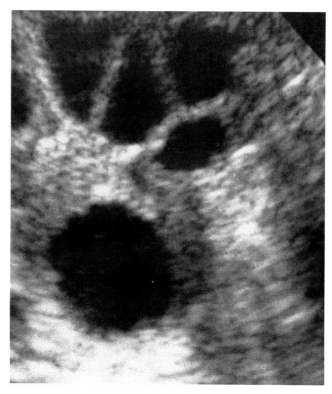

Figure 23–15. Ultrasound picture of an ovary, demonstrating multiple follicles within the ovary's substance. Note the dominant follicle inferiorly located, in contrast to the other anterior follicles.

are recognized in each ovary at any given day of the cycle[13] (Fig. 23–15).

Transvaginal ultrasonography visualizes 2- to 3-mm-sized ovarian follicles, and the normal developing follicle grows at a rate of about 2 mm per day.[14] The dominant follicle can be detected from day 8 of the normal regular cycle by its rapid growth compared with the other follicles.[15] The mean follicular diameter before ovulation varies in different studies from 20 to 25 mm. The average follicular growth from day 5 to ovulation is about 3 mm per day.[16]

Ultrasound can be used effectively to monitor follicular development in women undergoing ovarian stimulation with clomiphene citrate or gonadotropin. Additional monitoring by means of serum estradiol level, however, is usually recommended.[17] The correlation between follicular diameter and estradiol level is lower in induced cycles, when more than one follicle develops, than in a natural cycle. The total follicular volume seems to show the highest correlation with the serum estradiol level. The value of ultrasonography is in making the decision to administer human chorionic gonadotropin (HCG) at the appropriate time, that is, when the leading follicle reaches a diameter of 16 to 18 mm.[18]

The follicles, echo-free in appearance, have smooth borders. Ovulation can be detected by demonstrating previously nonexistent fluid in the cul-de-sac, the decrease in size or collapse of the follicle, the development of intrafollicular echoes, and the appearance of a corpus luteum.[19] To facilitate the demonstra-

tion of fluid in the pouch of Douglas, the patient must be positioned in the reversed Trendelenburg position, which allows the peritoneal fluid to pool in the cul-de-sac. This fluid, if present, creates a tissue–fluid interface with the uterus and, occasionally, the ovaries as well.[4]

The characteristic sonographic appearance of the corpus luteum is recognized shortly after ovulation. It is visualized as a spherical, predominantly cystic mass of 2 to 3 cm in diameter (Fig. 23–16), which may take one of several forms. It may contain a highly echogenic area inside the echo-free cystic mass, or it may appear as a septated cystic mass, or contain numerous components of different echogenicity. The septae may be solitary, trabecular, wheel–spoke shaped, or appear as a delineated network. The corpus luteum, in its diverse appearance, may imitate many ovarian abnormalities, thus imposing some difficulty in its recognition. Its development and regression involves dramatic changes. Blood clots and fluid content may appear as an irregular echogenic area. The diameter of a fully developed corpus luteum does not exceed 4 cm. In cases of a corpus luteum cyst, or hemorrhagic corpus luteum, it may attain the size of 8 cm or more.[20] Small follicles may still be identified within the ovary in the premenopausal period. The follicles cannot be seen in the menopausal period, while the normal ova-

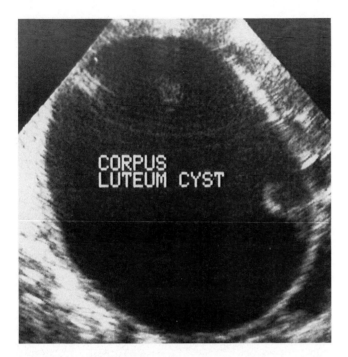

Figure 23–16. This is an ovarian cyst with echolucency throughout. These findings are consistent with a corpus luteum cyst, especially if such findings are identified at the time of midcycle.

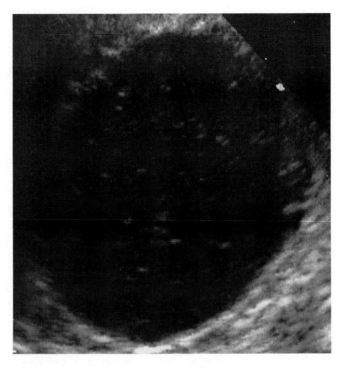

Figure 23–17. Ultrasound picture of an ovarian cyst with echolucency throughout and well-defined borders. These findings are consistent with a simple cyst.

ries are one half their size compared with the reproductive period.

SONOPATHOLOGY

Meire et al[21] have defined the sonographic characteristic features of a malignant ovarian cyst. These malignant cysts can be unilocular, or multilocular with thin septae, and papillae.

The Simple Cyst

This term is used when a large spherical sonolucent ovarian cyst is identified. This cyst may occasionally reach 10 cm, but most do not exceed 6 cm in size. The capsule appears smooth and without septae or papillae. Sonographic examination should be done after hormonal suppression (Fig. 23–17) to assess the outcome of the simple cyst.

The Polycystic Ovary

The polycystic ovary has typical sonographic features and can be recognized by its larger, spherical, multiple small follicles of 3 to 6 mm in size scattered along the surface. The image of the polycystic ovary becomes even more evident if the patient is hormonally stimulated (Fig. 23–18). The ovarian surface area, moreover, is always greater than 12 cm in cases of polycystic ovarian disease.[1] Ovaries with normal size and few

subcortical small follicles, however, are also found in women with polycystic ovarian disease. Typical sonographic findings of polycystic ovaries are not pathog-

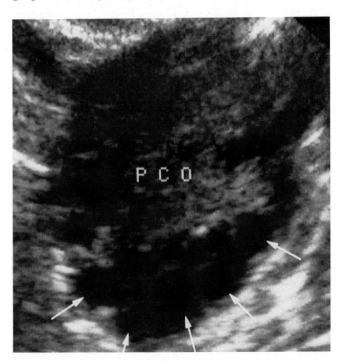

Figure 23–18. An ultrasound picture of an ovary with numerous small cysts throughout the substance of the ovary. The arrows indicate the cyst, particularly the outer edge of the ovary. These findings are consistent with a polycystic ovary.

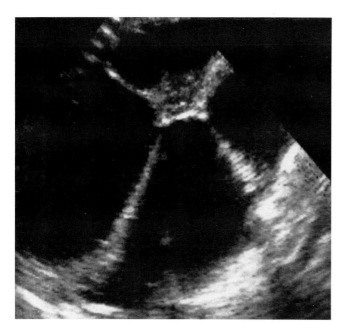

Figure 23–19. Ultrasound picture of an ovary demonstrating the wheel–spoke type of pattern representing multiple follicles within the ovary.

nomonic for polycystic ovarian disease, and clinical conditions can also be associated with multifollicular ovaries[22] (Fig. 23–19).

The Persistent Corpus Luteum

The corpus luteum occasionally may persist longer in the pregnant woman than its expected life span. An abnormal growth may form a corpus luteum cyst in such cases. This corpus luteum may appear as a trabecular, septated multicystic mass, or it may be wheel-like in its appearance.[4]

Dermoid Cyst

The dermoid cyst usually contains mucoid fluid, as well as solid structures such as hair, teeth, bones, or thyroid tissue. The mucoid fluid appears as a "snow storm," with areas of echodensity scattered throughout the cyst (Fig. 23–20).

Fallopian Tubes

SONOANATOMY

The fallopian tubes are not usually seen during a normal pelvic exam, even by transvaginal ultrasound. In some cases, however, where the fluid of various origins is collected in the pelvis, it reflects the image of the fallopian tubes. Longitudinal and cross-sectional

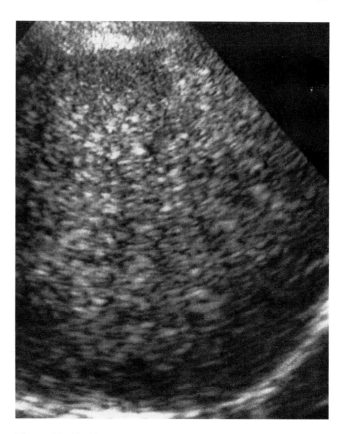

Figure 23–20. Ultrasound picture of an ovarian cyst with a hyperechoic and heterogenous pattern. These findings indicate intracystic contents of high viscosity; such findings suggest a dermoid cyst or a mucinous cystadenoma.

planes are obtained by rotating the transducer probe around the longitudinal axis. A push–pull motion of the probe, combined with the free-hand maneuver that

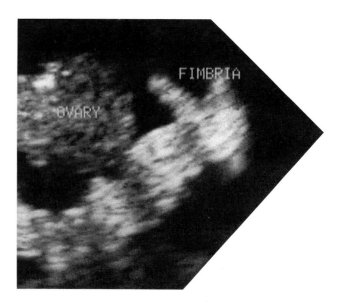

Figure 23–21. Transvaginal ultrasound exam of a female pelvis revealing the fallopian tube with the fimbria pointing toward the ovary. Note how the fallopian tube and the fimbria semiembrace the ovary.

pushes the lower abdomen toward the transducer, may increase visualization[1] (Fig. 23–21).

SONOPATHOLOGY

The fallopian tubes may be visualized sonographically in the presence of fluid in the cul-de-sac, in cases of ascites, or ectopic pregnancy accompanied by a ruptured fallopian tube, or with inflammatory disease in the pelvis.[23]

REFERENCES

1. Brown JE, Thieme GA, Shah DM, et al. Transabdominal and transvaginal endosonography: evaluation of the cervix and lower uterine segment in pregnancy. *Am J Obstet Gynecol.* 1986;155:721–726.
2. Lewit N, Thaler I, Rottem S. The uterus: a new look with transvaginal sonography. *J Clin Ultrasound.* 1990;18:331–336.
3. Miller EI, Thomas RH, Lies P. The atropic postmenopausal uterus. *J Clin Ultrasound.* 1977;4:261–263.
4. Timor-Tritsch IE, Rottem S, Taler I. Review of transvaginal sonography: a description with clinical applications. *Ultrasound Q.* 1988;6:1–34.
5. Fleischer AC, Pittaway DE, Beard LA, et al. Sonographic depiction of endometrial changes occurring with ovulation induction. *J Ultrasound Med.* 1984;3:341–346.
6. Chambers CB, Uis JS. Ultrasonographic evidence of uterine malignancy in postmenopausal uterus. *Am J Obstet Gynecol.* 1986;154:1194–1199.
7. Fleischer AC, Kalemeris GC, Machi JE, et al. Sonographic depiction of normal and abnormal endometrium with histopathologic correction. *J Ultrasound Med.* 1986;5:445–452.
8. Mendelson EB, Bohm-Velez M, Joseph N, et al. Endometrial abnormalities: evaluation with transvaginal sonography. *AJR.* 1988;150:139–142.
9. Fleischer AC, Gordo A, Stephe S, et al. Transvaginal scanning of the endometrium. *J Clin Ultrasound.* 1990;18:337–349.
10. Fleischer AL, Dudly BS, Etma SS, et al. Myometrial invasion by endometrial carcinoma: sonographic assessment. *Radiology.* 1987;162:307–310.
11. Forrest TS, Elyaderai MK, Muileburg MI, et al. Cyclic endometrial changes: US assessment with histologic correction. *Radiology.* 1988;167:233–237.
12. Malpai A, Siger J, Wolverso MK, et al. Endometrial hyperplasia: value of endometrial thickness in ultrasonographic diagnosis and clinical significance. *J Clin Ultrasound.* 1990;18:173–177.
13. Fleischer AC, Daniel JF, Rodier J, et al. Sonographic monitoring of ovarian follicular development. *J Clin Ultrasound.* 1981;9:275–280.
14. Itskovitz J, Boldes R, Levron J, et al. Transvaginal ultrasonography in diagnosis and treatment of infertility. *J Clin Ultrasound.* 1990;18:248–256.
15. Renaud RL, Macler J, Dervain I, et al. Echographic study of follicular maturation and ovulation during the normal menstrual cycle. *Fertil Steril.* 1980;33:272–276.
16. Kerin JF, Edmonds DK, Warnes GM, et al. Morphological and functional relations of graafian follicle growth to ovulation in women using ultrasonic, laparascopic, and biochemical measurements. *Br J Obstet Gynecol.* 1981;88:81–90.
17. Bryce RL, Shuter B, Siosich MJ, et al. The value of ultrasound, gonadotropin, and estradiol measurements for precise ovulation prediction. *Fertil Steril.* 1982;37:42–45.
18. O'Herlihy C, de Crespigny LC, Lopata A, et al. Preovulatory follicular size: a comparison of ultrasound and laparoscopic measurements. *Fertil Steril.* 1980;34:24–26.
19. Lade IM, Hill MC, Cosco FE, et al. Adexal and cul-de-sac abnormalities: transvaginal sonography. *Radiology.* 1988;166:325–332.
20. Rottem S, Levit N, Thaler I, et al. Classification of ovarian lesion by high-frequency transvaginal sonography. *J Clin Ultrasound.* 1990;18:359–363.
21. Meire HB, Farrant P, Guha T. Distinction of benign from malignant ovarian cysts by ultrasound. *Br J Obstet Gynecol.* 85:893–899.
22. Orsii LF, Venturoli S, Lorusso R, et al. Ultrasonic findings in polycystic ovarian disease. *Fertil Steril.* 1985;43:709–714.
23. Timor-Tritsch IE, Rottem S. Transvaginal ultrasonographic study of the fallopian tube. *Obstet Gynecol.* 1987;70:424–428.

24

Abnormal Gestations

INTRODUCTION

Abnormal gestations pose a significant dilemma for the clinician, since their presentation can be variable and atypical. Ultrasonography can aid in the diagnosis and management of abnormal early pregnancies. This chapter discusses the utility of ultrasound in the management of various types of abnormal gestations: anembryonic pregnancy, molar gestation, threatened abortion, missed abortion, inevitable or incomplete abortion, ectopic pregnancy, and pregnancy and uterine malformations.

ANEMBRYONIC PREGNANCY

An anembryonic pregnancy is represented by an empty gestational sac, which is usually abnormal in shape with a thin wall of variable size. The diagnosis is suspected, on the initial ultrasound exam, if a yolk sac is identified and the gestational sac is consistent with 7 weeks or more and the embryo is absent.[1] If there is doubt about the gestational age, the scan should be repeated in about 1 week. If an embryo cannot be visualized on follow-up examination, a presumptive diagnosis of anembryonic pregnancy or blighted ovum can be made.

Jouppila et al[2] reported that the initial human chorionic gonadotropin (hCG) values were normal for gestational age in 34% of the patients with anembryonic pregnancy and in 42% of the patients with missed abortions. They further observed a decline in the hCG curve as time progressed. Hence they concluded that the diagnostic accuracy of ultrasound was not improved by the use of hCG assays.

MOLAR GESTATIONS

Molar pregnancies have been divided into complete and incomplete moles. In the former there is no fetal tissue; it is usually associated with a chromosome complement of 46,XX. The incomplete mole usually coexists with a fetus or fetal tissue and the chromo-

some complement usually tends to be a triploid karyotype. Work by Kajii and Ohama[3] demonstrated that a hydatidiform mole may result from fertilization of an ovum without any active chromosome material. Apparently, the chromosome of the sperm reduplicates, resulting in a 46,XX pregnancy. These complete moles may have varying sequelae. Only about 20% of cases, however, will pursue a malignant course.[4]

The incomplete mole contains a small complement of fetal tissue such as placenta with membrane or even a developed fetus. These moles are almost always benign. The fetus often has congenital malformations as well as aneuploidy.

Patients with molar gestations tend to present with vaginal bleeding in over 90% of the cases. In approximately one half of these cases the bleeding may be severe and anemia may result. The traditional notion is that a large-for-date uterus is common in patients with molar gestation. This occurs, however, in only about 50% of cases. In other cases the patient may present with a uterus that is normal in size or even small for date. Early preeclampsia occurring before 24 weeks is considered a hallmark of molar pregnancy. This occurs in only 10% of molar pregnancies; nevertheless, the diagnosis ought to be considered when this clinical presentation is encountered.

Laboratory findings are usually diagnostic of molar gestation with a measurement of the beta-subunit of hCG, which almost always reveals a very elevated level.

Management and Outcome

As soon as the diagnosis of molar gestation is made, the uterus should be evacuated via dilatation and curettage. Medical evaluation prior to surgery should include a chest x-ray, a quantitative hCG level, and a hematocrit, as well as a blood type and cross-match. Additional workup should include an electrocardiogram, thyroid function test, and coagulation studies. Following uterine evacuation, beta-hCG should be obtained weekly to determine whether there is any remaining trophoblastic tissue. hCG levels are expected to return to normal within 12 weeks. Any evidence of persistent corpus luteum cyst, lack of involution of uterine size, slow decline of the hCG level, or rebound in hCG may indicate persistent trophoblastic disease, and further evaluation is required.

Sonographic Diagnosis

The diagnosis via sonography is characteristic, with echogenic intrauterine masses containing numerous areas of sonolucencies. The uterus is uniformly filled with variable and heterogenous echoes separated by small cystic spaces. The posterior wall is sometimes well defined due to the enhanced acoustic transmission to the fluid-filled vesicles. Sometimes these are described as a snowflake pattern within the uterus. The findings on ultrasound may occasionally be produced by other conditions. In missed abortion, for example, hydropic may sometimes be indistinguishable from molar gestations or a degenerated fibroid.

THREATENED ABORTION

A pregnancy showing signs of aborting, as evidenced by vaginal bleeding or uterine cramping is a threatened abortion. Approximately one third of all pregnancies will have a similar presentation. About one half of these women will abort, and the remainder will continue to have viable pregnancies.

Jouppila et al[2] reported that in patients with threatened abortions that fetal heart activity as established by ultrasound was associated with a viable outcome in 90% of the cases.[2] These findings were corroborated by Anderson,[5] who reported a good pregnancy outcome rate of 97% when fetal heart activity was observed in patients with threatened abortion presenting at 7 weeks of gestation.

Therefore, in patients who present with threatened abortion, ultrasound may be useful in establishing fetal heart activity and gestational age. A determination can be made from this basic examination about whether the patient has an incomplete abortion, inevitable abortion, and, by exclusion, a threatened abortion. If the latter is confirmed, a prognosis might be given, based on the presence or absence of fetal cardiac activity.

MISSED ABORTION

A missed abortion refers to early fetal demise, with the abortus retained within the uterine cavity. Patients with missed abortion usually present with uterine size four weeks behind their gestational age. There is also an inability to identify the fetal heart tones, either when they were previously identified or at a time when they were expected to be heard.

Ultrasound has proved useful in diagnosing this condition, since the diagnosis can be made simply by demonstrating the lack of fetal heart motion or fetal activity when it ought to be present.

Recent work by Goldstein et al[6] has provided data on developmental features of the fetus in the first trimester. In this cross-sectional study, transvaginal ultrasound was used to access 137 normal pregnancies, with gestational ages ranging from 5 to 12 weeks. The authors reported that when a gestational sac was identified at 5 weeks' gestation embryonic heartbeat was observed, and the mean gestational sac diameter measured 2 cm.

The embryonic body movements could be seen when the mean gestational sac diameter reached 3 cm. Furthermore, the embryonic heartbeat was identifiable after 6 weeks and 4 days, with a sensitivity of 100%, specificity of 93%, positive predictive value of 97%, and negative predictive value of 100%. Embryonic body movements were absent before 7 weeks' gestation, with a sensitivity of 100%, specificity of 93%, positive predictive value of 94%, and negative predictive value of 100%. These investigators concluded that by using these markers of normal embryo growth, a gestational sac diameter greater than 2 cm in the presence of embryo heart beat or a mean sac diameter measurement of greater than 3 cm in the presence of embryo movement confirmed normal embryonic development (Fig. 24–1).[6] With this information, the diagnosis of missed abortion can be made. Depending upon the size of the gestational sac and the abortus, the clinician can either opt for dilatation and curettage or conservative management.

INEVITABLE OR INCOMPLETE ABORTION

A diagnosis of inevitable abortion is made on clinical grounds and is usually characterized by the patient's presenting with excessive vaginal bleeding or excessive leakage of amniotic fluid or cervical dilation, with protrusion of the fetal part from the amniotic sac.

The ultrasound findings are variable, depending on the gestational age. For example, the uterus might be normal size or small for dates. The uterine cavity, however, will often demonstrate a gestational sac or an embryo or viable conceptus, with or without intrauterine echoes, suggestive of blood or blood clots within the cavity. Occasionally, the gestational sac will be seen untrasonically in the lower uterine segment, or it may protrude through the dilated cervical canal. The sonographic findings will be diagnostic of an inevitable abortion.

The diagnosis of incomplete abortion can be made clinically in patients presenting with bleeding, cramping, or passage of amniotic fluid with fetal or placental

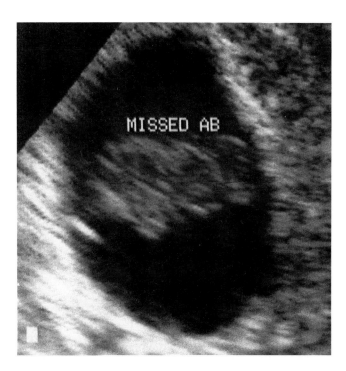

Figure 24–1. Transvaginal ultrasound of a pregnancy at 7 weeks' gestation by last menstrual period, depicting a large gestational sac with well-defined borders and internally the yolk sac is easily visualized. In addition, a small free-floating amniotic cavity can be seen but without an embryo. These findings are indicative of a missed abortion.

tissue. Sonographic findings are variable and may reveal either a uterus with heterogeneous echo densities indicative of retained tissue or a dilated cervical os with tissue trapped within the cervical canal, and usually with a uterus that is much smaller than the gestational age would predict.

VANISHING TWIN SYNDROME

Diagnosis of the vanishing twin syndrome is strictly ultrasonic and usually occurs in patients who present in early pregnancy with vaginal bleeding. These patients usually present with continued uterine growth and no overt clinical abnormalities, except for an initial episode of bleeding, cramping, or both.

Ultrasound examination often reveals a singleton fetus, with a second smaller sac containing echodense material suggestive of a prior fetal demise. If the sonographic findings are followed serially, within 4 to 6 weeks the second sac may be completely absent. Under other circumstances, a diagnosis of multiple gestation may be made early in pregnancy, with identifiable gestational sacs and fetal viability. Only a singleton pregnancy may be delivered at term, however. This has therefore become one explanation for the higher incidence of twin gestation diagnosed in early pregnancy compared with the delivery rate at term.

PREGNANCY AND UTERINE MALFORMATIONS

Various types of müllerian anomalies of the uterus might occur and result in a septum or complete duplication of the uterus or a uterus bicornis, bicollis, uterus bicornis unicollis, or the septate uterus (Fig. 24–2). Pregnancy may coexist with many of these uterine malformations. The overall pregnancy loss rate in women with congenital uterine fusion defects is in the range of 0.1% to 5%. Many of these patients are simply referred for dating scans or size greater than dates, or, very rarely, for an abnormal cervix based on clinical suspicion.

The chance of diagnosing a uterine anomaly decreases with gestational age. Ultrasonic findings consistent with either a bicornuate uterus or a uterus didelphia include a uterus with two separate cavities on transverse scans. Sometimes this is described as a dumbbell configuration, with a gestational sac appearing in either one of these compartments as a singleton pregnancy, or, rarely, in both compartments in twin gestations. In the case of the singleton pregnancy the gestation will appear on one side, with enlargement of the uterine cavity on the contralateral side as well. There will also be an increased echogenicity due to a residual response on the contralateral side. The septate uterus is more difficult to diagnose, since on transverse scan the septum may be missed.

When these uterine anomalies are recognized, pa-

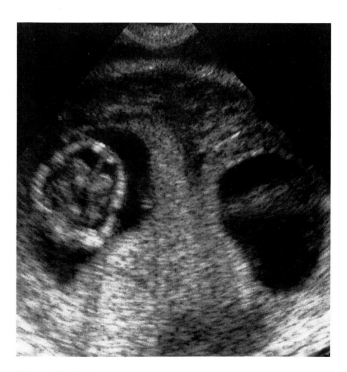

Figure 24–2. Transverse scan of the uterus in which a septum fully divides the uterine cavity into two compartments with a fetal head identified on the right side; the left side contains amniotic fluid only.

tients should be advised of the increased risk of spontaneous abortion and also the increased risk of preterm labor; therefore, surveillance or reduced activities may be advised during the course of pregnancy.

ECTOPIC PREGNANCY

The use of transvaginal ultrasound has significantly improved the evaluation of patients suspected of ectopic pregnancies. The presence or absence of an intrauterine gestation can be documented by as much as 7 to 10 days earlier than with transabdominal ultrasound (Fig. 24–3). Using a combination of transvaginal sonography and βhGC levels, the diagnostic accuracy of ectopic pregnancy may exceed 90%. Since ectopic pregnancies are currently responsible for as much as 10% of all maternal deaths, the use of ultrasound and these βhCG studies is critical for the evaluation, workup, and diagnosis of this disorder. A high suspicion ought to exist in patients who present with lower abdominal pain, vaginal bleeding, and amenorrhea. Relying on physical examination alone may cause the physician to miss up to two thirds of ectopic pregnancies.[7]

Vaginal sonography has recently improved the already high accuracy of transabdominal ultrasound

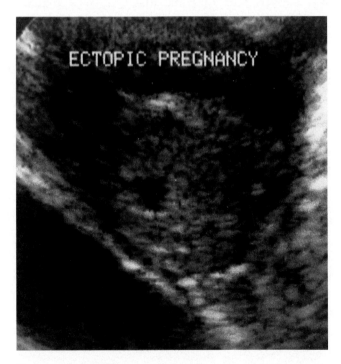

Figure 24–3. Transvaginal ultrasound exam of a pelvis showing to the right lower border the margin of the iliac vessel and anterior to it is a circular object with heterogeneous density and a central echolucent area. This adnexal structure strongly indicates an ectopic pregnancy.

diagnosis of ectopic pregnancy (unpublished data Gabrielli S, et al). The combination of transabdominal ultrasound findings combined with a beta-hCG titer of 6,500 mIU acts as a discriminatory zone for pregnancy. More recent work using transvaginal ultrasound and hCG levels has made the diagnosis possible even at earlier gestational ages. Work by Gabrielli et al on 127 patients with a clinical suspicion of ectopic pregnancy led to the following conclusions.

Of these 127 cases, 42 patients did have ectopic pregnancies (33.6%), 46 had spontaneous abortions (36.2%), and 36 pregnancies were continued uneventfully (28.3%). In three cases voluntary termination of pregnancy was chosen. In 60 cases (47.2%), an intrauterine gestational sac was clearly identified at the first ultrasound exam, whereas in the remaining 67 cases (62.8%) no sac could be seen. In this group, 42 ectopic pregnancies (62.6%) and 25 intrauterine pregnancies were later diagnosed.

Beta-HCG titers revealed that the cutoff value of 1,000 mIU previously established was most effective in discriminating between ectopic and intrauterine pregnancies, with an overall sensitivity of 65% and a false-positive rate of 20%. In this series, failure to identify with transvaginal ultrasound an intrauterine sac with an hCG level above 1,000 mIU was an excellent indicator of ectopic pregnancy. This criterion had a positive predictive value of 86% and specificity of 93%. These diagnostic indices were similar to those previously reported by transabdominal ultrasound using a threshold of 6,500 mIU. Furthermore, the detection of adnexal abnormality using transvaginal ultrasound was found in a very high proportion of ectopic pregnancies (Fig. 24–3).

REFERENCES

1. Longley JV, Sabbagha RE. Abnormal early pregnancy. In: Sabbagha RE, ed. *Diagnostic Ultrasound Applied to Obstetrics and Gynecology.* Philadelphia, Pa: JB Lippincott Co; 1987:465–466.
2. Jouppila P, Huhtaniemi I, Tapanainen J, et al. Early pregnancy failure: study by ultrasonic and hormonal methods. *Obstet Gynecol.* 1980;55: 42–47.
3. Kajii T, Ohama K. Androgenic origin of hydatidiform mole. *Nature.* 1977;168:633–634.
4. Reid MH, McGahan JO. Sonographic evaluation of hydatidiform mole and its look alike. *AJR.* 1983;140:307–311.
5. Anderson SG. Management of threatened abortion with real time sonography. *Obstet Gynecol.* 1980;55:259–262.
6. Goldstein I, Zimmer EA, Tamir A, et al. Evaluation of normal gestational sac growth: appearance of embryonic heart beat and embryo body movements using the transvaginal technique. *Obstet Gynecol.* 1991;77:885–888.
7. Halpin TF: Ectopic Pregnancy: The problem of diagnosis. *Am J Obstet Gynecol.* 1970;106:227–236.

Index

Page numbers followed by t and f refer to tables and figures, respectively.

Bladder (*cont.*)
  fetal, 108*f*
    normal, 131–132
  full, 9
Blebs, nuchal, 167
Blood flow
  cardiac, fetal, 85, 85*f*
  characterization of
    Doppler ultrasound in, 237–240, 238*f*
    intrauterine growth retardation and, 238–240
Blood pressure, maternal, fetal growth and, 192
Blood sampling, fetal, 226–228, 227*f*
Bodies of lateral ventricles, in fetal head evaluation, 36
Body mass measurement, ponderal index in, 195–196
Body movements, fetal, 219–221, 220*t*
Body stalk anomaly, 125
Body temperature, ultrasound-related increases in, 5–6
Bones, long. *See also* Limb bones
  fetal lung maturation and, 13
Bowel. *See* Colon; Gastrointestinal tract
BPD. *See* Biparietal diameter
BRA (bilateral renal agenesis), 133–134
Brachycephaly, craniosynostosis and, 61
Brain. *See* Head; *specific structures*
Bronchial development, 73, 74
Bronchogenic cysts, 79*f*, 79–80
Bronchopulmonary sequestration, 78–79, 79*f*
"Butterfly" appearance, in corpus callosum agenesis, 59

CAD (cerebroatrial distance), 37
Calcaneus, sonoanatomy of, 199, 200*f*
  clinical relevance of, 201, 201*t*
Calcification, intra-abdominal, 111
Calf circumference, macrosomia and, 196, 196*t*
Caliectasis, obstructive uropathy and, 135
Callosal agenesis, 52, 59
  syndromes with, 168–169, 169*f*
Calvarium, absence of, 62, 62*f*
Canalicular period of lung development, 73
Cancer, childhood, fetal ultrasound exposure and, 6–7
Cardiac malformations, 83. *See also* Echocardiography; Heart
  nonimmune hydrops fetalis and, 126
Cardiomyopathies, 92, 93*f*
Carotid vessels, Doppler flow in, intrauterine growth retardation and, 239–240
Cavitational mechanism, 6
Cell functions, ultrasound effects on, 6
Cell therapy, embryoscopy and, 232
Central nervous system. *See* Head; Spine
Cephalic index, 11, 43–44. *See also* Biparietal diameter (BPD); Occipitofrontal diameter (OFD)
  craniosynostosis and, 61
  gestational age and, 177

Cephalocele, 54*f*, 54–55
  cystic hygroma versus, 71
Cephalomeningocele, cystic hygroma versus, 71
Cerebellar vermis defect, in Dandy–Walker syndrome, 49
Cerebellum, 29, 30*f*, 41–42, 42*t*. *See also* Transverse cerebellar diameter (TCD)
  Arnold–Chiari type II malformation and, 98
Cerebral gyri, absence of, 60–61, 61*f*
Cerebroatrial distance (CAD), 37
Cerebrofrontal horn distance (CFHD), 36
Cerebroposterior horn distance (CPHD), 38
Cerebrospinal fluid (CSF), in hydrocephalus, 46. *See also* Hydrocephalus
Cervical–thoracic neural tube defect, 102*f*
Cervix, 245
CFHD (cerebrofrontal horn distance), 36
CHD. *See* Congenital heart disease
Chest circumference, 75*f*, 75–76. *See also* Thoracic circumference
Chiari type III deformity, 54
Children. *See also* Neonates
  behavior of, fetal ultrasound exposure and, 7
  cancer in, fetal ultrasound exposure and, 6–7
  polycystic kidney disease in, 133
Chondroectodermal dysplasia, 149
Chorionic villus sampling, 225, 225*f*, 226*f*
  advantages and disadvantages of, 226
  procedure for
    transabdominal, 226
    transcervical, 225–226
Choroid plexus, 29, 29*f*, 30*f*, 35*f*, 39–40
  cysts of, 62*f*, 62–63
    trisomy 18 and, 163, 164*f*
  papillomas of, 62–64, 64*f*
"Christmas tree" atresia, 117
Chromosomal abnormalities. *See also* Dysmorphology syndromes; Genetics
  choroid plexus cysts and, 63
  chylothorax and, 76
  corpus callosum agenesis and, 59
  cystic hygroma and, 70–71
  holoprosencephaly and, 57
  microcephaly and, 51
  neural tube defects and, 98
  nonimmune hydrops fetalis and, 127
  ultrasound exposure and, 6
Chylothorax, congenital, 76, 76*f*
Cingulate sulcus, corpus callosum agenesis and, 59
Cisterna magna, 42–43, 43*t*
  trisomy 21 and, 172
Clavicular length, 13, 142, 142*f*, 143*t*
Cleft lip, 68, 69*f*. *See also* Median cleft face syndrome
Cleft palate, 68, 69
Cloverleaf skull, 61
  thanatophoric dysplasia and, 148, 154*f*